# Injury Prevention and Public Health

## Practical Knowledge, Skills, and Strategies

Tom Christoffel, JD

Susan Scavo Gallagher, MPH

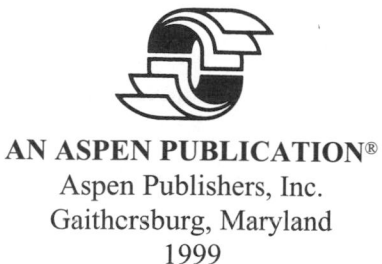

**AN ASPEN PUBLICATION®**
Aspen Publishers, Inc.
Gaithersburg, Maryland
1999

**Library of Congress Cataloging-in-Publication Data**

Christoffel, Tom.
Injury prevention and public health : practical knowledge, skills,
and strategies / Tom Christoffel, Susan Scavo Gallagher.
p. cm.
Includes bibliographical references and index.
ISBN 0-8342-0840-7
1. Wounds and injuries—Prevention. 2. Accidents—Prevention.
3. Personal injuries—Prevention. I. Gallagher, Susan Scavo.
II. Title.
RD93.C517   1999
617.1—dc21
98-49329
CIP

Orders: (800) 638-8437
Customer Service: (800) 234-1660

**About Aspen Publishers** • For more than 35 years, Aspen has been a leading professional
publisher in a variety of disciplines. Aspen's vast information resources are available in both
print and electronic formats. We are committed to providing the highest quality information
available in the most appropriate format for our customers. Visit Aspen's Internet site for more
information resources, directories, articles, and a searchable version of Aspen's full catalog,
including the most recent publications: **http://www.aspenpublishers.com**
**Aspen Publishers, Inc.** • The hallmark of quality in publishing
Member of the worldwide Wolters Kluwer group.

Editorial Services: Denise H. Coursey
Library of Congress Catalog Card Number: 98-49329
ISBN: 0-8342-0840-7

*Printed in the United States of America*

2   3   4   5

For Anne and Anna

"The landmarks of political, economic and social history are the moments when some condition passed from the category of the given into the category of the intolerable. . . . I believe that the history of public health might well be written as a record of successive re-definings of the unacceptable."

Geoffrey Vickers, "What sets the goals of public health?" *Lancet,* 1958

# Table of Contents

Step 5: Conduct Preliminary Data Analysis ....... 295
Step 6: Re-evaluate Objectives for the Surveillance System Based on Steps 3–5 .................. 296
Step 7: Consider Linking Information from Existing Data Sources ............................ 296
Step 8: Perform Validation Studies To Evaluate the Injury Surveillance System .................. 298
Step 9: Develop a Dissemination Plan for Sharing Data .................................. 299
Step 10: Tie Surveillance to Action and Funding ... 300
Conclusion ................................. 300
Appendix 12-A: An Injury Surveillance Example ............................... 305

**Chapter 13—Real World Evaluation Techniques ............ 309**
What This Chapter Is About .................. 309
Introduction ............................... 310
Evaluation Steps ........................... 311
Constraints on "Perfect" Evaluation ............ 327
Conclusion ................................. 330
Appendix 13-A: An Evaluation Case Study ....... 333

**Chapter 14—Barriers to Injury Prevention ............... 343**
What This Chapter Is About .................. 343
Introduction ............................... 344
Funding Limitations ......................... 344
Organizational Difficulties .................. 346
Turf Battles ............................... 347
Scientific and Policy Analysis and Data: Myths versus Reality ......................... 348
Economic and Political Aspects of Injury Prevention ............................. 349
Advocacy .................................. 355
Examples .................................. 361
Conclusion ................................. 365
Appendix 14-A: Developing a Comprehensive Injury Prevention Program: Selected Factors Contributing to Health Systems Problems ................ 369

# Acknowledgments

As is the case with all works on injury and injury prevention, this book rests on the shoulders of the theorists, scholars, researchers, and activists who have led all of us to our current understanding of how injuries occur and how they can be prevented. These individuals, and the conceptual revolution they guided, are described in Chapter 2. There is another group, however, to which we wish to pay even more direct tribute. These are the many people working actively at many levels to bring about reductions in our nation's injury rates. We are all indebted to the dedicated public health staff at local and state health departments and to the many other practitioners who continue to work to advance injury prevention policy and practice against strong odds and with very limited resources. Their commitment, enthusiasm, and persistence in adopting innovative approaches and their ability to refine and expand those programs that work best have made a difference in the reduction of injuries over the last 20 years. It is the work of these individuals that has inspired and guided the development of this book.

Sue Gallagher would particularly offer thanks for all that she learned at the Massachusetts Department of Public Health during her years of service, 1979–1986. She especially wishes to acknowledge Milt Kotelchuck and Bernard Guyer, who took a chance on a non-Ph.D. and provided her start in the injury prevention field. Special thanks are also due to David Heppel at the Maternal and Child Health Bureau, for his vision, understanding, and long-term support of the needs of practitioners. Finally, Sue wishes to thank her colleagues at the Children's Safety Network for their patience, their commitment to injury prevention, their enthusiasm on the job, and their continued spirit of teamwork. Very special thanks go to a good friend and colleague, Ilana Lescohier, for her wise counsel and encouragement.

On a more immediate level, we would like to thank all those who have offered useful comments and criticisms as we worked to bring this book into being—in particular Rebecca Atnafou, Susan Brink, Larry Cohen, Ed DeVos, Anara Guard, Murray Katcher, Susan Mallonee, Lenora Olson, Lotika Paintal, Carol Runyan, Rick Smith, Jon Vernick, and several anonymous reviewers. We gained from being able to work with Kalen Conerly, Denise Coursey, and Michael Brown at Aspen and have a special debt of gratitude toward Michel Ibrahim for initiating and supporting our efforts.

Finally, it is a gross understatement to note that completion of this work would not have been possible without the understanding and patience of Anne Guilfoile and Anna Scavo Gallagher. We gratefully and lovingly dedicate this work to them.

# Foreword

The role of public health and its concepts, methods, and values have recently received increased recognition by policy makers and those responsible for the financing and delivery of health care. This has resulted in numerous books and courses aimed at preparing students and practitioners of public health to respond to this increased demand and to give them the necessary skills and knowledge to do so. The general public health professional of the future will need to have a broad understanding of public health issues and critical insights into diverse health care topics in order to relate intelligently to the various segments of the health care sector.

This volume, *Injury Prevention and Public Health: Practical Knowledge, Skills, and Strategies*, presents complex information in an understandable and inviting manner. Topics are covered in self-contained chapters that begin with "what this chapter is about" and end with appropriate conclusions; yet the entire book is interwoven into a coherent whole.

The book provides an excellent synthesis of the three major elements of injury prevention: the nature and magnitude of injury, the basic concepts of prevention, and practical approaches for implementing prevention programs. The prevention of both unintential injury and violence deserves special mention as it is one of those measures that can make a difference by saving lives and reducing costs. Christoffel and Gallagher have combined injury prevention research with public health practice perspectives.

This book is targeted to public health students as well as public health practitioners for an engaging introductory review of injury prevention research and practices. All in all, this is a most welcome textbook on injury prevention for students and practitioners who are concerned with improving the health of the public.

*Michel A. Ibrahim, MD, PhD*
*Professor of Epidemiology and Social Medicine*
*University of North Carolina at Chapel Hill*

# Introduction

Each day it seems that the print and broadcast media seek to outdo one another in presenting a picture of the world as a place gone mad, a scary environment out of control. Random violence, religious wars, deadly epidemics, major disasters: these would seem to be the unstoppable mechanisms by which lives are ended in their prime, families and communities devastated, children traumatized . . . and media advertising sold.

Certainly life is fraught with risks, many of them—such as the AIDS virus and high powered assault weapons—are threats to life that were not concerns just a few decades ago, but it is important that such risks be kept in perspective and properly understood. The fact is that the world is, in many ways, a much better and safer place than it was a generation or two ago. Certainly this is the case in the economically richer nations.

In the United States, the average life has become significantly longer and fuller during this century. In 1900 the average American lived to age 45. Today, despite gun violence, AIDS, drugs, and other perils, the average American lives to age 76.[1] A small part of this 30-year addition to the life span—about five years' worth—can be attributed to modern medicine: the improved knowledge, technology, and pharmacology available to the health care delivery system. But most of the expanded life span—some 25 years of additional life—is the result of applied public health (i.e., improvements in living conditions and the environment and an understanding of risks to health and how to minimize them).[2,3]

Public health is the profession dedicated to extending and improving physical, mental, and emotional health and well-being for the population as a whole. By focusing on ways to control environmental risks, public health works to make the world a safer place in which to live. Much of public health's work is well established and well known, going back at least a century and including efforts to improve sanitation, screen the public for various contagious or preventable diseases, and immunize against diseases.[4] But one of the most important public health efforts is more recent in origin and less well understood. This is the field of injury prevention.

Injuries—both unintentional and intentional—are a major threat to the public's health and well-being. Each year 150,000 Americans die as the result of injuries, and an estimated 70 million suffer nonfatal injuries. "In the United States," notes the National Center for Health Statistics, "injury causes more deaths among children and young adults than does disease."[5(p15)] As one government study noted, injuries "kill more Americans aged 1–34 than all diseases combined."[6(p1),7] Injury ranks third among causes of death overall, and it constitutes the second most costly health problem in this country, after heart disease. More to the point, injuries result in more productive years of life lost than any other cause: more than four million potential years of life lost prematurely each year. Figure I–1 dramatizes the role unintentional injury deaths (motor vehicle, household, and the like) and intentional injury deaths (homicides and suicides) play in cutting short the lives of our fellow citizens, our friends, our children.

Figure I–1 is what this book is all about. If public health is about promoting health and preventing risks to health, then injury prevention would seem to call out as the number one priority of public health practice. Logic and common sense would dictate such a priority, such a focus . . . *unless* for some reason injuries were not preventable and not susceptible to the standard tools of public health.

But in fact, injuries are highly preventable. Rather than being random, unpredictable, and unavoidable occurrences, injuries can be understood and prevented. As injury prevention professionals are wont to say, "injury is not an accident." Injury prevention has become an important part of public health practice and an important goal of improved public health. Unintentional injury and violence prevention are key components of the National Health Promotion and Disease Prevention Objectives contained in *Healthy People 2000* (see the appendixes to Chapter 4: Unintentional Injury and Chapter 5: Intentional Injury). Indeed, the number of objectives specifically related to injury prevention increased from 19 for the 1990 health objectives (17 related to unintentional injuries and one each to homicide and suicide) to 45 for the Year 2000 Health Objectives (26 related

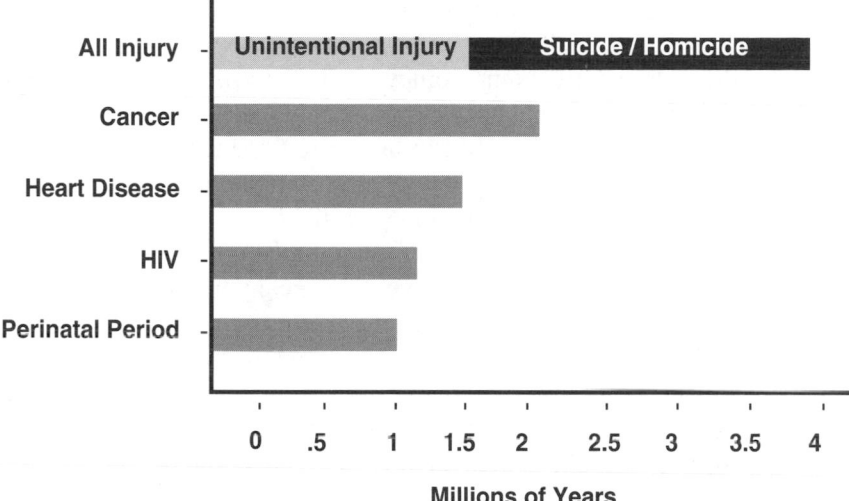

*Note.* HIV, human immunodeficiency virus.

**Figure I–1** Years of Potential Life Lost (YPLL) before Age 65, by Cause of Death—U.S., 1994. *Source:* Reprinted from http://www.cdc.gov/ncipc/pub-res/ypll94.jpg, National Center for Health Statistics Vital Statistics.

to unintentional injuries and 19 to violence). In addition, there are 30 injury-related objectives that appear under other priority areas, such as alcohol and other drugs, occupational safety and health, surveillance, and data systems.[8]

How do injury prevention objectives get put into action? A first critical step is the education and training of public health students and public health professionals in injury prevention. Injury prevention is a specialized field with its own distinct set of principles, techniques, and knowledge, which is the focus of this book. Given the significance and preventability of the injury problem, we would expect to find as much academic attention devoted to preparing public health professionals to implement injury prevention as is devoted to other aspects of public health education, such as acute and chronic disease prevention. This is not yet the case, however. Although the topic of injury is being taught increasingly in graduate schools of public health and included in some physician residency programs, most of these academic courses and texts have a research focus and do not prepare students for the difficulty of implementing proven prevention measures in real world settings. This may be because schools of public health have become isolated from the field of public health practice. The authors of *The Future of Public Health* noted that, "Many observers feel that some schools have become somewhat isolated from public health practice and therefore no longer place a sufficiently high value on the training of professionals to work in health agencies."[9(p15)] Comprehensive resources for incorporating injury prevention into the training of public health practitioners have not been widely available.

*Injury Prevention and Public Health: Practical Knowledge, Skills, and Strategies* focuses on what injury prevention means in the public health context. This book brings together the two basic parts of injury prevention—scientific information and practitioner implementation. Injury control encompasses many areas: epidemiology, prevention, behavioral sciences, biomechanics and engineering, acute medical care, rehabilitation, law, and policy. The authors each have close to 20 years of experience in public health, with the major focus on injury prevention. This book is shaped by our work in the implementation of community-based injury prevention interventions, injury surveillance, law, academia, government, and research.

There have been significant accomplishments in injury prevention and control during the past two decades. Violence, including firearm deaths, is now seen as a problem that can benefit from a public health approach. And the death toll from unintentional injuries continues to decline. Many proven strategies for prevention have been developed. The use of automobile child restraints has become the norm, at least for middle-class families. Bicycle helmets, seatbelts, and smoke detectors have come to be seen as customary practices for keeping children and adults safe. We have a National Center for Injury Prevention and Control as part of the U.S. Centers for Disease Control and Prevention (CDC). We have national data collected by the National Center for Health Statistics that include injury morbidity and injury causation. External cause of injury coding (i.e., E codes), critical to improving our understanding of injury causation and prevention, is required in more than 20 states. Many professional associations, including the American Public Health Association, American Academy of Pediatrics, American College of Emergency Physicians, American College of Physicians, American School Health Association, and American Health Information Management Association, now have sections, committees, and policy statements that deal with injury prevention. A State and Territorial Injury Prevention Directors Association has been established, with a designated public health representative in every state. A number of states have initiatives for injury prevention; initiatives exist not just in public health and traffic safety agencies, but also in state departments of education and labor and state attorneys general offices. Most of the 10 Public Health Service regions have formed injury prevention practitioner networks that host meetings, publish newsletters, operate list servers, conduct trainings, pool data, and otherwise collaborate to work more effectively and efficiently and to reduce the isolation often felt by practitioners.

We have more than enough data on which to base action to further reduce the toll of injury. The injury prevention literature has grown by leaps and bounds as research on injury and injury prevention continues to grow seemingly exponentially. Many public health and medical journals now include in nearly every issue articles relevant to injury and violence prevention. The journal *Injury Prevention* is in its fourth year of publication, with a focus of interest to practitioners, not just researchers. And the Institute of Medicine has selected injury control to be the focus of a second national assessment and report on the federal and state responses to the problem of injury, with recommendations for injury prevention programs, practices, and research in the decades ahead. What remains is for public health practitioners to play the necessary role in bridging the gap between research and policy implementation. We hope that this book will help in this endeavor.

Our goal has been to provide a comprehensive introduction to injury prevention without presenting the reader with an overwhelming and tedious tome. We could easily have made this text two or three times as long, but at the cost of readability and utility. Instead, we have attempted to provide succinct essays on key topics. The book is organized into three parts. Part I consists of a brief introduction to the injury problem: its magnitude, concepts, and epidemiology. Part II reviews the basics of injury prevention, including environmental, educational, and regulatory interventions. Part III, the largest component of the book, reviews programmatic efforts to reduce injury, focusing on how to be most effective in dealing with the injury problem. This is the "practical knowledge, skills, and strategies" of the book's subtitle. (Readers already familiar with the basics of injury prevention may wish to skim quickly over Parts I and II as a "refresher course" before focusing on Part III in greater depth.)

We do not assume that the reader is already expert in the sciences of public health, and so we present some basic background information on epidemiology, surveillance, and evaluation. But we obviously could not—and did not wish to—present a primer on any of these subjects. One area in particular is not presented: an international perspective on injury prevention. We have focused exclusively on the injury problem in the United States (although obviously the conceptual underpinnings of the discussion are universal in application). Economic conditions and varying stages of development have profound effects on a country's injury picture. The question for each nation is where to focus its prevention efforts and how to frame those efforts. It is interesting and instructive to compare both the data profiles and the differences in interventions between countries, but such an international review is beyond the scope of this introductory text. For the interested reader, there is a small but growing literature on injury and injury prevention from an international perspective.[10,11]

We have sought to use this text to inspire and assist students and public health practitioners in their efforts to effectively address the injury problem. We have sought to increase the reader's understanding, to point the reader toward useful sources of information, and to lay the groundwork for productive use of those sources. We hope that the result will meet with success.

---

## NOTES

1. Stolberg SG. U.S. life expectancy hits new high. *New York Times*, September 12, 1997, p. A12.

2. Bunker JP. Medicine matters after all. *J Royal Coll Physicians London.* 1995;29:105–112.

3. Leavitt JW, Numbers RL. Sickness and health in America: An overview. In: Leavitt JW, Numbers RL, eds. *Sickness and Health in America: Readings in the History of Medicine and Public Health*. Madison, WI: University of Wisconsin Press; 1985:3–10.

4. Fee E. History and development of public health. In: Scutchfield FD, Keck CW, eds. *Principles of Public Health Practice*. Albany, NY: Delmar Publishers; 1997:10–30.

5. Fingerhut LA, Warner M. Injury chartbook. In: *Health, United States, 1996–97 and Injury Chartbook*. Hyattsville, MD: U.S. Public Health Service; 1997.

6. Committee on Trauma Research, Commission on Life Sciences, National Research Council and the Institute of Medicine. *Injury in America: A Continuing Public Health Problem*. Washington, DC: National Academy Press; 1985:1.

7. Rivara FP, Grossman DC, Cummings P. Injury prevention (Part 1). *New Engl J Med.* 1997;337:543–548.

8. National Center for Health Statistics. *Healthy People 2000 Review, 1997*. Hyattsville, MD: U.S. Public Health Service; 1997.

9. Committee for the Study of the Future of Public Health. *The Future of Public Health*. Washington, DC: National Academy Press; 1988.

10. Barss P, Smith GS, Baker SP, Mohan D. *Injury Prevention: An International Perspective—Epidemiology, Surveillance, and Policy*. New York: Oxford University Press, 1998.

11. Berger LR, Mohan D. *Injury Control: A Global View*. Delhi: Oxford University Press; 1996.

# PART I

# Magnitude, Concepts, and Epidemiology of Unintentional and Intentional Injury

# CHAPTER 1

# The Importance of the Injury Problem: Magnitude, Cost, and Preventability

"Injury is the principal public health problem in America today."

William Foege, Preface to *Injury in America*, 1985

## WHAT THIS CHAPTER IS ABOUT

How and why has injury prevention become part of the public health agenda? How has a problem area that had been the purview of safety engineers and law enforcement personnel become a focus of local and state health departments and the U.S. Centers for Disease Control and Prevention (CDC)? And what exactly does it mean for the former director of the CDC to say, "Injury is the principal public health problem in America today"?[1]

In some ways the answers to these questions are straightforward. This chapter will review the magnitude and costs of injury for the United States, both in general terms and relative to other health problems. We will see that, by any measure we may choose to apply, injury is a critical component of the public's health profile. We will see that injury is a highly preventable source of morbidity and mortality. We will suggest factors that have contributed to injury being neglected as a public health problem. And we will see why it makes sense to deal with injury in the same ways we have dealt with acute and chronic diseases.

## INTRODUCTION

If today should turn out to be an average day in the United States

- 405 people will die of injuries
- 7,500 will be hospitalized because of nonfatal injuries
- 162,000 people will suffer injuries severe enough to restrict their usual activities and—in 92% of those cases—require that they seek medical attention[2(p18)]

Roughly one third of today's 400-plus injury deaths will be the result of motor vehicle injuries, one third the result of homicides and suicides, and one third the result of other types of "unintentional" injuries. Today, there may be a few more or a few less injuries than expected on an average day. Over the course of the year the nation will, tragically, average these numbers of injuries daily. Even more tragically, we know that many, if not most, of these injuries could be prevented.

Injury is damage or harm to the body resulting in impairment or destruction of health. More specifically, in *Injury Prevention: Meeting the Challenge*, the National Committee for Injury Prevention and Control defined injury as "any unintentional or intentional damage to the body resulting from acute exposure to thermal, mechanical, electrical, or chemical energy or from the absence of such essentials as heat or oxygen."[3(p4)] Injury, therefore, includes trauma from motor vehicle crashes, crushing and piercing by machines, falls, poisoning, burns, suffocation, and drowning. It also includes intentional acts like homicides, suicide, and assault. We usually define injury as occurring during a short period of time, as opposed to the effects of repeated exposures to chemical agents or cumulative damage from repetitive motions. Injuries can be fatal or nonfatal. (Injury may also be used to encompass psychological as well as physical trauma, such as that resulting from having witnessed a violent death or from being the victim of hate crimes. This is an important area of concern but one that is beyond the scope of this book.)

Injuries have always been a threat to the public's well-being, but until the mid-twentieth century, infectious diseases overshadowed the terrible contribution injury made to human morbidity and mortality. Public health's successes in other areas have left injury as a major public health concern, one that has been termed "the neglected epidemic." Public health improvements, particularly in the area of sanitation, have greatly reduced the prevalence of infectious diseases. As a result, injury's negative toll on the public's health has become more significant. Although heart disease and cancer continue as critical health problems in the United States, their combined contribution to premature deaths (measured as lost years of life before age 65) is less than that of injury because injury disproportionately affects a younger population, particularly children, teens, and young adults. Today injuries—both unintentional and intentional—constitute a major threat to public health. Unfortunately, this shift in significance has not yet been sufficiently reflected in the areas of research and prevention. Exhibit 1–1 shows the role of injury as a cause of death by age group.

Each year close to 150,000 Americans die as the result of injuries, a number roughly equivalent to the population of Fort Lauderdale, Florida. About one fourth of the U.S. population will fall victim to nonfatal injuries requiring some medical attention. More than two-and-one-half million people are hospitalized annually as the result of injuries, and 8% of all short-stay admissions are injury related.

In a perfectly rational world we would expect to find injury near the top of society's list of problems to be dealt with aggressively, but that is not the case. Why not? Why does injury not receive the public attention, the preventive resources, and the policy focus that problems of lesser impact receive?

The short answer is that we do not live in a perfectly rational world. In the real world—at least the United States at this time—injury as a social problem falls victim to several limiting factors. These factors, which are interrelated and synergistic, include the following:

- **Limitation #1**—Many people continue to consider injuries to be the result of random, uncontrollable factors that are largely beyond human control—so called "accidents" or "bad luck." As a result, the public seems to regard injury harm more stoically than other equally frightening personal disasters over which they (and the medical system) can exercise greater control—such as heart attacks and lung cancer. When it comes to the threat of a cancer slowly and uncontrollably destroying their bodies, however, the public seems to be more fearful and more demanding of solutions than for the tens of thousands of largely preventable motor vehicle deaths that occur in the United States each year. In fact, when it comes to injury risk, people seem to be rather resigned and accepting, reflecting the mistaken belief that injury is an

**Exhibit 1–1** Ten Leading Causes of Deaths by Age Group—1995

| Rank | <1 | 1–4 | 5–9 | 10–14 | 15–24 | 25–34 | 35–44 | 45–54 | 55–64 | 65+ | Total |
|---|---|---|---|---|---|---|---|---|---|---|---|
| | | | | | Age Groups | | | | | | |
| 1 | Congenital Anomalies 6,554 | Unintentional Injuries 2,280 | Unintentional Injuries 1,612 | Unintentional Injuries 1,932 | Unintentional Injuries 13,842 | Unintentional Injuries 13,435 | HIV 18,860 | Malignant Neoplasms 44,186 | Malignant Neoplasms 87,898 | Heart Disease 615,426 | Heart Disease 737,563 |
| 2 | Short Gestation 3,933 | Congenital Anomalies 695 | Malignant Neoplasms 523 | Malignant Neoplasms 503 | Homicide 7,284 | HIV 11,894 | Malignant Neoplasms 17,110 | Heart Disease 34,498 | Heart Disease 68,240 | Malignant Neoplasms 381,142 | Malignant Neoplasms 538,455 |
| 3 | SIDS 3,397 | Malignant Neoplasms 488 | Congenital Anomalies 242 | Homicide 405 | Suicide 4,784 | Suicide 6,292 | Unintentional Injuries 14,225 | Unintentional Injuries 9,261 | Bronchitis Emphysema Asthma 9,988 | Cerebrovascular 138,762 | Cerebrovascular 157,991 |
| 4 | Respiratory Distress Synd. 1,454 | Homicide 452 | Homicide 157 | Suicide 330 | Malignant Neoplasms 1,642 | Homicide 6,162 | Heart Disease 13,603 | HIV 8,179 | Cerebrovascular 9,735 | Bronchitis Emphysema Asthma 88,478 | Bronchitis Emphysema Asthma 102,899 |
| 5 | Maternal Complications 1,309 | Heart Disease 251 | Heart Disease 130 | Congenital Anomalies 207 | Heart Disease 1,039 | Malignant Neoplasms 4,875 | Suicide 6,467 | Cerebrovascular 5,473 | Diabetes 8,188 | Pneumonia & Influenza 74,297 | Unintentional injuries 93,320 |
| 6 | Placenta Cord Membranes 962 | HIV 210 | HIV 123 | Heart Disease 164 | HIV 629 | Heart Disease 3,461 | Homicide 4,118 | Liver Disease 5,247 | Unintentional injuries 6,743 | Diabetes 44,452 | Pneumonia & Influenza 82,923 |
| 7 | Perinatal Infections 788 | Pneumonia & Influenza 156 | Pneumonia & Influenza 723 | Bronchitis Emphysema Asthma 105 | Congenital Anomalies 452 | Cerebrovascular 720 | Liver Disease 3,705 | Suicide 4,532 | Liver Disease 5,356 | Unintentional Injuries 29,099 | Diabetes 59,254 |
| 8 | Unintentional Injuries 787 | Perinatal Period 87 | Benign Neoplasms 50 | HIV 66 | Bronchitis Emphysema Asthma 246 | Pneumonia & Influenza 622 | Cerebrovascular 2,772 | Diabetes 3,996 | Pneumonia & Influenza 3,458 | Alzheimer's Disease 20,230 | HIV 43,115 |
| 9 | Pneumonia & Influenza 492 | Septicemia 80 | Bronchitis Emphysema Asthma 38 | Benign Neoplasms 55 | Pneumonia & Influenza 207 | Diabetes 614 | Diabetes 1,844 | Bronchitis Emphysema Asthma 2,756 | Suicide 2,804 | Nephritis 20,182 | Suicide 31,284 |
| 10 | Intrauterine Hypoxia 475 | Cerebrovascular 57 | Anemias 31 | Pneumonia & Influenza 55 | Cerebrovascular 172 | Liver Disease 604 | Pneumonia & Influenza 1,480 | Pneumonia & Influenza 2,079 | HIV 2,320 | Septicemia 16,899 | Liver Disease 25,222 |

■ Unintentional Injuries
■ Homicide
■ Suicide

*Note:* HIV, human immunodeficiency virus; SIDS, sudden infant death syndrome.

*Source:* Reprinted from http://www.cdc.gov/ncipc/pub-res/101c95.gif, National Center for Injury Prevention and Control, U.S. Centers for Disease Control and Prevention.

inevitable part of life. This tends to be truer for men than for women (risk taking being "macho") and, unfortunately, especially the case for teenage males, who believe they are invulnerable. It also tends to be truer for certain causes of injury, such as sports, where risk taking is glorified and macho behavior is rewarded. (The long-term consequences of repeated injury from sports, such as arthritis, never seem to receive a second thought, suggesting that there is a critical need to come up with creative ways to reframe the public's perception of injury.)

- **Limitation #2**—Most people don't think about injury. When they do, they tend to focus their concern on dramatic, multiple-death injuries, such as those resulting from the crash of an airliner. Unfortunately, this obscures the fact that the greatest numbers of injuries occur in less newsworthy settings, such as falls or single-death motor vehicle crashes. An airplane crash with more than 100 deaths occurs in the United States perhaps once or twice a year; yet more than 100 people are killed in motor vehicle crashes every day (Exhibit 1–2). A critical task for the injury prevention community is to refocus the public's attention—and the federal government's response—onto these more common, much more deadly, and highly preventable kinds of injuries.
- **Limitation #3**—The media doesn't educate the public regarding injury. In fact, a major difficulty in refocusing the public's attention toward a clearer understanding of the injury problem comes from the print and broadcast media, which sensationalize injury events and focus on separate and unique injury events rather than patterns of injury and long-term trends in injury occurrence. Moreover, prevention doesn't make it into the headlines; the media rarely suggests possible preventive approaches. And too often the media conveys bad examples, such as picturing cyclists without helmets.
- **Limitation #4**  It is no "accident" that prevention is slighted. Prevention of injury—much more than a disease such as influenza—can present a problem and a challenge to powerful vested interests. This is because the vectors and environments that contribute to injury are largely manmade: motor vehicles, firearms, and consumer products. Making these vectors and environments safer—either voluntarily or through government regulation—can cut into profits. Thus the stakes can be high in fending off public efforts to enhance safety.

In a way, this is part of the magnitude of the injury problem. It is good news for public health if safety sells, but what if it doesn't sell—or manufacturers fear it won't sell? The automobile industry has a long history of resisting technological innovations to make cars more "crashworthy." Ironically, after decades of ridiculing Volvo's emphasis on safety over style, Detroit discovered that safety does indeed sell. Similarly, the technology exists to make firearms into safer consumer products, but the industry seems unwilling to incorporate this technology unless forced to do so. The drawback of such a situation—as seen

**Exhibit 1–2**  Investigation of Crashes

> When a plane goes down, it is not called an "accident," it's called a "crash." The National Transportation Safety Board investigates the cause and then works to prevent it from happening again. The Federal Aviation Administration employs about 40,000 people to accomplish its goals. In contrast, we lose more than 150 times as many people in car crashes. Each "crash" is called an "accident," we don't investigate them with the same level of attention, and we just hope it won't happen again.*
>
> –Chuck Hurley, noting that about 600 staff members at the National Highway Traffic Safety Administration work on reducing the number of car crashes.
>
> *Building Bridges Between Traffic Safety and Public Health—Proceedings of a Conference. Newton, MA: Education Development Center; 1991.

with airbags—is that when injury prevention principles based on scientific findings are forced on industry, the result can be a poorly executed, minimalist adoption of potential advances in safety technology.

- **Limitation #5**—Vested interests, with public relations support, often confuse the injury prevention issue. Industry, ably assisted by the media, continues to blame the victim and portray injury as largely a matter of individual fault—carelessness, stupidity, bad habits, or aberrant behavior—much more so than with heart disease, cancer, or infectious disease. Rather than exploring ways in which product designs can be improved to enhance safety, the victim is criticized for not using the product properly. This is especially true when it comes to firearms.

- **Limitation #6**—Injury prevention lacks the mystique and high-technology aura that excites the medical establishment and surrounds many other areas of disease prevention. A public that is acculturated to wonder drugs, coronary bypass surgery, and the much-publicized search for an acquired immune deficiency syndrome (AIDS) vaccine is understandably less excited by programs to lower hot water heater temperatures, encourage helmet use, and increase alcohol taxes. A helmet use program for all elementary schools in a city lacks the human interest of a desperate search to find a transplantable liver for a single, but therefore identifiable (i.e., more sympathetic) sick child in that same city. (Ironically, the organ donor for such a procedure is often a child who has died from a preventable injury, such as a head injury.)

- **Limitation #7**—A general lack of information and interest in injury prevention can be found not only among the public in general but also, unfortunately, within the medical profession, where prevention of any kind has long been give second (or third or fourth) place. As measured in terms of relative impact on morbidity and mortality, research dollars flow disproportionately away from injury prevention and toward more clinical disease entities. Injury prevention also is slighted in training programs for physicians and other health care professionals, and relatively few physicians are trained in injury causation and prevention. A recent survey of pediatricians indicated that only 18% received education on drowning prevention during their pediatric residency training, despite the fact that drowning is the second leading cause of unintentional injury death in the 0- to 19-year-old population.[4] The medical profession has been very slow to accept the fact that injury is a health problem with a supporting science that can be studied in much the same manner as the science that helps us deal more effectively with the disease-related areas of health.
- **Limitation #8**   Finally, injury surveillance and data are limited, especially at the local level—and especially when it comes to morbidity data. This makes it difficult to convince communities that there is an injury problem, to understand the problem and to develop effective preventive programs.

Despite these conceptual limitations, or irrationalities, on the part of the public, the media, and the health professions, much is known about how injuries occur and how injuries can be prevented. Much could be done with this knowledge. Various agendas for injury reduction exist, such as the injury prevention targets found in *Healthy People 2000* and the forthcoming *Healthy People 2010*.[5] The year 2000 objectives call for specific targets such as

- **7.11** Reduce by 20% the proportion of people who possess weapons that are inappropriately stored and therefore dangerously available. (Baseline data unavailable)
- **9.1** Reduce deaths caused by unintentional injuries to no more than 29.3 per 100,000 people. (Age-adjusted baseline: 34.7 per 100,000 in 1987)

- **10.1** Reduce deaths from work-related injuries to no more than 4 per 100,000 full-time workers. (Baseline: Average of 6 per 100,000 from 1983 to 1987)
- **9.24** Increase to 50 states laws requiring helmets for bicycle riders. (Baseline: 9 states in 1994)
- **9.12** Increase use of safety belts and child safety seats to at least 85% of motor vehicle occupants. (Baseline: 42% in 1988)
- **6.1** Reduce suicides to no more than 10.5 per 100,000 people. (Age-adjusted baseline: 11.7 per 100,000 in 1987)
- **7.16** Increase to at least 50% the proportion of elementary and secondary schools that teach nonviolent conflict resolution skills, preferably as a part of comprehensive school health education. (Baseline data unavailable)

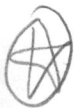

It is the task of public health professionals and public health agencies to make the argument for devoting collective attention and resources to injury prevention. What is that argument? It consists of two key points. First, the scope, magnitude, and social costs of injury should make injury and injury prevention leading public health concerns. Second, injury is indeed highly preventable and preventable in ways that are understood and achievable.

Injuries are not unpredictable, unavoidable events. To a large extent society chooses the injury rates it has. For example, it is a social choice to rely predominantly on automobiles and trucks to move people and goods and to do so at high speeds, despite the highly predictable injuries that will result. Similarly, it is a social choice to allow firearms to be readily accessible without any of the types of regulations applied to all other consumer products, despite their deadly consequences. And it is a social choice to have minimal protections, governmental and voluntary, for worker safety.

Public health professionals can help guide these social choices by providing clear information on the effectiveness of various interventions, so what is known to work can be put into action. Injury prevention professionals can also help counter misconceptions and objections that often serve as barriers to effective injury prevention efforts. These include such erroneous ideas as that motorcycle helmet use increases crash events, that the U.S. Constitution doesn't allow restrictions on gun possession, or that the decision not to wear a seatbelt affects only the individual making that decision.[6–9]

Public health professionals have a clear and important role in helping to reduce injury. It is a role that requires an understanding of the facts surrounding the injury problem. Let us therefore begin by looking more closely at the magnitude, costs, and preventability of injury to better understand why injury deserves major emphasis as a public health problem.

## MAGNITUDE

The scope of the problem is impressive and concerning. Baker et al note:

> Injury is important not only in relation to other health conditions but also in the absolute magnitude of the problem. More than six million people alive today in the United States can be expected to die from injuries. . . . The risk of injury while traveling, working, playing, or even sleeping is so great that most people sustain a significant injury at some time during their lives. Few escape the tragedy of a fatal or permanently disabling injury to a relative or friend.[10(p3)]

Injuries are the leading cause of death in the United States up to age 34 and, as one government study noted, "kill more Americans aged 1 to 34 than all diseases combined."[1(pp8–9)] Overall, injury ranks third among causes of death. Unlike heart disease and cancer, which primarily affect the old, injury deaths affect people of all ages, *especially* the young. "Injuries are the leading cause of death in the United States among children and teenagers. During this century, trauma has replaced infectious disease as the most important threat to our children. Injuries now claim almost 20,000 lives each year among the 0–19 age group."[11(p18)] In 1995, 77% of all deaths among 15 to 24 year olds were due to injuries, as were 52% of all deaths of 5 to 14 year olds.[2(p15)] Even for the elderly, despite their higher rates for heart disease and cancer, the death rate from injury remains higher than it is for young people. Minorities in the United States are also especially at risk for injury.

Injuries result in more productive years of life lost than any other cause: about three-and-one-half million potential years of life lost prematurely each year as compared to less than two million each for cancer, heart disease, and AIDS, and only 0.3 million each for liver disease and strokes. Baker et al note:

From age 1 through 4, injuries cause almost half of all deaths and result in more than three times the number of deaths from congenital anomalies, the second leading cause. Injury deaths exceed deaths from all other causes combined from age 5 through 34 and are most prominent at ages 15–24, when they cause 78% of all deaths. From age 35 through 44, they continue to outnumber deaths from any other single cause.[10]

As discussed in later chapters—particularly Chapter 12: Injury Surveillance—most injury data consists of mortality data. It is much harder to collect reliable information on nonfatal injuries—i.e., morbidity—and on the severity of injuries. Thus the total number of injuries—fatal and nonfatal—can only be approximated. Fingerhut and Warner, drawing on National Health Interview survey data for 1994, report "approximately 59 million episodes of injuries involving 62 million acute injury conditions" occur among the civilian noninstitutionalized population of the United States.[2(p18)]

Injury rates and causes vary according to age, sex, race, income, and geography. Injury death rates are highest for the very old, reflecting their much higher overall death rate. Prior to that the highest injury death rates are for those between 15 and 24 years old (Figure 1–1). Injury death rates are also higher for males than for females. Race also has an impact: "Native Americans (Indians, Eskimos, and Aleuts) have the highest death rates from unintentional injury; blacks have the highest homicide rates; and whites and Native Americans have the highest suicide rates."[10(p24)] These racial differences reflect dramatic differences in death rates based on economic class.

> For unintentional injuries, the death rate varies inversely with per capita income, decreasing from 61 per 100,000 in the lowest-income areas to 27 in the highest income areas. . . . For suicide, there is little relationship between death rate and per capita income; for homicide, residents of the wealthiest areas have much lower rates than those in other areas."[10(p26)]

Unintentional injury death rates are highest in rural areas, while homicide rates are highest in urban central city areas. There are also regional differences. For example, drowning rates are highest in the Southern and Western states and in Alaska. Motor vehicles and firearms are the most

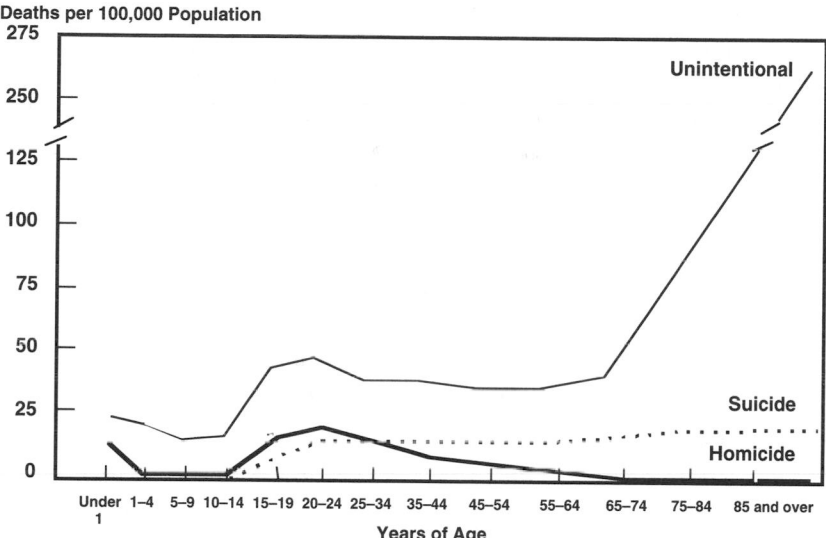

*Note:* Excludes ICD-9 codes E870–E879 and E930–E949.

## Intent

*Unintentional* injury comprised the largest portion of fatal injuries, about 61 percent, ranging from 50 percent at ages 20–24 years and 25–34 years to 79–91 percent for persons 1–10 years of age and 75 years and over. In 1995, 90,402 persons died as a result of an unintentional injury, at a crude rate of 34.4 per 100,000. . . . *Suicide* accounted for 21 percent of injury mortality, ranging from about 8 percent of all injury among those aged 85 years and over to 28 percent at 45–54 years. In 1995, 31,284 suicides were completed at a crude rate of 11.9 per 100,000 population. . . . *Homicide* accounted for 15 percent of all injury deaths, about 23-28 percent of injury deaths for infants and teens and young adults 15–34 years of age. In 1995, 22,552 persons were victims of homicide, at a crude rate of 8.6 per 100,000 population. . . . Intent was not determined for 2 percent of injury deaths in 1995.

**Figure 1–1** Injury Death Rates by Age and Manner of Death: United States, 1995. *Sources:* Graph, reprinted from Centers for Disease Control and Prevention, National Center for Health Statistics, National Vital Statistics System. Text, reprinted from L.A. Fingerhut and M. Warner, Injury Chartbook, in *Health, United States, 1996–1997*, p. 20, 1997, National Center for Health Statistics, U.S. Public Health Service.

likely causal agents to be involved in injury deaths for the young, while falls are the most common cause of fatal injuries for the old.

The impact of injury on the nation's health care resources is dramatic. In 1995, some 35 million emergency department visits were injury related, or 13.2 injury-related visits per 100 persons.[12] In 1995, more than 2.5 million hospital discharges were related to the treatment of injury.[2(p18)] Injury has long been a leading cause of physician contacts. "There were an estimated 126.1 million injury-related ambulatory care visits in 1995, representing 14.7% of the total number of visits."[13(p5)] Each year in the United States close to half a billion days are lost from work, school, or usual daily activities due to injury, affecting close to one third of Americans each year, with another quarter of a billion days lost from long-term disability associated with injury.[14] The Committee on Trauma Research has noted that

> Injury is also a leading cause of short- and long-term disability. In 1981, people spent 144 million days in bed because of injuries. With respect to long-term disability, more than 75,000 Americans each year sustain brain injuries that result in long-term disability including 2,000 who remain in persistent vegetative states. In addition, over 6,000 persons who were injured are discharged from hospitals with paraplegia or quadriplegia.[1(pp19–20)]

The numbers are so staggering that they may be held in disbelief and result in numbness on the part of policy makers. Yet injury holds important implications for the trend toward managed care in the United States. With such a significant portion of health care service delivery being devoted to dealing with the results of injury, it is apparent that the health care industry has a vital interest in seeing the number and the severity of injuries reduced. Injuries disproportionately affect the poor and the uninsured for many specific causes of injury, such as firearm and motorcycle injuries, and thus cause a major drain on health resources.

A discussion of the magnitude of injury should not end without saying something about long-term trends. As discussed above, the bad news is that injury is a leading public health problem resulting in serious morbidity and mortality. The good news is that in many ways the picture is improving (although not all the trends are toward improvement). Baker et al note that:

> For the United States as a whole, there was a 7.6% decrease in the overall injury death rate [between 1980 and 1985 and between

1986 and 1992]. Among the various causes of injury, the greatest decreases in death rate were for deaths related to farm machinery (–44%) and motorcycling (–43%) and the greatest increase nationwide was for firearm homicide (66%)."[11(p2)]

In several states, the number of firearm fatalities now equals the number of motor vehicle fatalities. The decreases in injury have been dramatic in some states with longstanding state health agency injury prevention programs. For example, childhood injury fatality rates in Massachusetts declined from 23.1 per 1,000 in 1985 to 14.3 per 1,000 in 1994, giving Massachusetts one of the lowest rates of any state. The number of unintentional injury fatalities among children age 19 and under dropped 53% during this period.[15] They must be doing something right.

## COSTS

The economic costs to society resulting from injury are high. "Injuries are the second leading cause for direct medical costs in the civilian, non-institutionalized population," after circulatory ailments.[16(p456),17] Injury accounts for 12% of medical spending in the United States.[17] However, measuring the overall cost of injury is not easy. Some costs are measurable, some are not. Some are economic, some are not. Deaths and hospital admissions, for example, are more readily measured than are lost future wages or the costs associated with permanent disfigurement. And as Fingerhut and Warner point out, "some very large number of injuries are not part of any data system because they were not medically treated and thus impose an unmeasured burden on society."[2(p15)] We also know that injury, especially sudden traumatic deaths from firearms or motor vehicle crashes, have social and psychological costs affecting the victims, the victims' families, and society as a whole.

There is a much more extensive literature on the cost of infectious disease than there is on injury costs. Only in recent years has much been done to develop cost information on injury.[18,19] So what do we know? We know, in the words of a 1989 report to Congress on the *Cost of Injury in the United States,* that:

> For the 57 million persons injured in 1985, the cost amounts to $157.6 billion, or $2,772 per injured person. . . . Direct expenditures for hospital and nursing home care, physician services,

drugs, and other medical and rehabilitation services amount to $44.8 billion or $790 per injured person. . . .

The direct cost is only the beginning. Disability from injury results in loss of output. Taking into account members of the labor force, housekeepers, and others unable to attend to their usual activities, more than 5 million life years are lost, 9 years per 100 injured persons, valued at $64.9 billion. The morbidity cost amounts to $1,145 per injured person.

Other losses result from premature injury fatalities. Approximately 143,000 premature deaths from injury occurred in 1985 and an additional 13,000 deaths occurred in later years due to injury sustained in 1985. Premature death due to injury is extremely costly to the nation, amounting to an estimated annual loss of 5.3 million life years, or 34 years per death. The loss to the economy amounts to $47.9 billion at a 6% discount rate, or $307,636 per death.[18(p38)]

This report to Congress can now be seen as an underestimate of injury costs. By the mid-1990s the estimated cost of injury had risen to more than $224 billion (a 42% increase in a decade). Public sources (federal, state, and local) pay about 28% of this cost.[20] Injury economist Ted Miller provides an even higher estimate for 1995: $325 billion spent on injury and its consequences (including medical costs, work lost, and insurance claims processing expenses).[21]    Wow!!!!

## PREVENTABILITY

Former CDC Director Dr. William Foege has noted that:

Injury is a problem that can be diminished considerably if adequate attention and support are directed to it. Exciting opportunities to understand and prevent injuries and to reduce their effects are at hand. The alternative is the continued loss of health and life to predictable, preventable, and modifiable injuries.[1(pv)]

Yet there exists a wide disparity between what is known about injury prevention and what is actually done to prevent injury. This disparity is greater than in any other major health problem area, including human immunodeficiency virus and AIDS. Thus while the grim injury picture shows some signs of improving in the face of mounting evidence that many if not most injuries are not inevitable, the improvement lags far behind where it could be. The challenge is to close the gap between knowledge and action as effectively as possible. This is where the time-tested tools of public health can come into play.

If injuries are viewed as "accidental"—random, unpredictable and unavoidable occurrences— or as events resulting from individual carelessness, then there is little reason or opportunity for societal interventions. Instead, injuries are viewed as isolated problems of the individual victims, rather than as public concerns. Until recently this was largely the conventional outlook. The prevention efforts that did exist focused on the supposed shortcomings of the victims, and interventions were almost entirely aimed at modifying the individual. For example, motor vehicle crashes were seen as almost entirely matters of individual driver fault. The government therefore could limit its involvement to legislating who could drive, prohibiting drunk driving, and punishing recklessness and other poor performance. Few people thought of automobile crashes as a public health problem that required broader intervention to protect all drivers through redesign of roads and motor vehicles.

During the past three decades, the science of injury prevention has moved away from such a highly individualistic approach to one that more readily relies on socially based policies. There are a variety of reasons for this change, including that injury prevention has drawn the attention of a continually broadening range of disciplines. This interdisciplinary collaboration has fostered a number of significant conceptual advances. Epidemiological studies have altered the overall picture of injury, shifting it from a single-cause view toward a multiple-causation model. There has been growing recognition of the fact that the public health tools and methods used effectively against infectious and other diseases can also be applied to injury prevention. As a result, attention is paid not only to individual victims, but also to the environment and to the products used by the public.

This is where public health comes into play, by offering the tools and expertise that can effectively organize preventive interventions. These things do not happen by themselves. As Baker et al note: "Sometimes people in positions to make changes that could reduce injury risks do not know that effective remedies are available, or they are unaware of their power to implement or promote them."[11(p1)] Implementation requires

- assessing the specific injury problem via data collection and risk factor identification
- facilitating the formation of multidisciplinary groups in the community to coalesce around the problem
- developing injury prevention interventions
- evaluating these early injury prevention programs
- replicating proven programs

One version of this process has been graphically portrayed by the National Center for Injury Prevention and Control. Its representation of the "public health approach" appears as Figure 1–2.

Public health can bring the approach outlined in *The Future of Public Health*—assessment, policy development, and assurance—to injury prevention. *Assessment* requires that "every public health agency regularly and systematically collect, assemble, analyze, and make available information on the health of the community, including statistics on health status, community health needs, and epidemiologic and other studies of health problems." *Policy development* requires that "every public health agency exercise its responsibility to serve the public interest in the development of comprehensive public health policies by promoting use of the scientific knowledge base in decision-making about public health and by leading in developing public health policy." And *assurance* requires that "public health agencies assure their constituents that services necessary to achieve agreed upon goals are provided, either by encouraging actions by other entities (private or public sector), by requiring such action through regulation, or by providing services directly."[22(pp7–8)] How can this approach be organized? One useful blueprint can be found in *Injury Prevention: Meeting the Challenge*, a collaboration of more than 30 injury prevention experts and 3 federal agencies.[3] This report, to which the reader is referred for useful advice and examples, underscores the theme that injury occurrences are understandable, predictable, and preventable. The *Meeting the Challenge* report concludes that:

> Were we to apply the lessons of the science of injury prevention in a truly comprehensive way, we would see an enormous reduction in death, disability, and cost to individuals, government, and the private sector.[3(pp4–9)]

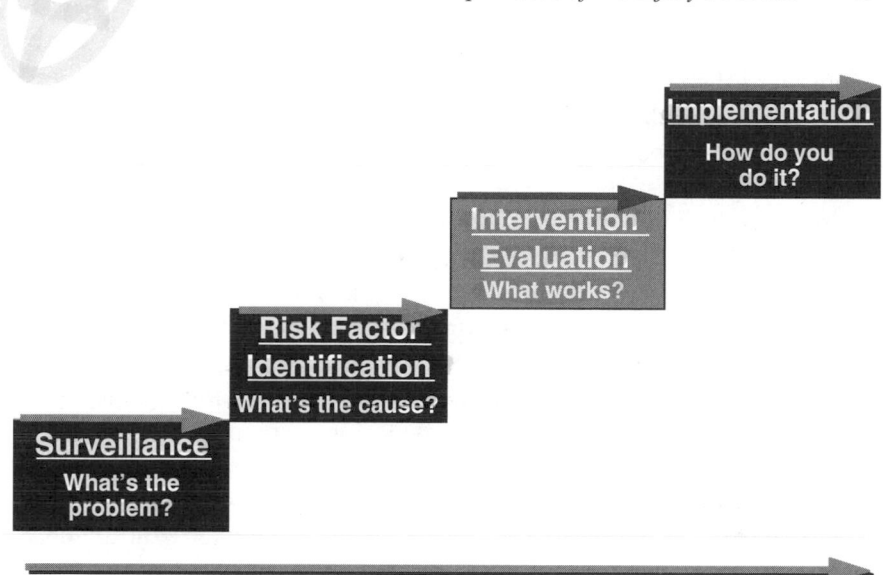

**Figure 1–2** Public Health Approach. *Source:* Reprinted from http://www.cdc. gov/ncipc/pub-res/mr930d.htm, National Center for Injury Prevention and Control, U.S. Centers for Disease Control and Prevention.

Public health can contribute to reducing injury in the United States by drawing on expertise in advocacy, surveillance, data analysis, research, training, needs assessment, public education, and intervention. These are some of the key areas of expertise that agencies in the Public Health Service  like the National Center for Injury Prevention and Control and the Maternal and Child Health Bureau—have tried to foster through their grant funding mechanisms, either through those specific to injury prevention or through the state formula block grant process.

Misinformation and misunderstanding regarding any public health problem needs to be overcome. Ignorance should not deter public health practitioners and public health agencies from dealing with the problem of injury in a rational manner. In fact, it is the task of those charged with protecting the public's health to bring about the perceptional changes necessary in order for society to respond adequately to injury as a social problem of significant magnitude.

AIDS prevention has a constituency of advocates. There are also associations concerned with many chronic and infectious diseases (such as heart, lung, kidney, and diabetes associations) that are able to capture the attention of the public for the resources needed to seek solutions, cures, and services. But although there are victims groups for specific subgroups of injury, with a focus on after-injury service provision, and groups that focus on important parts of the injury problem—such as childhood injuries or drunk driving injuries—there is no overall advocacy group to focus public attention on all of injury prevention. Public health practitioners involved in injury prevention must therefore play this role, raising awareness about injuries and their prevention, mobilizing the support of communities and policy makers, and fostering collaborative efforts with those disciplines with a history of working to make safety an issue. Public health practitioners must also highlight the need for training in injury control. And, finally, they must ensure that existing injury data, albeit imperfect, is actively made use of to drive and guide programs and policies, rather than waiting for the perfect data set before resources are directed at injury problems.

## CONCLUSION

Injuries have always been with us, although over time the nature of the leading types of injury has changed. In the United States today, with a heavy reliance on the automobile, it is certainly not surprising that motor vehicle injuries predominate. Nor should it be surprising that in the United States, where handguns are so unusually plentiful and accessible, firearm death rates are tragically high.

The significance of injury as a public health problem has received increasing attention during recent years. This is particularly dramatic when it comes to children, for whom injury is today the leading cause of death. Fortunately the conceptual approach to injury is becoming less fatalistic and more scientific. There has been progress—albeit painfully slow—in reducing the imbalance between the significance of injury as a public health problem and the amount of attention and resources directed at the problem by health departments, research programs, foundations, academia, the private sector, and others. But much remains to be done, especially in public health education and in public health agencies.

Injury continues to be the leading public health problem in the United States. It is a problem of tremendous magnitude in terms of mortality, morbidity, disability, and costs. At the same time, injury is better understood as a highly preventable occurrence. Public health can and should play the critical role in injury prevention. The pages that follow are intended to guide public health practitioners in optimizing their abilities to deal with this important problem and in integrating injury prevention into their work in an effective manner.

---

## NOTES

1. Committee on Trauma Research, Commission on Life Sciences, National Research Council and the Institute of Medicine. *Injury in America: A Continuing Public Health Problem.* Washington, DC: National Academy Press; 1985.

2. Fingerhut LA, Warner M. Injury chartbook. In: *Health, United States, 1996–97 and Injury Chartbook.* Hyattsville, MD: U.S. Public Health Service; 1997.

3. National Committee for Injury Prevention and Control. *Injury Prevention: Meeting the Challenge.* New York: Oxford University Press (Published as a supplement to the *Am J Prev Med.* 1989;5:4).

4. O'Flaherty JE, Pirier PL. Prevention of pediatric drowning and near drowning. *Pediatrics.* 1997;99:169–174.

5. See the most recent update of the Healthy People objectives in National Center for Health Statistics. *Healthy People 2000 Review, 1997.* Hyattsville, MD: U.S. Public Health Service; 1997.

6. For information on helmet use, see the World Health Organization Helmet Initiative Web site at http://www.sph.emory.edu/Helmets.

7. On seatbelts, helmets, and "liberty rights" see *Simon v. Sargent,* 346 F.Supp. 277 (D.Mass.), *aff'd* 409 U.S. 1020 (1972).

8. *People v. Kohrig,* 113 Ill.2d 384, 498 N.E.2d 1158 (1986); *State v. Hartog,* 440 N.W.2d 852 (Iowa 1989).

9. The U.S. Supreme Court and the lower federal courts have consistently adhered to this interpretation, which is why those gun laws that have been enacted have withstood Second Amendment challenges. For a useful summary of the extensive literature on this subject, see Henigan DA, Nicholson EB, Hemenway D. *Guns and the Constitution: The Myth of Second Amendment Protection for Firearms in America.* Northampton, MA: Aletheia Press; 1995.

10. Baker SP, O'Neill B, Ginsburg MJ, Li G. *The Injury Fact Book.* 2nd ed. New York: Oxford University Press; 1992.

11. Baker SP, Fingerhut LA, Higgins L, Chen LH, Braver ER. *Injury to Children and Teenagers: State-by-State Mortality Facts.* Baltimore: The Johns Hopkins Center for Injury Research and Policy; 1996.

12. McCaig LF, Stussman BJ. National ambulatory medical care survey: 1996 emergency department survey. *Advance Data.* Hyattsville, MD: National Center for Health Statistics; December 17, 1997. No. 293.

13. Schappert SM. Ambulatory care visits to physician offices, hospital outpatient departments, and emergency departments: United States, 1995. *Vital Health Statistics.* 1997;13:5.

14. Smith GS, Falk H. Unintentional injuries. In: *Closing the Gap: Health Policy Project.* Atlanta: The Carter Center of Emory University; 1984:144.

15. Injury Prevention and Control Program. *Injury Fatalities and Hospitalizations among Massachusetts Children and Youth, 1985–1994.* Boston: Massachusetts Department of Public Health; 1997.

16. Harlan LC, Harlan WR, Parsons SE. The economic impact of injuries: A major source of medical costs. *Am J Public Health.* 1990;80:453–459.

17. Miller TR, Lestina DC, Galbraith MS, Viano DC. Medical-care spending—United States. *MMWR* 1994;43:581–586.

18. Rice DP, MacKenzie EJ, and Associates. *Cost of Injury in the United States: A Report to Congress.* San Francisco: Institute for Health and Aging, University of California and Injury Prevention Center, The Johns Hopkins University; 1989.

19. Miller TR, Pindus NM, Douglass JB, Rossman SB. *Databook on Nonfatal Injury: Incidence, Costs, and Consequences.* Washington, DC: The Urban Institute; 1995.

20. See http://www.cdc.gov/ncipc/about/about.htm.

21. Miller TR. Children's Safety Network Economics and Insurance Resource Center. Landover, MD: National Public Services Research Institute; 1995.

22. Committee for the Study of the Future of Public Health. *The Future of Public Health.* Washington, DC: National Academy Press; 1988.

# CHAPTER 2

# Conceptual and Historical Underpinnings of Injury and Injury Prevention

"Measures to reduce injuries have been used since ancient times. . . . Many have worked so well that they have been used for millennia."

William Haddon, Jr., *Landmarks in American Epidemiology*, 1980

## WHAT THIS CHAPTER IS ABOUT

What are injuries? How and why has injury prevention become part of the public health agenda? Is it realistic to focus traditional public health research and program tools on the injury problem? Is intentional injury really a public health problem? These are important questions, the answers to which require some understanding of the conceptual and historical underpinnings of injury and injury prevention.

This chapter will trace the evolution of the modern-day conceptual understanding of injury. This is important because the way we think about injury is what has brought injury prevention into the public health arena more than anything else has. And it is the way that we think about injury that will determine how effective we are in reducing the toll of injury in America.

## INTRODUCTION

Until not too many years ago, unintentional injuries (intentional injuries are discussed later) were viewed as either "accidental"—random, unpredictable, and unavoidable occurrences—or events resulting from individual carelessness or "accident-prone" lack of coordination. This viewpoint made them isolated misfortunes experienced by individual victims, rather than public health concerns that could be understood and dealt with on a population basis. Working from such a conceptual approach it made little sense to devote limited public health resources to dealing with injury. For example, motor vehicle crashes were seen almost entirely as matters of individual driver fault. Society could legislate who could drive, prohibit drunk driving, and punish reckless driving behavior, but few people thought of automobile crashes as a public health problem. At most the public health community's injury prevention focus consisted of admonitions to the public to "be careful."

Viewing a social problem in individualistic terms centering on the shortcomings of the victim is not unique to injury. Many people (particularly politicians and leaders of the religious right) have portrayed acquired immune deficiency syndrome (AIDS) as being the result—and also the just desserts—of the "shortcomings" of those who are gay or intravenous drug users. This focus on individual deficits was, for a long time, well received as a framework for understanding the injury problem. Sylvia Noble Tesh notes that science itself has long been permeated with value judgments and that one of the most important has been individualism, which:

> makes the individual the basic unit of social analysis. It supports a politically conservative predisposition to bracket off questions about the structure of society . . . and to concentrate instead on questions about the behavior of individuals within that (apparently fixed) structure. One consequence is the assumption that health education is the best way to prevent disease. Unhealthy behavior results from individual choice, the ideology implies, so the way to change such behavior is to show people the error of their ways and urge them to act differently.[1(pp161–162)]

It is of great significance therefore that over the past several decades the theoretical focus on injury has shifted from a biological and behavioral emphasis on the individual to a concern with the environmental context within which injury occurs. This conceptual shift was connected to another theoretical advance: the growing awareness that single-cause explanations of injury events are incomplete and misleading. For example, it is not sufficient to say that a motor vehicle fatality was the result of "drunk driving." Such an explanation obscures a variety of surrounding questions. Why did *this* drunk driver crash while another did not? Why did he or she crash during *this* trip and not during any previous drunk driving episodes? Why did he or she crash at *this* place and not a mile earlier? Why was *this* crash fatal? Why was it fatal to *this* driver but not the passenger? In short, was *this* fatality inevitable and, if not, what could have prevented it? As Julian Waller has pointed out, because injury events are relatively rare occurrences, it is easy for people to fall into the trap of associating the event with a single characteristic—such as drunk driving—and then infer causation.

During this century, and especially during the past three decades, the science of injury prevention has moved away from a highly individualistic approach to one that is more amenable to socially based (i.e., public health) interventions. There are a variety of reasons for this change, including the fact that injury prevention has drawn the attention of a growing number of disciplines, and that this interdisciplinary collaboration inspired conceptual advances. Intentional violence was once seen solely as a law enforcement and criminal justice issue, suicide was viewed as a mental health problem, and unintentional injury prevention was primarily the purview of safety engineers and psychologists. A public health approach has made injury the focus of research and programmatic concerns by a wide range of disciplines, not only those just mentioned but also epidemiologists and biostatisticians, maternal and child health officials, environmental and biomechanics experts, public health lawyers, and policy analysts. The public health approach to preventing both unintentional and intentional injuries is one in which, as Garen Wintemute stated, "We examine more of the variables, and we don't insist that we have to change the fundamental nature of people in order to do something about a health problem. And unlike the other disciplines, we take the results of our scientific work to the public and into the legislative arena."[2(p48)]

There has been growing recognition that public health tools and methods used effectively against infectious and other diseases also can be applied to injury prevention. The National Center for Injury Prevention and Control, part of the U.S. Centers for Disease Control and Prevention (CDC), is staffed by an interdisciplinary group of public health experts drawn from the traditional areas of public health expertise. These CDC experts point out that interventions designed to reduce the impact of injury, such as bicycle or motorcycle helmets, can be considered an injury "vaccine," making the vaccinated public more resistant to injury. And as with any vaccine, its use must be fostered through a combination of education and legal requirements and its impact must be measured through surveillance and epidemiological analysis. A result of this heightened public health awareness regarding injury is that preventive interventions concentrate not only on individual victims, but also on the environment and on the products used by the public.

## HIGH POINTS IN THE CONCEPTUAL EVOLUTION OF INJURY

The preventability of injuries is not a late twentieth-century notion. Julian Waller notes that, in 1788, Johann Peter Frank described injury prevention activities as a desirable part of comprehensive public health programs.[3] But Waller also notes that this message did not fall on fertile ground in highly individualistic, noninterdependent frontier America.

The science of modern injury prevention has evolved during this century along with the social realization that individuals are often in a poor position to perceive and control injury risks. The standard history of this evolution focuses on several people who played critical roles in advancing understanding. The first of these individuals was Hugh De Haven, a World War I pilot who survived a plane crash and went on, as a physiology researcher, to attempt to better understand the reasons why. This pioneer in biomechanics concluded that "Structural provisions to reduce impact and distribute pressures can enhance survival and modify injury within wide limits in aircraft and automobile accidents."[4(p6)] In other words, the fact that a crash or other injury event occurs is but the first step in a process that may or may not result in an injury. The injury event is only the beginning of understanding the injury process.

Another critical figure in injury prevention history was John Gordon, an epidemiologist at Harvard at midcentury, who studied the distribution and causes of injury in the same way as classic infectious diseases were studied. Disease had long been the subject of scientific scrutiny and rarely did such scrutiny focus on the "disease-prone" behaviors and shortcomings of victims (only much more recently has AIDS become an unfortunate exception). Epidemiology, as the scientific study of diseases among populations, focuses on patterns and distributions of disease in order to tailor preventive measures to reduce disease by focusing on populations. Gordon was interested in applying the same approach to injury. His studies of injury distribution patterns, according to such factors as age, place, time, and the like, demonstrated the nonrandomness of injury events. Gordon focused epidemiological techniques not only on injury patterns, demographics, and trends, but also on the classic triad of epidemiology. Rather than concentrating on single-cause explanations of injury, Gordon described injuries as being the result of "forces from at least three sources . . . the host . . . the agent . . . and the environment in which host and agent find themselves."[5] This approach parallels that of infectious disease prevention, where the host might be protected via immunization, environmental transmission interrupted by sanitary engineering, and the agent dealt with through antibiotics. In terms of injury, the host might be a curious, mobile 2 year old; the agent might be a potentially poisonous bottle of cleaning fluid that looks similar to a drink—such as apple juice—that the toddler likes; and the environment might be a screw-top bottle in an accessible area at the toddler's level, such as under the kitchen sink. Taken together, this scenario could result in a serious, unintentional injury. But intervention to prevent such an injury could occur at several points to secure the host, agent, and/or environment.

This insight was critically important because it showed the full power of an epidemiological approach to a study and understanding of injuries. But while the injury host and the injury environment could be understood in terms comparable to that of the disease model, it was not clear how to approach and understand the agent of injury. Unlike a virus or toxin associated with a disease, the agents of injury seemed innumerable and varied: knives and explosives, cars and fires, or ladders and machinery. In 1961 James Gibson advanced the concept of injury in classic epidemiological terms by suggesting that "energy interchange" was the agent of injury harm. Today injury is commonly defined as the transfer of energy to human tissues in amounts and at rates that damages the cellular structure, tissues, blood vessels, and other bodily structures. This includes mechanical (kinetic), thermal, chemical, electrical, or radiation energy: *mechanical energy,* as when an unrestrained motor vehicle occupant's head strikes the windshield during a crash; *thermal energy,* as when the heat and flames of a house fire; *chemical energy* as with the aforementioned cleaning fluid attacks the toddler's metabolic process; *electrical energy* as from contact with accessible high-voltage power lines; *radiation energy*, as with a serious sunburn.

Gibson's definition didn't fit perfectly, for it ignored injuries such as death by drowning or freezing. William Haddon, a physician and engineer who is considered the "founding father" of modern-day injury prevention, took Gibson's insight further, showing that the few injuries that did not fit this pattern of physical energy transfer involved the absence of necessary energy elements—such as oxygen or heat occurring in drowning or hypothermia. By 1989, the National Committee for Injury Prevention and Control would define injury as "any unintentional or intentional damage to the body resulting from acute exposure to thermal, mechanical, electrical, or chemical energy or from the absence of such essentials as heat or oxygen."[4]

## INJURY BIOMECHANICS

Of the various forms of energy—kinetic, thermal, chemical, electrical, and radiation—kinetic (or mechanical) energy transfer is the biggest contributor to injury. It is useful for public health injury prevention specialists to understand the biomechanics of kinetic energy injuries (just as it is important for them to understand the epidemiology of injury). Injury texts by Leon Robertson[6] and Julian Waller[7] provide useful explanations of the physics (and chemistry) of injury. No injury prevention library would be complete without these two basic texts, along with the latest edition of *The Injury Fact Book*.[8]

Mechanical injury results from the "deformation of tissues beyond their failure limits."[9(p48)] In *Injury in America*, the Committee on Trauma Research noted that:

> Injury biomechanics research uses the principles of mechanics to explore the mechanisms of physical and physiologic responses to mechanical forces . . . by penetrating or nonpenetrating blows to the body. . . . Research in biomechanics involves a variety of disciplines, including engineering, physiology, medicine, biology, and anatomy.[9(p48)]

The Committee on Trauma Research also noted that mechanical injuries can be caused in three ways:

1. Crushing deformation of the body, such as through chest compression, rib fracture, and aortic laceration.
2. Impulsive impact, such as by violent sternal motion that deforms the heart beyond its viscous tolerance and causes contusion and rupture.

3. Acceleration of the skeleton and tearing of internal organs, because of their inertia; for example, during head impact, the skull accelerates and the loosely attached brain lags, so injury is due in part to deformation of brain tissues beyond their limit of recovery. . . . As long as the energy delivered to the tissue is below the limit of injury—whether it be the crush limit, the viscous limit, or the acceleration limit—the energy will be absorbed without causing injury. . . . The two main types of strain . . . that can damage tissue are tensile strain and shear strain; a third type is compressive strain, which is responsible for crushing injuries.[9(pp49–51)]

Regardless of whether the kinetic energy results from a motor vehicle crash, a shooting, or a fall, the force to which human tissue will be subjected is the product of the mass and the velocity involved. The basic formula—force equals one half of mass multiplied by the square of velocity—illustrates that the effect of velocity is greatly enhanced as velocity increases. This force will cause more or less damage to the host depending upon the shape and the rigidity of the colliding surface or object, but velocity usually plays the most critical role.

The physics and biomechanics of injury has been of concern primarily to the engineers who design the environment in which injury occurs, whether it be automotive design, highway design, building design, or other designs. The resulting designs affect all people, so in some cases government controls those designs (e.g., federal motor vehicle safety standards or local building codes). In other cases the market influences the designer (for example, in terms of whether cars are larger—with more "crush space" to absorb dangerous energy—or smaller). Certainly biomechanics has made a broad contribution to injury prevention, ranging from determining the best bike helmet design for minimizing head impact to developing hip pads to reduce the effect of falls by the elderly to defining human tolerance limits for injury among very young children, women, and the frail elderly.

For the public health practitioner, understanding the physics and biomechanics of injury is important not only in helping to educate the men and women who design these environments, but also in educating the public who must interact with (i.e., be subjected to) energy transfers within these environments. For example, it is important to educate parents on why holding a baby in their arms is not a way of providing protection in a crash and on why a child restraint system offers protection in a crash. In a crash, an unrestrained object—such as a child—travels with a force equal to one half of the product of its mass times the square of its velocity. If a car is traveling at 35 miles per hour and crashes into a rigid object, a 20-pound baby will travel with a force of as much as 800 pounds (depending on the amount of energy absorbed by the car's "crush space"). It would be as easy to hold such a baby securely as it would be to lift 800 pounds a foot off the ground. As one commentator has noted, "Crashing an automobile at 30 miles per hour is like diving headfirst off a three-story building."[10(p9)]

It is not difficult to imagine the result of forces of this magnitude striking some part of a car's interior (the so-called "second collision"). A child restraint system allows for a more uniform "ride down" of such a crash, so that the force is distributed more uniformly over time, and also spreads the load, so that the force is distributed more uniformly over the body.

## INJURY PREVENTION

William Haddon, Jr., of the New York State Health Department, also extended John Gordon's epidemiological insights by noting that injury host, agent, and environment can be analyzed temporally in terms of a preinjury phase, an injury phase, and a postinjury phase. The preinjury phase is when primary prevention approaches can be implemented (such as conflict resolution programs, divided highways, or enforcement of speed limits). The injury phase is when secondary prevention is possible (such as the deployment of airbags in crashes or the installation of breakaway signposts). The postinjury phase is the time to focus on tertiary prevention (such as effective emergency medical services, minimal trauma response times, or rehabilitation programs). This systematic breaking down of the injury problem into temporal as well as epidemiological components is often represented in what has come to be known as the Haddon Matrix (Exhibit 2–1).

Haddon continued this systematic conceptualization of injury by identifying 10 basic categories of injury prevention countermeasures, also arranged temporally. These approaches or strategies represent the various ways in which energy transfer can be controlled, modified, or interrupted. They are

1. Prevent the initial creation of the hazard by banning the manufacture and sale of inherently unsafe products or prohibiting inherently un-

**Exhibit 2–1**  The Haddon Matrix

| Factors / Phases | Human Factors | Agent or Vehicle | Physical Environment | Sociocultural Environment |
|---|---|---|---|---|
| Pre-event | | | | |
| Event | | | | |
| Post-event | | | | |

safe practices (e.g., don't produce firecrackers, three-wheeled all-terrain vehicles, or various poisons; eliminate "spearing" in high school football).

2. Reduce the amount of energy contained in the hazard (e.g., limit the muzzle velocity of guns and the amount of gunpowder in firecrackers; limit the horsepower of motor vehicle engines; package toxic drugs in smaller, safer amounts).

3. Prevent the release of a hazard that already exists (e.g., store firearms in locked containers; close pools and beaches when no lifeguard is on duty).

4. Modify the rate or spatial distribution of the hazard (e.g., require safety valves on boilers; use seatbelts to control the deceleration of occupants in motor vehicle crashes; use short cleats on football shoes so feet rotate rather than transmit sudden force to knees).

5. Separate, in time or space, the hazard from that to be protected (e.g., provide pedestrian overpasses at high volume traffic crossings; do not have play areas near unguarded bodies of water).

6. Separate the hazard from that which is to be protected by a material barrier (e.g., install fencing to enclose all four sides of swimming pools; insulate electrical cords; provide protective eyewear for racquet sports; build highway medians; make use of bulletproof barriers).

7. Modify relevant basic qualities of the hazard (e.g., provide padded dashboards in motor vehicles; make crib slat spacing too narrow to strangle a child; adopt use of safer baseballs and breakaway baseball bases; install nonslip surfacing in bathtubs).

8. Make what is to be protected more resistant to damage from the hazard (e.g., encourage calcium intake to reduce osteoporosis and brittle bones in case of falls; encourage musculoskeletal conditioning for athletes; prohibit alcohol sales and consumption near recreational water areas).
9. Begin to counter the damage already done by the hazard (e.g., provide emergency medical care on-site at car crashes; employ systems to route injured persons to appropriately trained trauma care providers; develop school protocols for responding to injury emergencies).
10. Stabilize, repair, and rehabilitate the object of the damage (e.g., develop rehabilitation plans at an early stage of injury treatment; make use of occupational rehabilitation for paraplegics).

The conceptual advances of Haddon and others were introduced into the policy and political arenas by Haddon himself, Ralph Nader (beginning with *Unsafe at Any Speed*), and Daniel Patrick Moynihan, among others. Their efforts—and those of many others—led to legislative enactments such as the National Traffic and Motor Vehicle Safety Act of 1966, which incorporated a system of motor vehicle safety standards organized according to preinjury, injury, and postinjury phases.

Public health practitioners can educate the public regarding the nature of injury and the logic of injury prevention mechanisms. Public health also helps increase the body's tolerance to injury forces by helping the public deal with alcohol abuse, osteoporosis, hypertension, arteriosclerosis, and other health problems that lower the body's tolerance to mechanical forces.

It is hard to overemphasize the importance—from a public health perspective—of the conceptual shift from single-cause, behavioral explanations of injury to multiple-cause, environmental explanations. It is only from within the later conceptual framework that it is possible to apply the strengths of the public health approach to the injury. If injuries are "accidents," there is little society can do to prevent them. If injuries result from individual shortcomings, there is little other than heightening awareness through education that society can do to reduce injury risks. As the authors of *Injury Prevention: Meeting the Challenge* put it:

> The contributions of De Haven, Gordon, Gibson, Haddon, and others helped to shift injury prevention away from an early, naive preoccupation with distributing educational pamphlets and post-

ers and toward modifying the environments in which injuries occur. By developing new laws and enforcement mechanisms and through new technologies and engineering changes in products, injury experts from a broad range of disciplines sought to protect people from coming into contact with injurious amounts of energy.[4(p7)]

The goal of the environmental approach to injury prevention is to structure the physical environment so as to minimize the injurious release of energy. This approach, if aggressively implemented, can significantly reduce the toll of injury. An example is the dramatic decrease in U.S. motor vehicle deaths during the past three decades, resulting from environmental modifications—particularly federal motor vehicle safety standards to improve vehicle crashworthiness and safer highway design with fewer roadside hazards. There have also been important changes in the "psychosocial environment." For example, even those individuals whose attitudes regarding drinking and driving may be irresponsible must now function in an environment in which those around them are less likely to tolerate and facilitate drinking and driving behavior.

Environmental modification obviously cannot provide perfect protection from injury. So education and behavioral approaches, once the mainstay of injury prevention, continue to play a role in preventing injury. It is a more meaningful role today, because behavioral interventions are a complement to environmental modifications, rather than the sole approach to injury prevention. Moreover, behavioral modifications no longer rest solely on the shoulders of the potential injury victim. Waller emphasizes the important point that injury events occur when performance levels—driving performance, for example—fall below task demands.[7] These can occur less frequently by not only improving individual performance levels but also by lowering task demands either behaviorally—as convincing people not to drive in unfavorable conditions—or by re-engineering the task itself. As a result, for most of us most of the time performance has become increasingly more than a match for task demand.

The significance of the Haddon Matrix and Haddon's 10 injury prevention countermeasures is that they make clear that not only can society intervene to reduce injury, but that such intervention can occur at many different points. As Haddon and Susan Baker have pointed out, the goal is to be most effective in reducing the overall toll of injury.[11] This may or may not mean that intervention at the preinjury phase is the most effective approach. The beauty of having a variety of intervention points, as highlighted in Haddon's work, is that it allows for a mixed preventive approach, incorporating several intervention options. Haddon and Baker emphasize that having several intervention points allows for selection of the strategies likely to provide the greatest efficacy at lowest cost. They argue that:

> *First,* the choice of countermeasures should <u>not</u> be determined by the relative importance of causal or contributing factors or by their earliness in the sequence of events. . . . Rather, priority and emphasis should be given to measures that will *most effectively* reduce injury losses. . . . *Second*, a "mixed strategy" should usually be employed, incorporating countermeasures addressed to each of the three phases of the injury-control sequence. . . . *Third*, preference should be given to "passive" measures, i.e., those that protect the individual automatically, without any action on his part.[11]

Just as the line between "injury" and "disease" is often vague (compare an "injury" caused by a crushing weight falling on a person to a "disease" of the back caused by years of lifting heavy weights), the line between "intentional" and "unintentional" injury can be more apparent than real.

Intentional injuries—homicides and suicides—are no more unpredictable and random than are "unintentional" injuries. Nor is intent a clear distinguishing characteristic. Just how intentional or unintentional are drunk driving deaths, "shaken baby" injuries, or copycat suicides? During the past decade it has begun to dawn on the public health community that intentional injury is a public health problem amenable to interdisciplinary public health surveillance, analysis, and interventions similar to those employed to reduce "unintentional" injuries. From a prevention perspective it is not at all clear that "intent" is the critical factor in reducing injury occurrence and severity. It is clear, however, that the same prevention approaches can have an impact on injury regardless of intent. For example, parenting courses or home visits for pregnant teens can help reduce both child abuse and falls from infant furniture. And the modification of firearm design to produce safer, personalized "smart" guns can reduce unintentional deaths from firearms as well as suicides and homicides.

## CONCLUSION

In recent years many public health agencies have added injury prevention to their agendas. Fortunately, this increased responsibility for protecting the public has been accompanied by increased insights into how to apply public health approaches to the task. There is still a long way to go, however. Individual behaviors are still overemphasized in the public's understanding of injury. And much of injury prevention is still focused on making injury-creating environments more survivable, rather than on changing the nature of these environments through broader social change. For example, a massive changeover from individual automobile use to effective public transportation use would substantially reduce motor vehicle injury. Organizations such as the Campaign to Make America Walkable need to be promoted as part of a public health approach to reducing motor vehicle injuries. From a public health perspective it would be better if we moved people out of cars, rather than focusing almost solely on making automobile travel safer. Yet in practical terms this is not an approach currently amenable to public health agency intervention.

Still, the way we look at and deal with injuries has changed significantly in the last decade or two. Even the term "accident" does seem to be in decline. It has never been the case that the public or the media would refer to an airliner "accident." Today, through organized efforts by the injury prevention community, the word "accident" is used less and less in any injury context. More important, "injury prevention" is more and more the focus of organized public health—at the federal level with the National Center for Injury Prevention and Control and at state and local levels with injury prevention programs or divisions within health departments. As with other major public health problems, the pace of prevention may seem too slow, but it is steady and its momentum is growing.

---

### NOTES

1. Tesh SN. *Hidden Arguments: Political Ideology and Disease Prevention.* New Brunswick, NJ: Rutgers University Press; 1989.
2. Meredith N. The murder epidemic. *Science 84. December* 1984:48.
3. Waller JA. Reflections on a half century of injury control. *Am J Public Health.* 1994;84:664–670.

4. National Committee for Injury Prevention and Control. *Injury Prevention: Meeting the Challenge*. New York: Oxford University Press (Published as a supplement to the *Am J Prev Med*. 1989;5:4–8).

5. Gordon JE. The epidemiology of accidents. *Am J Public Health*. 1949;39:504–515.

6. Robertson LS. *Injuries: Causes, Control Strategies, and Public Policy*. Lexington, MA: Lexington Books; 1983.

7. Waller JA. *Injury Control: A Guide to the Causes and Prevention of Trauma*. Lexington, MA: Lexington Books; 1985.

8. Baker SP, O'Neill B, Ginsburg MJ, Li G. *The Injury Fact Book*. 2nd ed. New York: Oxford University Press; 1992.

9. Committee on Trauma Research, Commission on Life Sciences, National Research Council and the Institute of Medicine. *Injury in America: A Continuing Public Health Problem*. Washington, DC: National Academy Press; 1985.

10. Allman WF. Staying alive in the 20th century. *Science 85*. October 1985:31.

11. Haddon WJ Jr., Baker SP. Injury control. In: Clark D, MacMahon B, eds. *Preventive and Community Medicine*. Boston: Little Brown & Co; 1981:109–140.

# Overview of Landmark Injury Prevention Events in the United States, 1937–1997

1937 Godfrey publishes one of the first statements in the United States on the need for public health involvement in accident prevention in the *American Journal of Public Health*.

1942 DeHaven publishes breakthrough work describing structural environments as a primary cause of injury in falls from heights.

1943 American Public Health Association (APHA) Committee on Administrative Practice appoints a subcommittee on accident prevention. Subcommittee reports accident prevention programs in six state and two local health departments.

*Note:* Reflecting the realities of the day, the term *accident* is used above—instead of *injury*—until events of the 1980s. This timeline expands upon earlier work by one of the authors and others. See Dana A & Gallagher SS. *Overview of injury prevention events in the United States, 1937–1990*. Boston, MA: Childhood Injury Prevention Resource Center, Harvard School of Public Health; 1990; Fisher L. Childhood injuries—causes, preventive theories and case studies—An overview of the role of sanitarians and other public health workers. *J Environ Health*. 1988;50:355–360; and *Injury Control and Emergency* Health Services. *A timeline of the history of injury prevention*. Poster presented at the 125th anniversary of the American Public Health Association. Indianapolis, IN, November 1997.

1945    Federal Children's Bureau, American Academy of Pediatrics (AAP), National Safety Council, and Metropolitan Life Insurance Company sponsor national child safety campaign.

APHA Subcommittee on Accident Prevention develops program guidelines for accident prevention. Subcommittee reports accident prevention programs in 9 state and 25 local health departments.

1948    WK Kellogg Foundation awards first home accident prevention demonstration grant (Kalamazoo, Michigan).

1949    Gordon formalizes concept that epidemiology could be used as a theoretical foundation for accident prevention in health departments.

1950    AAP forms Committee on Accident Prevention.

1951    Kellogg Foundation funds three- to six-year home accident prevention demonstration projects in Michigan, Massachusetts, California, Ohio, North Carolina, Kentucky, Georgia, Kansas, and Oregon.

1953    First conference on home accident prevention held at the University of Michigan School of Public Health, with sponsors including the National Safety Council, APHA, U.S. Public Health Service, and the Kellogg Foundation.

First poison control center opens (Chicago).

1954    AAP Committee on Accident Prevention creates Subcommittee on Accidental Poisonings.

1955    McFarland publishes "Epidemiological Principles Applicable to the Study and Prevention of Child Accidents" in the *American Journal of Public Health.*

APHA surveys 1,556 state, local, and provincial health departments to assess the scope and effectiveness of health department programs in accident prevention. A total of 33 state, 3 provincial, and 296 local health departments report having an accident prevention program. Sixty-two report a full-time position in place for public health safety.

1956    APHA policy statement urges health agencies to assume an active role in all types of accident prevention programs. Recommends the development of a national accident prevention center within the federal government to coordinate activities among various accident prevention agencies.

U.S. Public Health Service establishes an accident prevention program. Program grows to division status, only to be discontinued in the early 1970s.

1957    APHA policy statement urges that state and local health departments give high priority to training staff in accident prevention principles and techniques and to developing accident prevention programs.

1958    Department of Health, Education and Welfare publishes uniform definitions of home accidents.

1959    APHA policy statement recommends that state health departments develop and maintain accident prevention programs and designate a full-time director.

1960    APHA public policy statement recommends that accident prevention be recognized as a major public health problem and that all units of APHA cooperate to improve accident prevention efforts at the local, state, and national levels. Recommendations are made concerning roles for state and local health departments, research initiatives, collaboration among national organizations, and funding for injury prevention programs.

1961    Gibson publishes theory of injury produced by energy exchange.

The *Journal of Trauma* begins publication.

APHA publishes *Accident Prevention: The Role of Physicians and Public Health Workers.*

Health sanitarians and educators in Philadelphia initiate four-year research demonstration project on home injuries ("Accident Control through Small Group Discussion").

1962    The *Journal of the American Medical Association* publishes article on "Battered Child Syndrome."

1963    Haddon publishes pioneering paper on "accident theory."

1964    Twenty-four state health departments report having accident prevention programs.

Eleven schools of public health develop training programs in injury prevention with funding from the U.S. Public Health Service.

1965    U.S. Public Health Service publishes *A Guide to the Development of Accidental Injury Control Programs.*

1966    National Research Council, National Academy of Sciences recommends the development of a national coordinating council on accident prevention in a report entitled *Accidental Death and Disability: The Neglected Disease of Modern Society.*

National Highway Safety Bureau, later the National Highway Traffic Safety Administration (NHTSA) established as part of the U.S. Department of Transportation.

1968    American Trauma Society established.

APHA publishes monograph by Iskrant and Joliet on *Accidents and Homicide.*

U.S. Department of Transportation authorized to promulgate motor vehicle safety standards.

1969    Insurance Institute for Highway Safety founded.

*Accident Analysis and Prevention* begins publication.

1970    Occupational Safety and Health Act enacted by Congress, creating the Occupational Safety and Health Administration within the U.S. Department of Labor and elevating the Bureau of Occupational Safety and Health to national institute status as the National Institute for Occupational Safety and Health.

Report of the National Commission on Product Safety.

National Institute on Alcohol Abuse and Alcoholism established.

1972    Consumer Product Safety Act, Flammable Fabrics Act, Hazardous Substances Act, and Poison Prevention Packaging Act passed by Congress.

Highway Loss Data Institute established.

1973    Congress enacts Emergency Medical Services Systems Act, establishing a systems approach to emergency medical care.

National Center on Child Abuse and Neglect established by Congress.

National Institute on Disability and Rehabilitation Research founded.

The Robert Wood Johnson Foundation funds 44 EMS projects in 32 states.

1974    Congress passes Child Abuse Prevention and Treatment Act.

1976    APHA issues policy statement on handguns as a public health hazard.

1977    Federal Mine Safety and Health Act established the Mine Safety and Health Administration.

1978    National Coalition against Domestic Violence founded.

Tennessee becomes the first state to enact a child passenger safety law.

1979    Federal Division of Maternal and Child Health established in the U.S. Department of Health and Human Services.

The Center for Disease Control, later the Centers for Disease Control and Prevention (CDC), establishes a violence epidemiology branch to track the incidence of interpersonal violence.

1980    AAP publishes *Handbook on Accident Prevention.*

First population-based emergency room injury surveillance systems implemented (Massachusetts and Ohio).

Mothers Against Drunk Driving (MADD) founded.

1981    First national conference on injury control held, sponsored by the CDC and Johns Hopkins University.

National Child Passenger Safety Association established.

Survey by the National Environmental Health Association finds that 12 state health departments have injury prevention programs.

1982    CDC publishes *Injury Control and Implementation Plan for State and Local Governments.*

1983    CDC hosts an invitational injury program management course for state health agency officials.

Division of Maternal and Child Health publishes *Developing Childhood Injury Prevention Programs: An Administrative Guide for Maternal and Child Health (Title V) Programs.*

Center to Prevent Handgun Violence founded.

1984    Division of Maternal and Child Health funds Massachusetts injury prevention implementation project.

Congress enacts the Health Services, Preventive Health Services, and Home and Community Based Services Act, establishing the Emergency Medical Services for Children program.

Contra Costa County, California, adopts isolation fencing ordinance for new home swimming pools (calling for pool covers, pool alarms, and/or self-latching, self-closing devices on all exits to pools).

1985    *Injury in America: A Continuing Public Health Problem* published by the National Academy of Sciences.

First regional injury control network established (New England Network to Prevent Childhood Injuries).

Division of Maternal and Child Health funds five childhood injury and violence prevention demonstration projects (Ohio, New England, New Mexico, North Carolina, and Wisconsin).

Surgeon General hosts Workshop on Violence and Public Health.

U.S. Department of Transportation provides $10 million to CDC to fund injury prevention research.

1986    CDC funds 5 Injury Prevention Research Centers and 31 injury prevention research projects.

1987    First Injury in America conference.

National Safe Kids campaign founded.

California enacts first legislation requiring helmets for child bicycle passengers 4 years old and under.

1988    *Injury Control*, an outside review of the CDC injury control program, published by National Academy of Sciences as follow-up to *Injury in America.*

Childhood Injury Prevention Resource Center releases national assessment of injury prevention programs in state health departments.

Congress enacts Child Abuse Prevention, Adoption and Family Services Act.

Violence Policy Center founded to reduce gun death and injury in America.

1989    *Injury Prevention: Meeting the Challenge* published by a national committee of experts assembled by the Division of Maternal and Child Health, CDC, and NHTSA.

Report to Congress on *Cost of Injury* is released.

All states now have occupant protection laws covering children less than 4 years of age.

Advocates for Highway Safety founded.

1990    Six states (Arizona, California, New York, Rhode Island, Virginia, and Washington) mandate E coding.

CDC sponsors forum on youth violence in minority communities, "Setting the Agenda for Prevention."

CDC releases report to Congress on *Childhood Injuries in the United States.*

Howard County, Maryland, adopts law requiring children 16 years and younger to wear helmets while riding as either passengers or operators of bicycles.

1991    CDC sponsors national injury control conference to set a national agenda for injury control.

World Health Organization Helmet Initiative begun.

Institute of Medicine publishes *Disability in America: Towards a National Agenda for Prevention.*

National Committee on Vital and Health Statistics recommends national plan for collection of E code data with release of *Report on the Need To Collect External Cause of Injury Codes in Hospital Discharge Data.*

1992    CDC establishes the National Center for Injury Prevention and Control.

1993    Congress passes the Handgun Violence Prevention Act (the Brady Bill).

Institute of Medicine releases *Emergency Medical Services for Children.*

National Research Council releases *Understanding and Preventing Violence.*

President Clinton declares violence to be a public health emergency.

1994    National Academy of Sciences publishes *Violence in Urban America: Mobilizing a  Response.*

1995    *Injury Prevention*, the journal of the International Society of Child and Adolescent Injury Prevention, is initiated with a practitioner focus.

1996    National Academy of Sciences publishes *Violence in Families: Assessing Prevention  and Treatment Programs.*

National Rifle Association succeeds in getting Congress to prohibit firearm violence research by the CDC or its grantees, contractors, or researchers.

1997    Institute of Medicine convenes panel of experts to review injury prevention in America 12 years after *Injury in America* report.

NHTSA follows earlier lead of CDC by officially abandoning use of the word "accident."

E coding mandated in 23 states.

# CHAPTER 3

# Epidemiology of Injury

"A prerequisite for the scientific study of injury is the acquisition of data on which to base priorities and research."

Committee on Trauma Research, Commission on Life Sciences, and the National Research Council and Institute of Medicine, *Injury in America*, 1985

## WHAT THIS CHAPTER IS ABOUT

You are a public health professional—or training to become one. You may have worked in public health for several years, developing and administering prevention programs. You have some understanding of the basics and uses of epidemiology. You've probably used epidemiological input to better target and tailor your intervention programs. You may have worked on preventing epidemics of influenza and food poisoning or you may have worked on breast cancer screening and prevention, on senior wellness, and—most recently—on human immunodeficiency virus and acquired immune deficiency syndrome prevention. Now you approach the new public health concern of injury prevention. How will injury epidemiology help you better understand and target your injury prevention efforts? This chapter will show how the classic tools of epidemiology are being applied to injury and injury prevention. Since a mere chapter cannot provide a full primer on the science of epidemiology, readers completely new to the subject may wish to consult one of the many general epidemiology texts.[1–7]

## INTRODUCTION

Early epidemiology focused on the infectious diseases. It was not until the twentieth century, as methods of epidemiological investigation evolved, that noninfectious acute and chronic diseases became a subject of epidemiological study. Most recently epidemiology has been used to better understand and respond to injury as a public health problem, primarily to elucidate the chain of causation—the etiology and mechanisms—of injuries and subsequent disabilities. Chapter 2 explained how applying epidemiological methods to injury distribution patterns and causes began at midcentury by understanding injury in terms of the classic epidemiological triad of host, agent, and environment, and how this conceptual understanding was advanced by viewing "energy interchange" as the agent of injury harm. Table 3–1 shows the parallel between the epidemiological conceptualization of injury and of disease.

Epidemiology often provides the information necessary to identify the interventions most likely to reduce injury occurrence or minimize injury disability and to target these interventions at the populations at greatest risk. Epidemiology also provides an evaluation tool to ascertain the effect of known interventions on injury morbidity and mortality and on their associated costs (although it should not be used in isolation from other sources of evaluation information, such as the behavioral sciences). The potential for injury epidemiology is great, but unfortunately reality is slow in catching up to that potential. Most epidemiological training and practice still focuses on disease entities—often diseases of far lesser impact and potential for prevention than injury problems. An example is suicide, which accounts for more than 30,000 deaths annually and is studied less than many diseases with a small fraction of that mortality level.

What are the most frequent causes of injury in a community? Why do local data differ from national patterns? What does this suggest about potential preventive interventions? It would be possible to approach injury prevention efforts without the input of epidemiology and epidemiologists, but the result would be a cruder, hit-and-miss effort that used general injury knowledge to develop and target interventions to reduce injuries. Injury rates are far from uniform among subpopulations; state-specific death

**Table 3–1** Injury Etiology: Malaria versus Fractured Skull

| Human Damage | Agent | Vector/Vehicle | Exposure Event |
|---|---|---|---|
| Malaria | P. Vivax | Mosquito | Mosquito bite |
| Fractured skull | Kinetic energy | Motor vehicle | Crash |

Courtesy of Education Development Center and Johns Hopkins Injury Prevention Center, 1990, Newton, Massachusetts.

rates for causes of injury can vary by a factor of 10 or more. In and of themselves, however, these variations may be a poor guide to prevention efforts, for they may simply reflect other factors, such as differences in demographics, exposure to injury risk, or confounding factors. In a sense, epidemiology provides a systematic method to look at such variations and suggestive patterns of injury in a way calculated to avoid erroneous conclusions. Information about the circumstances, location, nature, and severity of injury, and of the impact of various protective devices and approaches, are key variables for epidemiologic study. The result can often be a useful *local* picture—essential for convincing a community to deal with a particular injury problem—and a useful contrast to national data. As Cummings et al stated:

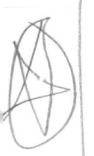
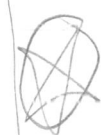

> Public health agencies seeking to reduce injuries need methods for counting injuries, calculating injury rates, identifying the causes of injuries, and measuring outcomes of interventions. . . . Epidemiologists in public health agencies and their academic colleagues increasingly are involved in injury research, in the belief that a public health approach can decrease injury morbidity and mortality.[8(p381)]

## WHAT IS EPIDEMIOLOGY?

"Epidemiology is the study of the distribution and determinants of health-related states and events in specified populations and the application of this study to the control of health problems."[9] The epidemiological method has been described as consisting of "[c]areful clinical observation, precise counts of well-defined cases, and demonstration of relationships between cases and the characteristics of the populations in which they occur."[10(p11)] Most people in public health are familiar with the ways in which epidemiology is used to better understand traditional public health problems. For example, epidemiology can identify clusters of cancers that exceed expected rates and which may suggest an unusual problem or need for a specific intervention. Similarly with injury, epidemiology can increase our public health knowledge in important ways. The authors of *Injury in America* note:

> Drowning is an example of a phenomenon on which more refined epidemiologic knowledge than is now available is needed, if bet-

ter prevention strategies are to be developed. To prevent drowning, information is needed about the bodies of water involved, the activities of the drowned persons and others in their company at the time of the drownings, and the environmental conditions.[11(p35)]

Environmental conditions could include the availability and use of protective equipment such as personal flotation devices or the absence of four-sided swimming pool fencing of sufficient height with a self-locking entry point.

Why is epidemiology such a powerful tool? It is a well established science that, being population based in its focus, is more powerful than anecdotal reports, clinical studies, or statistical risk assessment. As the scientific study of the distribution and determinants of disease, epidemiology is the interrelated investigation of population patterns (distribution) and "causal" factors (determinants) associated with injury occurrence. Investigating the distribution of injury means looking at population patterns and injury risks as they are distributed among the population.

Epidemiology can focus on *description* or on *analysis*. In the injury field, the use of epidemiology has focused in particular on descriptive studies that identify the distribution of injuries according to a specific cause or demographic characteristics. Much of public health departments' work has been confined to this very basic "descriptive epidemiology" approach, focusing on identification of the host's characteristics, examining state-level snapshots of the leading causes of injury, making comparisons to national data or to the Year 2000 Health Objectives, and identifying geographic hot spots that exceed statewide rates. Public health professionals need to understand this baseline epidemiologic information before moving on to the more challenging area of testing hypotheses using the tools of analytic epidemiology. Leon Robertson notes:

> To understand the impact of injuries in a population, it is necessary to classify them into relatively homogeneous subsets, to count them, to measure severity, and to specify the population in which they occur. Descriptive studies may be devoted to the identification of all injuries in a population, based on some minimum severity criteria, or may be focused on place of occurrence (e.g., roads), particular types of disability (e.g., spinal cord), a subset of the population (e.g., children), those associated with a given activity (e.g., swimming), or any number of other categories.[12(p23)]

Investigating the determinants of injury means looking at factors associated with injury occurrence in terms of the classic epidemiological triad of host, agent, and environment.

For example, the schematic in Figure 3–1 shows the interaction of factors in childhood poisoning. The potency of the bleach (agent), its packaging in a white plastic jug that resembles a milk container and storage in an environment that facilitates access (environment), and the developmental characteristics of a toddler (host) all play important roles. Interruption at any one point could prevent an unintentional poisoning. Interventions could be directed at host, agent, or environmental factors to reduce the risk of poison ingestion. By studying the injury host or victim on a population basis, we can learn which subgroups of the population are most at risk for particular types of injuries and thereby target our interventions. By studying the agent of injury, which we know to be the various forms of energy, and the vehicles and vectors that deliver that energy to the host, we can

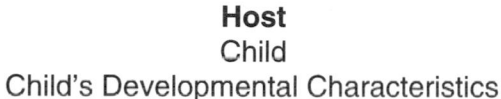

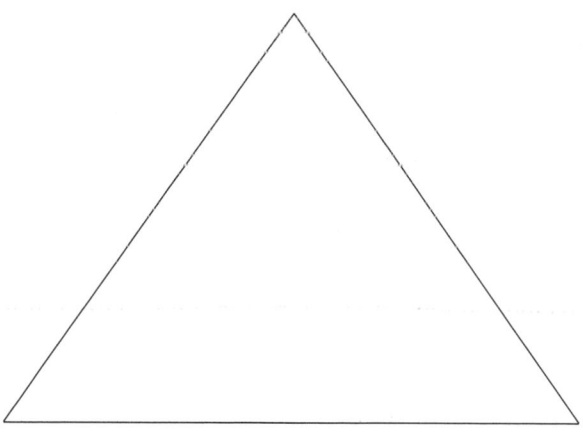

**Figure 3–1** Factors in Childhood Poisoning

better understand which countermeasures are likely to be most effective in holding energy transfer to tolerable levels. And by studying the environments in which this energy transfer occurs, we can better work to eliminate injury hazards from that environment.

"Analytic epidemiology" takes our understanding of injury problems a step further than simple description. Analytic epidemiology has been a particularly useful tool in determining exposure to factors that may increase or decrease the risk of injury and death. In analytic study designs, groups of fatal or nonfatal cases will be identified and studied for the purpose of systematically determining whether or not the risk of injury is different for individuals exposed or not exposed to a given risk factor (e.g., absence of a bike helmet, presence of a firearm, or exposure to driver education). An appropriate comparison group that allows testing of a hypothesis is a critical component of analytic epidemiology. A number of design options are available including randomized controlled trials, case-control studies, cohort studies, and cross-sectional studies. Studies can be retrospective or prospective. These different methodologies are described later in this chapter.

One important use of epidemiology is to assess what amount of a particular type of injury is associated with a particular exposure within a population. This is called the *attributable risk* (or *attributable fraction*), or the maximum proportion of an injury (or disease) "that can be attributed to a characteristic or etiologic factor; alternatively, it is considered the proportional decrease in the incidence of [the injury or disease] if the entire population were no longer exposed to the suspected etiological agent."[13(p217)] Attributable risk, for example, is a way to estimate how many motor vehicle injuries are prevented by laws requiring seatbelt use. Measurement of attributable risk is useful in planning injury prevention programs, since it allows one to predict the effectiveness of a program to eliminate categories of exposure to injury.

In their basic description of epidemiology, Tyler and Last explain:

> Epidemiological reasoning is based on a group of fundamental and straightforward actions. First, the epidemiologist defines the events or clinical cases to be studied, using careful, specific, and objective observations. Next, these events or cases must be counted and oriented to time, place, and person. After this orientation, the epidemiologist determines the population at risk and

calculates rates using methods little more complicated than long division, that is, putting the events or cases in the numerator according to their relevant characteristics and using a denominator of (the portion of) the population at risk characterized in a manner similar to that of the numerator. These rates are then compared with the rates of occurrence in other population groups. Finally, using this information, the epidemiologist draws inferences about the events that define the health problem, the agent or agents that cause it, the host and environmental factors that influence the risk or its occurrence, and the means by which it is transmitted. Using this information and collaborating with other health professionals, the epidemiologist proposes control measures and then continues the observations required to assess the proposed control program.[10(p13)]

This is the process of study underlying the public health model. It is a process based on detailed surveillance, an analysis of distributions of a problem (injury) and identification of particular types of risks, followed by the development and implementation of intervention strategies, and the subsequent evaluation of the effectiveness of these interventions. Leon Robertson, a leading export in this field, has written a textbook on *Injury Epidemiology* that is a particularly useful source of information on the topic and to which the interested reader is referred. In it Robertson notes that:

Causal analysis of injury can inform preventive approaches when it specifies factors that are substantially changeable and that account for a proportion of a given type of injury and rules out factors that are spuriously correlated to injury. Attention to the nature of types of causes gives guidance to the extent that a given injury might be reduced if a given factor were changed.[14(p87)]

## DATA

Effective epidemiological analysis requires adequate data. As explained in the discussion of injury surveillance in Chapter 12, such data may be quite limited, if not altogether lacking, in most areas other than motor vehicle injuries. This is especially true regarding information on severity of injuries and on exposure to particular injury hazards. Large numbers of a

particular injury present a less pressing case for intervention if most require only a Band-Aid. On the other hand, a seemingly modest number of
motor vehicle occupant injuries in a low-income community may be more
significant than first appears to be the case if it turns out that few people in
the community have access to motor vehicles. Thus the first injury prevention task for public health departments will often be to access data and
upgrade injury surveillance systems. This is particularly important because the injury picture will vary from state to state and locality to locality.
Fires and burns constitute the leading cause of injury death for children
ages 1 to 4 in many states, but in some other states motor vehicle injuries or
drowning may be the leading injury threat for this age group.

Critical to the epidemiology of injury is the ability to understand, classify, and analyze injury data in a consistent way. The International Classification of Diseases,[15] the official world classification of medical conditions, diseases, and injuries, provides systems for epidemiologists to
identify both (1) the nature of an injury (e.g., skull fracture) and (2) how
the injury occurred (e.g., fall from playground equipment). Information on
the nature of an injury is captured with N codes; information on the external cause of an injury is captured with E codes. See Exhibit 3–1 for N code
and E code examples. E codes are especially important for epidemiologists
and injury prevention practitioners in assessing a community's injury
problem, tailoring prevention efforts, and evaluating these efforts. It is
therefore a matter of some importance as to whether or not hospitals routinely collect E code information.

The E code system, albeit not perfect, has many potential benefits for
public health professionals. The Injury Control and Emergency Health
Services Section of the American Public Health Association has pointed
out that:

> E codes may be grouped into large categories to classify falls,
> motor vehicle–related crashes, fires, drowning, poisonings, as-
> saults, and firearm injuries. E codes may also be very precise. For
> example, several E codes apply to the "falls" classification alone,
> including: E880.9—fall on or from steps or stairs other than an
> escalator; E881.1—fall from scaffolding; E882—fall on or out of
> building; E884.0—fall from playground equipment; E884.1—
> fall from a cliff; E885—fall on the same level, such as slipping,
> tripping, or stumbling; E886.0—fall in sports due to pushing,
> shoving, colliding, or tackling.[16]

E CODES

**Exhibit 3–1** Example of Coding of Injuries, International Classification of Disease, 9th Revision, Effective 1979

---

**Nature of Injury**
**(N Codes 800–999)**

| | |
|---|---|
| Fractures | 800–829 |
| Fracture of humerus | 812 |
| Fracture lower end, open | 812.5 |

**External Cause of Injury**
**(E Codes E800–E999)**

| | |
|---|---|
| Accidental falls | E880–E888 |
| Fall one level to another | E844 |
| Fall from playground equipment | E844.0 |

---

The E code classification scheme is required on all death certificates.[17] For nonfatal injuries, E codes provide a standardized set of information categories that can be used to group what physicians, nurses, paramedics, social workers, and others may document in the medical record.[15] Unfortunately, there is presently no national requirement for hospitals to report E codes on their hospital discharge data forms and such coding has been sporadic at best. It is up to public health professionals to bring this issue to the attention of the hospital associations and data organizations that house such statewide data, to the medical information specialists who code such data, and to the clinicians who can document such data. E codes have aptly been called the missing link in injury prevention. External causes of injury are classified into several hundred categories that enable epidemiologists to examine both the mechanism of the injury (e.g., fall, motor vehicle crash, poisoning, firearm) and the intent (e.g., intentionally self-inflicted, intentional inflicted by another, unintentional, intent undetermined). E codes may be grouped into large categories to classify all drownings or all assaults or more precisely to distinguish drowning incidents involving boats or drowning in a pool or bathtub or distinguishing unarmed assaults from armed assaults with a weapon such as a cutting instrument or firearm. E codes also allow for the identification of the location of occurrence (e.g., industrial place, public building, home, farm, recreation and sport setting), but this is less often used because it requires a second field on a data form and proper documentation of the location in the medical record. In one study, only about 50% of medical records included enough information to code the place of occurrence.[18]

The potential of E codes for injury epidemiology is tremendous. A collaboration among the National Center for Health Statistics, the National Center for Injury Prevention and Control, and the Injury Control and Emergency Health Services Section of the American Public Health Association has produced "Recommended Framework for Presenting Injury Mortality Data." This publication presents standard E code groupings in a matrix that categorizes mechanisms of injury according to intent (e.g., poisoning-related [mechanism] suicide [intent] rather than the traditional tabulation categories that solely emphasize the manner of death [homicide, suicide, unintentional]). The Centers for Disease Control and Prevention note that this new framework "can provide the basis for comparison of national and state injury-mortality statistics for use in identifying external causes of injury death needing priority public health attention in jurisdictions."[19(p28)] Before the matrix was developed, there was no uniformity in definition and presentation of grouped E-coded injury data and state-by-state comparisons were not valid. Appendix 3–A presents the proposed matrix and Appendix 3–B shows how matrix categories can display basic data on injury deaths and crude death rates for epidemiologic analysis. A similar framework is under development for nonfatal injuries.

Today the "Recommended Framework for Presenting Injury Mortality Data" is important primarily for establishing a system goal and demonstrating what E code data collection can achieve when the full potential of this approach is finally realized. (Progress in fully establishing the E code system is discussed in Chapter 12: Injury Surveillance.) Public health professionals need to ensure that state epidemiologists and others involved with health statistics use the framework in analyzing vital statistics data for injury program staff.

Two other important data issues affecting injury epidemiology involve injury severity and exposure to injury risks. Both are discussed in Chapter 12, but a few observations regarding exposure should be made here. The selection of an appropriate denominator is a particular challenge for injury epidemiologists. Incidence rates are usually defined as the number of new cases in a given population over a set period of time. The population denominators for injury rates must be refined to reflect the population at actual risk of injury, such as those participating in a specific activity. Guyer and Gallagher note:

> when motor vehicle occupant injury rates to low income urban adolescents are calculated on the denominator of the population alone, they may underestimate the true injury risk because relatively few of these adolescents have access to motor vehicles. An alternative denominator might include a measure of exposure resulting in a rate of adolescent motor vehicle injuries per 10,000 passenger miles driven.[20]

The same is true for rates of work-related injuries among teens, which substantially underestimate the risk to teens at work unless injury rates use hours of work expressed as full-time equivalents as the denominator,[21] and for risks of sports-related injuries without denominators based on the number of participants or number of hours at play.[22]

## METHODOLOGY

Epidemiology should not be a black box affair—data in one end and results miraculously appear out the other. Quite the contrary. If done properly, epidemiology should be open and visible, so that anyone reviewing study results can see what was done and how it was done, what assumptions were made and what techniques were used. It is possible to share and compare methodologies in this way because there are a limited number of standard study designs that can be employed. Individuals may disagree as to which types of study design to use to answer a particular question, but there will be agreement as to which study designs are available. Epidemiological studies can be either experimental or observational (see Figure 3–2). The standard study designs are described below.

### Randomized Controlled Trials

Ideally, studies of any public health problem would be undertaken with a randomized controlled experiment, which allows the researcher to assign hosts, vehicles, or environments to experimental and control groups. But in the real world this is rarely feasible, because this type of prospective study requires a degree of control that is not often possible (or ethical), particu-

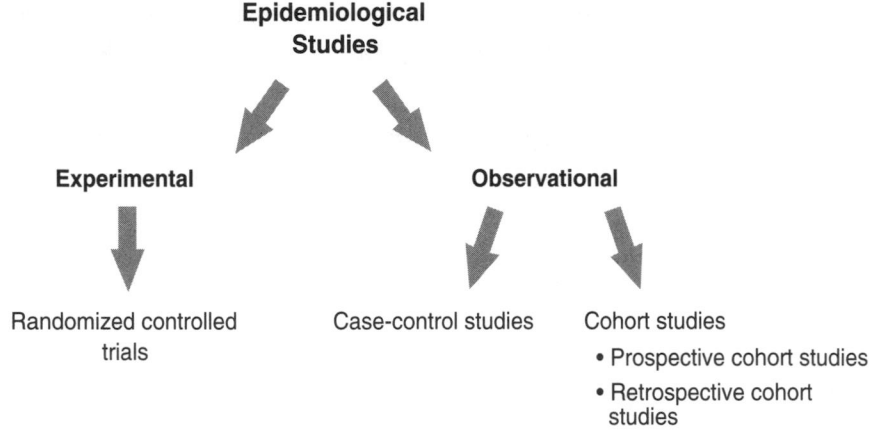

**Figure 3–2** Major Study Designs

larly in the injury field. There have been studies, for example, where police domestic violence calls were randomly assigned to one of three response techniques—automatic arrest, removal of the perpetrator, or "standard" assessment and mediation—but the results have been inconclusive. Random assignment of any protective device would raise serious ethical questions.

## Case-Control Studies

Unlike randomized controlled trials, observational studies involve assignment without control over which hosts, vehicles, or environments will be exposed to the factors under study. An important observational design in injury epidemiology is the case-control study, in which a group of individuals or events are chosen according to whether they do or do not have a characteristic or risk factor of which the cause is to be studied (cases) and are compared with controls who share important characteristics with the cases. Either existing or past characteristics judged to be of possible relevance are compared in the two groups. Robertson explains that:

> A case may be an injured person, a vehicle that rolled over, a section of road where a vehicle hit a tree, and so on. The analogous control would be persons not injured, vehicles that did not roll over, sections of road that the vehicle traversed without hit-

ting trees. The research question is how relevant individual, vehicle, or environmental factors differ between cases and controls.
The controls may be matched on certain factors (age, sex, time,
place) or unmatched.[14(pp94–95)]

Retrospective data is collected on cases and controls. For example, in a
case-control study of the effectiveness of bicycle safety helmets, the cases
were bicyclists who sought care for a bicycle-related head injury in one of
five emergency rooms during a one-year period. The study had two separate control groups: (1) bicyclists who sought care at the same emergency
rooms for bicycle-related injuries other than head injures and (2) a population-based control group of bicyclists who experienced cycling mishaps
(whether or not they were injured or sought medical care). Information
was collected from cases and controls using detailed questionnaires. The
researchers concluded that bicycle helmets were highly effective in preventing head injuries.[23]

Case-control studies allow us to develop *odds ratios* (i.e., a representation of the odds in favor of incurring a particular type of injury when an
associated factor—such as installation of smoke detectors—is present as
compared to when the same factor is absent) This term is sometimes used
synonymously with *relative risk* (i.e., "the ratio of the risk of [injury]
among the exposed to the risk among the unexposed"[9(p91)]).

Case-control studies have been especially effective in the injury prevention field. For example, a population-based case-control study was carried
out in two distinct cities to determine if access to firearms in the home
increased the risk of suicide. In this study, 803 suicides were identified
through police and medical examiner data and interviews were conducted
with a person close to the deceased suicide victim and with neighborhood
controls matched to the deceased by sex, race, and age range. The hypothesis under study was that the rate of suicide should be higher in homes with
guns than in homes without guns. The results offered strong evidence that
the presence of a gun in the home increases the risk of suicide in the home
(by a factor of 4.8).[24] In a study of risk factors for fatal residential fires,
researchers looked at single-dwelling fires in North Carolina during a 13-
month study period. They compared all fatal fires (cases) with fires where
someone was home but no one died (controls). They found that while
"heating incidents were the leading cause of fires, fatal fires were more
likely to have been caused by smoking."[25] This same study also provided

odds ratio information on other risks for fatal fires: mobile home (1.7), older home (2.0), mobile home with two or fewer exits (2.6), no telephone (3.2), absence of a smoke detector (3.4), person less than 5 years old or older than 64, impaired or disabled (6.5), and presence of an alcohol-impaired person (7.5). The latter was the strongest risk factor for death from a fire (i.e., fires with an alcohol-impaired person present were 7.5 times more likely to be associated with fatal than with nonfatal fires). The same study also indicated characteristics that did not appear to be related to fatal fires, for example, fire response system items like lack of 911 (0.9) or an all-volunteer fire department (0.7).

As Cummings et al note: "Although a case-control study does not directly yield information about absolute risk in persons with or without exposure to some factor, it does allow estimation of the risk of injury or illness in persons with a given exposure relative to that of unexposed persons."[26]

Case-control studies often require substantial resources and expertise, which may not be readily available to public health agencies. But even when such studies are carried out by trained epidemiologists in an academic setting, practitioners have a role in identifying the potential risk factors to be studied.

### Cohort Studies

Another type of observational study is the cohort study, either prospective or retrospective. In a cohort study, a group of individuals with a common characteristic (e.g., age) or exposure (e.g., head injury or an injury prevention intervention) are observed over time. In cohort studies, the case group is exposed to the injury problem and the comparison group is not exposed. Prospective cohort studies follow similar groups with difference exposures into the future for the occurrence of a specified event or outcome, whereas retrospective cohort studies reconstruct records of exposure and outcome. Cohort studies involve larger numbers than do case-control studies and over a period a time are therefore more expensive and take longer to complete, but injury research would benefit from having more of this type of study done.

Cohort studies allow us to develop an *incidence rate*, a measure of the rate at which new injury events occur in the population (i.e., "new cases . . . reported during a defined period of time is the numerator, and the number of persons in the stated population in which the cases occurred is the denominator" [9(p49)]).

Regardless of the specific study design, a major goal of an epidemiological study is to assess levels of association. When we look at relationships between cause and effect, we look at association. "Events are said to be associated when they occur more frequently together than one would expect by chance. Association does not necessarily imply a causal relationship."[9(p5)]

Readers interested in the methodological details of these study designs should consult basic epidemiology texts or epidemiology courses, some of which are available on the World Wide Web.[27]

## Cross-sectional Studies

One other study design—perhaps of more limited potential than those discussed—is the cross-sectional study (or survey), which involves observations of a group made during a cross-sectional slice in time. The cross-sectional study can be used to examine the relationship between injury events and other relevant variables as they exist in a defined population at one particular point in time.[9(p24)] This often involves measures of exposure. Cross-sectional studies are easy and rapid to do, but although they can indicate the maximum magnitude of possible correlations, they cannot be used to establish the temporal sequence of cause and effect necessary for drawing causal inferences.

Cross-sectional studies are essentially prevalence studies. They can be used to determine *prevalence rates* (or ratios), which are defined in *A Dictionary of Epidemiology* as:

> The total number of all individuals who have an attribute . . . at a particular time (or during a particular period) divided by the population at risk of having the attribute . . . at this point in time or midway through the period. A problem may arise with calculating period prevalence rates because of the difficulty of defining the most appropriate denominator.[9(p82)]

It would be worthwhile to review Chapter 4 (Causal Analysis and Its Uses) in the second edition of Robertson's *Injury Epidemiology*.[14] Robertson discusses a variety of study design approaches, noting that:

> The choice of study designs to investigate a given set of factors is affected by numerous considerations. What is the unit of analysis

(people, vehicles, environments)? In what population should the study be conducted? To what population of people, vehicles, or environments will the results be generalizable? What measurements of the factors are available or could be obtained? How reliable and valid are the measurements? Can the data be collected without violating ethical guidelines? How can the study isolate the effects of given factors independent of, or in combination with, other relevant factors? How much time will be needed to complete the study? How much will the study cost?[14(p93)]

Regardless of the study design used, injury epidemiology must deal with several methodological difficulties. The major difficulties include

- Determining the appropriate denominator—the amount of exposure to a particular injury risk. Did the injuries under study occur at a high rate in a low-frequency activity (e.g., parasailing) or did they involve extensive exposures (e.g., motor vehicle travel)? Are motor vehicle injuries most meaningfully viewed in terms of total population? Number of vehicles? Vehicle miles traveled? Passenger miles traveled? How are passenger miles traveled to be calculated?
- Measuring the numerator. Nonfatal injuries can range from profound disability to a mere cut finger. Would it be at all meaningful to lump such widely disparate levels of severity together?
- Determining intentional and unintentional injury. This provides the two basic categories of injury type, but intent is an amorphous factor. Did a person who killed another in a barroom brawl intend death as an outcome? Does the company that decides not to install known safety devices on their assembly line intend for some injuries to result?
- Determining "statistical significance" and "causal inference." Is statistical significance simply a matter of whether an arbitrary decision-making convention has been attained? Could it be that "causal inference is not a part of science at all, but lies strictly in the domain of public policy"[28(p550)]?
- Determining whether identifying all of an epidemiological study's risk factors is necessary to be useful. Is Robertson correct that "[f]ocusing on multiple risk factors in causal webs may lead astray rather than toward injury control"[14]?
- Establishing if selection bias, limitations in sampling, and/or problems in measurement distort the potential success of study designs.

These all are important and interesting questions that need to be addressed as part of injury epidemiology. They are, however, beyond the scope of this brief review of the nature of injury epidemiology today. The serious student will need to consult appropriate texts and draw upon appropriate expertise. It would be just as imprudent for an injury prevention specialist to undertake analytical epidemiology without consulting with a trained epidemiologist as it would be imprudent for an epidemiologist to undertake injury epidemiology without consulting with an experienced injury prevention practitioner.

Over the past several decades we've learned much from injury epidemiology, but there is much more still to be learned—especially at state and local levels. Public health department personnel charged with injury prevention at the state level must obtain the input and commitment of departmental epidemiologists. This may mean educating them regarding the state of epidemiological knowledge on injury. It may mean working with them to develop priorities for injury epidemiological studies or to get injury data presented in greater detail (e.g., according to developmental stage) or in less aggregated form (e.g., breaking out various unintentional injury causes). Perhaps most important, it may mean persuading them that injury is a health problem that is highly preventable and for which their expert input can mean significant progress in protecting the public's health. Injury epidemiology provides a different context for the classical epidemiology in which many epidemiologists have been trained. The message needs to be conveyed that this makes for an interesting challenge, not a problem. There is a body of work to build on,[18,29–36] there are specialists to provide assistance, and there is a constantly growing body of published, peer-reviewed literature.

## CONCLUSION

Epidemiology investigates, analyzes, and helps control health problems. As Tyler and Last note, "[e]pidemiology, as the scientific basis for the practice of public health, has important applications to the resolution of high-priority contemporary health problems."[10(p37)] As the newest major category of health problem on the public health agenda, injury particularly is in need of the illumination, guidance, and direction that the science of epidemiology can provide. A successful linkage of surveillance, epidemiological analysis, and prevention has the potential to significantly reduce the toll of injury.

## NOTES

1. Gerstman BB. *Epidemiology Kept Simple: An Introduction to Classic and Modern Epidemiology.* New York: John Wiley & Sons; 1998.

2. Gordis L. *Epidemiology.* Philadelphia: W. B. Saunders Co; 1996.

3. Friedman GD. *Primer of Epidemiology.* New York: McGraw Hill; 1994.

4. Friis RH, Sellers TA. *Epidemiology for Public Health Practice.* Gaithersburg, MD: Aspen Publishers; 1996.

5. Lilienfeld DE, Stolley PD. *Foundations of Epidemiology.* 3rd ed. New York: Oxford University Press; 1994.

6. MacMahon B, Trichopoulos D. *Epidemiology: Principles and Practice.* 2nd ed. Philadelphia: Lippincott-Raven Publishers; 1996.

7. Rothman KJ, Greenland S. *Modern Epidemiology.* 2nd ed. Philadelphia: Lippincott-Raven Publishers; 1998.

8. Cummings P, Koepsell TD, Mueller BA. Methodological challenges in injury epidemiology and injury prevention research. *Annu Rev Public Health.* 1995;16:381.

9. Last JM. *A Dictionary of Epidemiology.* New York: Oxford University Press; 1983.

10. Tyler CW Jr, Last JM. Epidemiology. In: Last JM, Wallace RB, eds. *Maxcy-Rosenau-Last: Public Health and Preventive Medicine.* Norwalk, CT: Appleton & Lange; 1992: 11–37.

11. Committee on Trauma Research, Commission on Life Sciences, National Research Council and Institute of Medicine. *Injury in America: A Continuing Public Health Problem.* Washington, DC: National Academy Press; 1985.

12. Robertson LS. *Injury Epidemiology.* New York: Oxford University Press; 1992.

13. Lilienfeld AM, Lilienfeld DE. *Foundations of Epidemiology.* 2nd ed. New York: Oxford University Press; 1980.

14. Robertson LS. *Injury Epidemiology: Research and Control Strategies.* 2nd ed. New York: Oxford University Press; 1998.

15. *International Classification of Diseases, 9th Revision, Clinical Modification.* U.S. Department of Health and Human Services, Public Health Service, Health Care Financing Administration; October 1996.

16. *E Codes: The Missing Link in Injury Prevention.* Prepared by the Education Development Center for the Injury Control and Emergency Health Services Section of the American Public Health Association; 1994.

17. *Manual of the International Classification of Diseases, Injuries and Causes of Death.* 9th rev. Geneva: World Health Organization; 1977.

18. Gallagher SS, Finison MA, Guyer B, Goodenough S. The incidence of injuries among 87,000 Massachusetts children and adolescents: Results of the 1980–81 Statewide Childhood Injury Prevention Program surveillance system. *Am J Public Health.* 1984;74:1340–1347.

19. Recommended framework for presenting injury mortality data. *MMWR*, Recommendations and Reports. August 29, 1997;46, No. RR-14:28.

20. Guyer B, Gallagher SS. An approach to the epidemiology of childhood injuries. *Pediatr Clin North Am*. 1985;32:5–15.

21. Brooks DR, Davis LK, Gallagher SS. Work-related injuries among Massachusetts children: A study based on emergency department data. *Am J Ind Med*. 1993;24:313–324.

22. Lescohier I, Gallagher SS. Unintentional injury. In: DiClemente RJ, Hansen W, Ponton LE, eds. *Handbook of Adolescent Health Risk Behavior*. New York: Plenum Press; 1996.

23. Thompson RS, Rivara FP, Thompson DC. A case-control study of the effectiveness of bicycle safety helmets. *New Engl J Med*. 1989;320:1361–1367.

24. Kellerman AL, Rivara FP, Somes G, et al. Suicide in the home in relation to gun ownership. *New Engl J Med*. 1992;327:467–472.

25. Runyan CW, Bangdiwala SI, Linzer MA, Sacks JJ, Butts J. Risk factors for fatal residential fires. *New Engl J Med*. 1992;327:859–863.

26. Cummings P, Koepsell TD, Weiss NS. Studying injuries with case-control methods in the emergency department. *Ann Emerg Med*. 1998;31:99–105.

27. For example, at http://www.pitt.edu/~super1.

28. Rothman K. *Modern Epidemiology*. Boston: Little, Brown; 1986:20, citing Lanes S. Causal inferences is not a matter of science. *Am J Epidemiol*. 1985;122:550.

29. Scheidt PC, Harel Y, Trumble AC, Jones DH, Overpeck MD, Bijur PE. The epidemiology of nonfatal injuries among U.S. children and youth. *Am J Public Health*. 1995;85:932–938.

30. Barancik JI, Chatterjee BF, Greene YC, et al. Northeastern Ohio Trauma Study: I. Magnitude of the problem. *Am J Public Health*. 1983;73:746–751.

31. Fife D, Barancik JI, Chatterjee BF. Northeastern Ohio Trauma Study: II. Injury rates by age, sex, and cause. *Am J Public Health*. 1984;74:473–478.

32. Davidson, LL, Durkin MS, O'Connor P, et al. The epidemiology of severe injuries to children in Northern Manhattan: Methods and incidence rates. *Pediatr Perinat Epidemiol*. 1992;6:153–165.

33. Grisso JA, Wishner AR, Schwarz DF, et al. A population-based study of injuries in inner-city women. *Am J Epidemiol*. 1991;134:59–68.

34. Schwarz DF, Grisso JA, Miles CG, et al. A longitudinal study of injury morbidity in an African-American population. *JAMA*. 1994;271:755–760.

35. Durkin MS, Davidson LL, Kuhn L, et al. Low-income neighborhoods and the risk of severe pediatric injury: A small area analysis in Northern Manhattan. *Am J Public Health*. 1994;84:587–592.

36. Braddock M, Lapidus G, Gregorio D, et al. Population, income, and ecological correlates of child pedestrian injury. *Pediatrics*. 1991;88:1242–1247.

# Appendix 3–A

## Proposed Matrix Table with Assignment of E Codes for Injury Mortality Data

| Mechanism/Cause | Manner/Intent | | | | |
|---|---|---|---|---|---|
| | Unintentional | Suicide | Homicide | Undetermined | Other[1] |
| Cut/pierce | E920.0–.9 | E956 | E966 | E986 | E974 |
| Drowning/submersion | E830.0–.9, E832.0–.9, E910.0–.9 | E954 | E964 | E984 | — |
| Fall | E880.0–E886.9, E888 | E957.0–.9 | E968.1 | E987.0–.9 | — |
| Fire/burn | E890.0–E899, E924.0–.9 | E958.1, .2, .7 | E961; E968.0, .3 | E988.1, .2, .7 | — |
| Fire/flame | E890.0–E899 | E958.1 | E968.0 | E988.1 | — |
| Hot object/substance | E924.0–.9 | E958.2, .7 | E961, E968.3 | E988.2, .7 | — |
| Firearm | E922.0–.9 | E955.0–.4 | E965.0–.4 | E985.0–.4 | E970 |
| Machinery | E919.0–.9 | — | — | — | — |
| Motor vehicle traffic[2] | E810–E819 (.0–.9[3]) | E958.5 | — | E988.5 | — |
| Occupant | E810–E819 (.0, .1) | — | — | — | — |
| Motorcyclist | E810–819 (.2, .3) | — | — | — | — |
| Pedal cyclist | E810–E819 (.6) | — | — | — | — |
| Pedestrian | E810–E819 (.7) | — | — | — | — |
| Unspecified | E810–E819(.9) | — | — | — | — |
| Pedal cyclist, other | E800–E807 (.3); E820–E825 (.6); E826.1, .9; E827–E829 (.1) | — | — | — | — |
| Pedestrian, other | E800–E807 (.2), E820–E825 (.7), E826–E829 (.0) | — | — | — | — |
| Transport, other | E800–E807 (.0, .1, .8, .9), E820–E825 (.0–.5, .8, .9), E826.2–.8, E827–E829 (.2–.9), E831.0–.9, E833.0–E845.9 | E958.6 | — | E988.6 | — |

*Source:* Reprinted from "Recommended Framework for Presenting Injury Mortality Data," Recommendations and Reports, *MMWR*, Vol. 46, No. RR–14, pp. 6–7, 1997.

| Mechanism/Cause | Manner/Intent | | | | |
|---|---|---|---|---|---|
| | Unintentional | Suicide | Homicide | Undetermined | Other[1] |
| Natural/environmental | E900.0–E909, E928.0–.2 | E957.3 | — | E988.3 | — |
| Bites and stings | E905.0–.6,.9; E906.0–.4,.9 | — | — | — | — |
| Overexertion | E927 | — | — | — | — |
| Poisoning | E850.0–E869.9 | E950.0–E952.9 | E962.0–.9 | E980.0–E982.9 | E972 |
| Struck by, against | E916–E917.9 | — | E960.0, E968.2 | — | E973, E975 |
| Suffocation | E911–E913.9 | E953.0–.9 | E963 | E983.0–.9 | — |
| Other specified, classifiable | E846–E848, E914–E915, E918, E921.0–.9, E923.0–.9, E925.0–E926.9, E929.0–.5 | E955.5–.9; E958.0,.4 | E960.1, E965.5–.9; E967.0–.9, E968.4 | E985.5; E988.0,.4 | E971, E978, E990–E994, E996, E997.0–.2 |
| Other specified, not elsewhere classifiable | E928.8, E929.8 | E958.8, E959 | E968.8, E969 | E988.8, E989 | E977, E995, E997.8, E998, E999 |
| Unspecified | E887, E928.9, E929.9 | E958.9 | E968.9 | E988.9 | E976, E997.9 |
| All injury[4] | E800–E863, E880–E929 | E950–E959 | E960–E969 | E980–E989 | E970–E978, E990–E999, E870–E879, E930.0–E949.9 |
| Adverse effects | — | — | — | — | E870–E879, E930.0–E949.9 |
| Medical care[5] | — | — | — | — | E870–E879 |
| Drugs[6] | — | — | — | — | E930.0–E949.9 |
| All external causes | — | — | — | — | E800–E999 |

*Note:* "—" represents categories in which no E codes are assigned.

**Notes**

[1]Includes legal intervention (E970–E978) and operations of war (E990–E999).

[2]Three fourth-digit codes (.4—"occupant of street car," .5—"rider of animal," and .8—"other specified person") are not separated because of the minimal number of deaths in these categories. However, because they are included in the overall "motor vehicle traffic" category, the sum of these categories can be derived by subtraction.

[3]This parenthetical notation implies that the decimal should be applied to each individual three-digit E code in the grouping.

[4]Adverse effects have been excluded from the "all injury" category but are included in the "all external causes" category.

[5]Includes (1) adverse effects to patients during surgical and medical care and (2) surgical and medical procedures as the cause of abnormal reactions or later complications without mention of negative events at the time of procedure.

[6]Includes drugs and medicinal and biological substances causing adverse effects when used therapeutically.

# Number of Deaths and Crude Death Rate per 100,000 Population, by Mechanism-by-Intent Categories—United States, 1993

| Mechanism/Cause | Unintentional Number | Unintentional Rate | Suicide Number | Suicide Rate | Homicide Number | Homicide Rate | Undetermined Number | Undetermined Rate | Other[1] Number | Other[1] Rate | Total Number | Total Rate |
|---|---|---|---|---|---|---|---|---|---|---|---|---|
| Cut/pierce | 108 | 0.04 | 537 | 0.2 | 3,204 | 1.2 | 5 | —[2] | — | — | 3,854 | 1.5 |
| Drowning/submersion | 4,390 | 1.7 | 355 | 0.1 | 52 | 0.02 | 262 | 0.1 | — | — | 5,059 | 2.0 |
| Fall | 9,788 | 3.8 | 605 | 0.2 | 24 | 0.01 | 56 | 0.02 | — | — | 10,473 | 4.1 |
| Fire/burn | 4,030 | 1.6 | 188 | 0.1 | 227 | 0.1 | 102 | 0.04 | — | — | 4,547 | 1.8 |
| Fire/flame | 3,900 | 1.5 | 187 | 0.1 | 214 | 0.1 | 97 | 0.04 | — | — | 4,398 | 1.7 |
| Hot object/substance | 130 | 0.1 | 1 | —[2] | 13 | —[2] | 5 | —[2] | — | — | 149 | 0.1 |
| Firearm | 1,521 | 0.6 | 18,940 | 7.3 | 18,253 | 7.1 | 563 | 0.2 | 318 | 0.1 | 39,595 | 15.4 |
| Machinery | 999 | 0.4 | — | — | — | — | — | — | — | — | 999 | 0.4 |
| Motor vehicle traffic[3] | 40,899 | 15.9 | 108 | 0.04 | — | — | 14 | —[2] | — | — | 41,021 | 15.9 |
| Occupant | 24,586 | 9.5 | — | — | — | — | — | — | — | — | 24,586 | 9.5 |
| Motorcyclist | 1,927 | 0.7 | — | — | — | — | — | — | — | — | 1,927 | *0.7* |
| Pedal cyclist | 789 | 0.3 | — | — | — | — | — | — | — | — | 789 | 0.3 |
| Pedestrian | 5,978 | 2.3 | — | — | — | — | — | — | — | — | 5,978 | 2.3 |
| Unspecified | 7,583 | 2.9 | — | — | — | — | — | — | — | — | 7,583 | *2.9* |
| Pedal cyclist, other | 116 | 0.04 | — | — | — | — | — | — | — | — | 116 | 0.04 |
| Pedestrian, other | 941 | 0.4 | — | — | — | — | — | — | — | — | 941 | 0.4 |
| Transport, other | 1,829 | 0.7 | — | — | — | — | — | — | — | — | 1,829 | 0.7 |
| Natural/environmental | 1,544 | 0.6 | 8 | —[2] | — | — | 7 | —[2] | — | — | 1,559 | 0.6 |
| Bites and stings | 89 | 0.03 | — | — | — | — | — | — | — | — | 89 | 0.03 |
| Overexertion | 19 | —[2] | — | — | — | — | — | — | — | — | 19 | — |
| Poisoning | 8,537 | 3.3 | 5,271 | 2.0 | 59 | 0.02 | 1,903 | 0.7 | — | — | 15,770 | 6.1 |

*Source:* Reprinted from "Recommended Framework for Presenting Injury Mortality Data," Recommendations and Reports, *MMWR*, Vol. 46, No. RR–14, p. 10, 1997.

**Manner/Intent**

| Mechanism/Cause | Unintentional | | Suicide | | Homicide | | Undetermined | | Other[1] | | Total | |
|---|---|---|---|---|---|---|---|---|---|---|---|---|
| | Number | Rate | Number | Rate | Number | Rate | Number | Rate | Number | Rate | Number | Rate |
| Struck by, against | 901 | 0.3 | — | | 368 | 0.1 | — | | 4 | —[2] | 1,273 | 0.5 |
| Suffocation | 4,178 | 1.6 | 4,627 | 1.8 | 554 | 0.4 | 76 | 0.03 | — | | 9,835 | 3.8 |
| Other specified, classifiable | 1,626 | 0.6 | 308 | 0.1 | 363 | 0.1 | 25 | 0.01 | 31 | 0.01 | 2,353 | 0.9 |
| Other specified, not elsewhere classifiable | 109 | —[2] | 117 | 0.05 | 1,093 | 0.4 | 121 | 0.05 | 9 | —[2] | 1,449 | 0.6 |
| Unspecified | 6,063 | 2.4 | 38 | 0.01 | 1,356 | 0.4 | 285 | 0.1 | 2 | — | 7,444 | 2.9 |
| All injury | 87,598 | 34.0 | 31,102 | 12.1 | 25,653 | 10.0 | 3,419 | 1.3 | 364 | 0.1 | 148,136 | 57.5 |
| Adverse effects | — | | — | | — | | — | | — | | 2,925 | 1.1 |
| Medical care | — | | — | | — | | — | | — | | 2,724 | 1.1 |
| Drugs | — | | — | | — | | — | | — | | 201 | 0.1 |
| All external causes | — | | — | | — | | — | | — | | 151,061 | 58.6 |

*Note:* "—" denotes that no applicable deaths have occurred with the respective ICD-9 E codes. Rates are given to two decimal places when the rate is ≤0.05.

**Notes**

[1]Includes legal intervention (E970–E978) and operations of war (E990–E999).

[2]The crude death rate would have been based on <20 deaths.

[3]Three fourth-digit codes (.4—"occupant of streetcar," .5—"rider of animal," and .8—"other specified person") are not separated because of the minimal number of deaths in these categories. However, because they are included in the overall "motor vehicle traffic" category, the sum of these categories can be derived by subtraction.

# CHAPTER 4

# Unintentional Injury

"In 1995 unintentional injury accounted for 61 percent of all injury deaths."

National Center for Health Statistics, *Health, United States, 1996–97*

## WHAT THIS CHAPTER IS ABOUT

Injuries can be prevented; this is a goal of public health agencies, but injury prevention programs are not implemented in a generic, undifferentiated manner. Instead, to be effective, injury prevention programs must target specific categories of injury such as childhood poisonings or falls among the elderly. To do so effectively, injury prevention professionals must understand something about each of the leading types of injuries. How do they compare in terms of frequency? What subgroups of the population are at greatest risk? How do the various types of injuries occur (i.e., what circumstances surround particular types of injuries)? These are questions that need to be explored in terms of data specific to your particular area, because geographic variation in injury rates is extremely wide and extremely important. This chapter will provide some context for approaching and using the information your local injury surveillance provides you. We will review some of the most frequently occurring types of unintentional injuries and provide brief summaries of each. In short, we will outline what is known about the leading types of unintentional injuries. We wish to emphasize, however, that our goal is to provide an overview and an introduction, *not* a reference work. For the most up-to-date data on any aspect of unintentional injury, readers should consult the most recent publications of the National Center for Health Statistics, the National Center for Injury Prevention and Control, and other sources listed in the notes to this chapter, as well as the data-related World Wide Web sites included in Appendix A at the end of this book.

Julian Waller defines unintentional injury events as

> events in which (1) injury occurs over a relatively short period of time—at most, seconds or minutes, (2) the harmful outcome was not sought, and (3) the injury resulted either from one of the forms of physical energy in the environment (kinetic, chemical, thermal, electrical, or ionizing radiation) or because normal body mechanisms for using such energy were blocked by external means (such as by drowning).[1(p8)]

The conceptual distinction between "unintentional" and "intentional" injuries is in many ways more apparent than real. Certainly not all suicides and homicides are entirely "intended," no more than drunk driving deaths, boxing deaths, or occupational deaths are purely "unintentional." From a prevention perspective, intent is only one relevant factor, along with access to the means of injury, injury countermeasures, medical response, and the like. But for ease of presentation we will limit the discussion in this chapter to those types of injuries commonly viewed as unintentional and reserve the discussion of homicide, suicide, and nonfatal assaults—"intentional" injuries—to the next chapter.

## INTRODUCTION

Those injuries commonly considered to be unintentional constitute about two thirds of all injury deaths, which are about equally divided between transportation (motor vehicle) injuries and other unintentional injuries. The "other" category is often labeled home and leisure or home and recreation to reflect the circumstances surrounding most of the injury occurrences, but many occur in occupational settings or schools. According to the injury chartbook in *Health, United States, 1996–97 and Injury Chartbook:*

> *Unintentional* injury comprised the largest portion of fatal injuries, about 61%, ranging from 50% at ages 20–24 years and 25–34 years to 79–91% for persons 1–9 years of age and 75 years and over. In 1995, 90,402 persons died as a result of an unintentional injury, at a crude rate of 34.4 per 100,000.

> Age-specific unintentional injury death rates follow a pattern similar to that of all injury—relatively higher in infancy than for young children, rising through the early to mid-twenties, then declining through middle age, and rising again among the elderly.[2(p20)]

Injuries differ greatly in terms of their distribution within the population. The same is true of injury trends. But as a group, unintentional injuries have been declining. Baker et al note that "[f]rom 1930 to 1986, the overall death rate from unintentional injuries declined by more than half, from 81 to 40 per 100,000 population, with a further decline to 35 per 100,000 in 1988. This decline, however, has been far from uniform."[3(p58–59)]

The remainder of this chapter will look at the leading categories of unintentional injury: motor vehicle, falls, poisonings, fires and burns, drowning, and aspirations. It should be noted that these categories are not entirely composed of injuries that are unintentional. Practically all motor vehicle and aspiration fatalities are indeed unintentional, as are most deaths from falls (93%), drowning (86%), and fires and burns (89%),[2(p24)] but only a little over one half of all deaths due to poisoning were unintentional (see Figure 4–1). Before going further, however, it should be noted that the top 5 (or 10) unintentional injury death categories are not the same as the top 5 (or 10) nonfatal unintentional injury categories. For example, injuries in the home account for about one fifth of all unintentional injury deaths and about two fifths of all unintentional nonfatal injuries. The same relationship is found with sports injuries. But a converse relationship is found for drowning, where deaths predominate. Nor is an overall listing of the top 5 (or 10) unintentional injury categories the same for Whites as for Blacks, men as for women, or children as for the elderly.

Also, it should be noted that this discussion uses categories based on the type of injury event. Another approach would be to categorize according to settings of the injury event—occupational, home, or school. This might be helpful from the perspective of interventions by public agencies, but it creates a complicated way to sort out injury categories. For example, motor vehicle crashes are the most common cause of occupational injury deaths. And not all injuries fit neatly into these categories: are bicycle injuries transportation or recreation injuries? Are swimming pool drownings home or recreation injuries? Rather than worry about neatly compartmentalizing every injury into its proper category, however, we will use the standard categories of types of injuries in order to structure an overview of unintentional injury.

This discussion is based on national data. There are large variations between states and local areas. Obviously your primary concern will be with the types of injuries that present the biggest problems *in your area*. Thus the discussion of injury surveillance in Chapter 12 should become the critical starting point in understanding the nature of the injury problem you

**Number of Deaths**

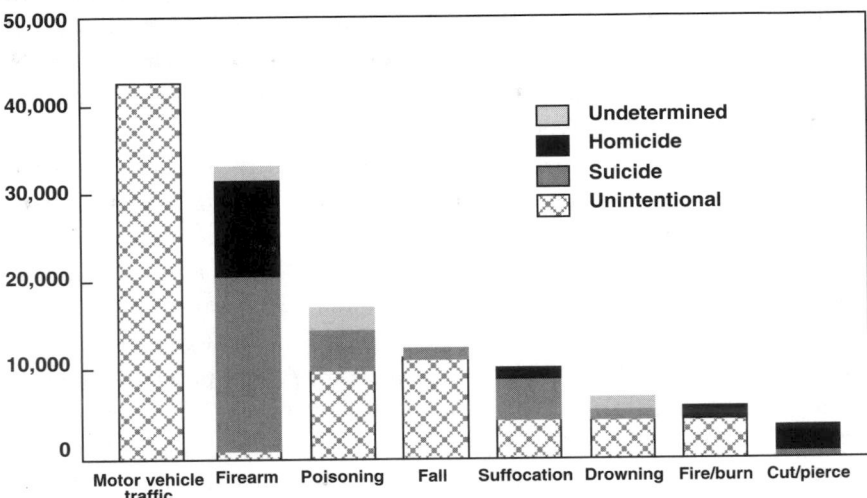

*Note:* In this figure, firearm homicide includes the 284 firearm deaths due to legal intervention.

**Figure 4–1** Leading Causes of Injury Death by Manner of Death: United States, 1995. *Source:* Reprinted from L.A. Fingerhut and M. Warner, Injury Chartbook, in *Health, United States, 1996–1997*, p. 24, 1997, National Center for Health Statistics, U.S. Public Health Service.

confront. The discussion that follows provides short sketches of the unintentional injury problem. The information is drawn primarily from the injury chartbook in *Health, United States, 1997–96 and Injury Chartbook[2];* Baker et al, *The Injury Fact Book, Second Edition[3];* and Waller, *Injury Control: A Guide to the Causes and Prevention of Trauma.*[1] The reader should peruse these and other sources of injury data[4,5] for the fullest, most up-to-date details on unintentional injury numbers. To develop an appreciation for unintentional injury in terms of prevention goals, explore the listing of unintentional injury-related *Healthy People 2000* Health Objectives in Appendix 4–A at the end of this chapter.

## MOTOR VEHICLE INJURIES

"Motor vehicle injury" encompasses several different types of injury situations and can be categorized according to single-vehicle crashes, multiple-vehicle crashes, truck-automobile crashes, and the like. They also can be categorized according to whether the victim is an occupant, a pedestrian, a motorcyclist, or a pedal cyclist. Motor vehicles account for 29% of all injury deaths in the United States (and 47% of all unintentional injury deaths), with 42,331 deaths in 1995 alone. Motor vehicle crashes are the third leading cause of significant years of life lost in the United States after heart disease and cancer. More people have died in motor vehicle crashes in the United States than have died in all of this nation's wars. More than 80% of motor vehicle crash deaths involve vehicle occupants, the remainder being pedestrians, bicyclists, and motorcyclists. Motor vehicle crashes are the leading cause of death in the U.S. from age 1 through age 34 and account for more than one fifth of all deaths in the 5 to 29 age range. And motor vehicle crashes are the leading cause of work-related deaths. More than a half million hospitalizations each year in the United States are the result of motor vehicle crashes, as are close to 5 million nonhospitalized injuries. Motor vehicle crashes are responsible for 44% of the country's brain injuries and constitute the major cause of serious permanent head and spinal cord disabilities. In 1985 dollars, the annual cost of U.S. motor vehicle injuries is close to $50 billion. Rivara et al note that motor vehicle occupant injuries are related to "the mass of the vehicle, its speed at the time of the crash, the extent to which the occupant's movement was restrained, whether the occupant was ejected, and the extent to which the occupant was protected from the impact of vehicle parts against the body."[5(p544)]

The gruesome picture presented by motor vehicle injuries affects the population unevenly, particularly regarding age. Two fifths of all motor vehicle injury deaths involve those in their late teen years, and males have three times the motor vehicle death rate of females. As a group, males 15 to 24 years of age suffer by far the highest rates of motor vehicle trauma. At the other end of the age spectrum, the elderly—due to their greater fragility— have the highest ratio of motor vehicle deaths to motor vehicle injuries. Motor vehicle deaths also vary significantly by race and income and by geographic location. Fatal motor vehicle injury rates are twice as high in rural areas as in cities, while the reverse relationship is true of nonfatal motor vehicle injuries. Motor vehicle death rates are highest in the Southern and Western states, perhaps the result of more rural roads and higher speeds.

Pedestrian injuries affect school-age children in particular.[6] There were 5,412 pedestrian deaths in the United States in 1996—one such death every 97 minutes—and 82,000 nonfatal pedestrian injuries.[7] A variety of factors are associated with pedestrian injury, including the pedestrian's developmental stage, traffic volume and speed, density of curbside parking, and driver attentiveness.[5,8] Pedestrian injuries have been declining, primarily because there are fewer pedestrians (i.e., people—especially children—are walking less).

The motor vehicle injury picture is improving, with the most dramatic improvements occurring in the 1980s and 1990s. These improvements have been the result of advances in several areas. Federal legislation has resulted in more crashworthy automobiles (including important advances in occupant protection). Federal legislation has also focused on improving roadway safety and reducing the role of drugs (particularly alcohol) in traffic crashes. The states have also focused on reducing impaired driving. In the past two decades, there have been important improvements in trauma care, which enable motor vehicle crash victims to receive critical on-site care and faster transport to hospitals during the "golden hour" (the crucial period for lifesaving trauma care). The decline in the size of the teenage population has also been reflected in an improved motor vehicle injury picture.

For many years motor vehicle injury was primarily the concern of transportation safety professionals who tended to focus their efforts on the precrash phase of the motor vehicle injury event, in particular the behavior of drivers. More recently public health has become more involved with motor vehicle injury, particularly that of infants and children. This has heightened the focus on the crash phase of the motor vehicle injury event. The goal is to make crashes more survivable, particularly by distributing the mechanical energy of the crash over time and space to reduce the impact on the occupants through use of infant car seats, seatbelts, and airbags. The role of health departments in dealing with motor vehicle injury is discussed more fully in Chapters 10 and 11. The major focus of these departments remains getting the higher-risk target populations to use seatbelts, to properly restrain children in car seats, and to get children to ride restrained in the rear of the vehicle (regardless of whether or not there is an airbag).

Significant work remains to be done to further reduce motor vehicle injuries. Two fifths of all motor vehicle deaths are alcohol related.[9] Yet despite clear evidence that alcohol use is highly sensitive to tax increases, governments have been extremely hesitant to increase these taxes. Despite clear evidence that motorcycle helmets and helmet use laws reduce deaths, states have been unwilling to pass and maintain such laws. And despite clear evidence that increased speeds increase crash fatalities, Congress opened the door in 1996 so that states could raise interurban highway speed limits. At the same time, politicians intent on attacking government as the enemy of the people have created an environment in which adherence to and enforcement of traffic laws seems to be disintegrating, with potentially dire consequences. And the United States remains heavily reliant on automobile and truck traffic. This is a public policy choice that could be changed; but as long as it is not, motor vehicle injury will continue to be a major cause of mortality and morbidity.

## FALLS

Falls account for 8% of all injury deaths in the United States, which meant 11,275 deaths in 1995—93% of them unintentional. This makes falls the second leading cause of unintentional injury death after motor vehicles. The nonfatal injury rate associated with falls is higher than for any other single type of injury. Each year 1 of every 20 people in the country receives emergency room treatment for a fall injury. Falls occur in many settings, including infants from furniture, children from windows and playground equipment, and the elderly on stairs or while walking on the same level. The majority of fall events resulting in death occur in the home, especially for children and the elderly. One third of fall events involve people more than 85 years of age, and 87% of fractures suffered by the elderly are the result of falls. Three fifths of all fall-related deaths involve people 65 years old or older. The trend has been downward for fall fatalities, perhaps due to improvements in the medical care system's ability to deal with complications related to fall injuries.

Information on the circumstances surrounding falls is limited, although it would seem that only one third involve falls from heights. Waller notes that "extreme youth, alcohol, aging, and impairment . . . are important factors" for fall injuries. Factors associated with falls among the elderly include "a history of one or more prior falls, cognitive impairment, chronic illness, balance and gait impairment, a low body-mass index, female sex, general frailty, use of diuretics, use of psychotropic drugs, and hazards in the home."[5(p613)]

For the elderly, strategies to prevent fall injuries can include weight-bearing exercise and other physical activities to increase strength, mobility, and flexibility; minimization of psychotropic drug use; environmental modifications; and adequate calcium uptake and hormone replacement therapy for women.[5(pp613–614),10] For children, preventive approaches include installation of window guards in high-rise buildings, gates on stairways, energy-absorbing surface materials in playgrounds, and counseling of parents.

## POISONINGS

Poisonings account for 11% of all injury deaths in the United States. This meant 16,307 deaths in 1995, of which 9,072 (or 56%) were unintentional. The largest portion of intentional poisonings was suicide. There are about one quarter of a million hospital admissions annually associated with poisoning. The most common cause of unintentional poisonings is legal and illegal drugs; the most common cause of intentional poisonings is carbon monoxide. Waller[1] suggests that many poisoning deaths classified as unintentional may also be suicides.

A major preventive approach to decrease childhood poisoning is the sale of medications and other hazardous substances in childproof packaging. In large part as the result of the Poison Prevention Packaging Act of 1970, childhood poisoning is no longer the major problem it once was. Of the childhood poisoning deaths that do occur, 94% occur in the home and usually involve cosmetics, personal care products, and household cleaning products. For individuals of all ages, poisonings may be reduced by attention to prescribing medications in the least toxic forms and with clear labeling to minimize overmedication and mismedication by the elderly.

## FIRES AND BURNS

Fires and burns account for 3% of all injury deaths in the United States, which meant 4,345 deaths in 1995, 89% of them unintentional. This makes fires and burns the fourth leading cause of unintentional injury deaths, with someone in the United States dying about every two hours in a fire. Fatal and nonfatal injuries result from flame, scald, contact, electrical, chemical, and ultraviolet radiation burns, and from smoke inhalation. About 60,000 people are hospitalized for burns each year. House fires were the location for 80% of all unintentional fire deaths. The majority of fire deaths occur during the winter months, when heating and lighting sources are most in use. The most common cause of residential fires is cooking and heating equipment. Alcohol impairment contributed to 40% of residential fire deaths. Cigarettes caused about one fourth of all fire deaths. As with injury in general, social class was a strong factor in fire deaths; these deaths were five times more likely to occur in low-income areas than in high-income areas. As with injury deaths in general, the human factors involved in fire deaths are extreme youth, aging, and medical impairments, as well as abuse of alcohol.

On the individual level, fire and burn prevention includes installation and maintenance of smoke detectors; having and practicing a home fire-escape plan; ensuring attention to burning cigarettes, stovetops, and ovens[11,12]; and setting hot water heaters in the 120 to 125° F range. On the community level, fire and burn prevention could include smoke detector ordinances and giveaways,[13] laws requiring that hot water heaters be preset at 125° F,[14] and introduction of "fire-safe" cigarettes.[15]

## DROWNING

Drowning accounts for 3% of all injury deaths in the United States, which meant 5,071 deaths in 1995, 86% of them unintentional. This makes drowning the third leading cause of unintentional injury deaths for all ages and the second leading cause for children and young adults. In 10 states, drowning is the leading cause of unintentional injury death for children under 15 years old. Males have four times the drowning rate of females. Drowning rates are particularly high for Asian Americans and Native Americans, and overall drowning rates among Blacks are twice that for Whites. Drowning is by definition fatal. But for every 10 drownings, 36 near-drowning victims are admitted to hospitals and 140 near-drowning victims are treated in emergency departments.

The data on circumstances surrounding drowning is rather limited, even as compared to other types of injury; however, roughly one fifth of drownings are related to boating. Swimming pools account for 60% to 90% of drownings of 0 to 4 year olds. Alcohol may be involved in as many as half of all drownings. Drowning rates have decreased considerably since 1930, although the reasons are unclear.

Drowning prevention strategies involve fencing to enclose all four sides of swimming pools and use of personal flotation devices. It is not known what role swimming training has,[5(p615)] nor—given that it is rarely done—

what role anticipatory guidance by pediatricians and others could play.[16] Preventive efforts aimed at the alcohol-drowning connection would certainly seem worth pursuing.[17]

## ASPIRATIONS

Aspirations are part of the broader category of asphyxiation injuries. This broader category consists of intentional asphyxiation (usually referred to as suffocation) and unintentional asphyxiation (usually referred to as aspiration or choking). To complicate the terminology, suffocation is sometimes used to refer to the entire category of unintentional and intentional asphyxiations.

In 1995 suffocation (the term used by the National Center for Health Statistics) accounted for 7% of all injury deaths in the United States, or a total of 10,376 deaths. Of these, 50% were suicides (primarily by hanging), 8% homicides, and the remaining 41% were unintentional, of which one half involved nonfood obstructions—such as toy parts, balloons, coins, and other objects—in the respiratory tract and one quarter involved inhalation or ingestion of food (including regurgitated food) leading to respiratory obstruction. Most of the remainder involved mechanical suffocation. Among children under 1 year of age, 40% of all unintentional deaths were caused by aspiration.

A major focus for prevention of childhood aspirations must be consumer products. The Hazardous Substances Act of 1972 provides for a test of object size in articles intended for children younger than 3 years. The Consumer Product Safety Commission performs the testing using the small parts test fixture, but this approach seems too limited to be fully effective.[18] Increasing the size of the test instrument, extending coverage for toys intended for older children, and focusing regulatory attention on other objects—such as balloons[19]—seem promising. New product design standards also seem called for to reduce pediatric window cord strangulations.[20] For adult aspiration, training in the Heimlich Maneuver and requiring aspiration-dislodging devices in restaurants have received attention.

## SPORTS INJURIES

Sports injuries constitute a category determined by setting rather than by cause (although the same point might also be made regarding motor vehicle injuries). Compared to other categories of injury, data on sports injuries are quite poor, with little known about relative risks and exposure. But from what we do know, this is an injury category that must not be ignored—not only because it primarily involves the young but also because, while deaths are few, the number of nonfatal injuries is considerable.[21] According to Bijur et al:

> Sports activities account for a large number and substantial proportion of all injuries to children. . . . The estimated annual number of all injuries from sports and recreation in US children and adolescents is 4,379,000 . . .; from serious sport injuries, 1,363,000.[22(p1009)]

Football accounts for the bulk of high school sports injuries; basketball also has a high injury rate, as do gymnastics, wrestling, and ice hockey. The majority of sports injuries result from falls, from being struck by an object, or from overexertion. In the Massachusetts Statewide Childhood Injury Prevention Project data system, sports injury rates were second only to motor vehicle occupant injury rates among all causes of injury—for both inpatient and outpatient injury treatment settings.[23]

Prevention of sports injuries will require, first of all, much better data collection.[24] Currently only one third of sports injuries can be identified as such by current E code categories.[25] Still, experience to date suggest that alterations in the rules of various sports to prohibit particularly dangerous practices (such as "spearing" in football), requiring protective equipment (such as mouthguards), and ability grouping can all contribute to injury reduction. The medical role is also important, both in overseeing conditioning practices and in ensuring adequate emergency response when injuries do occur.[26]

## CONCLUSION

Not all unintentional injuries can be prevented, but many can. These are not "accidents." They are predictable events with known causes and risk factors. There is much that public health agencies can do to reduce unintentional injury.

There are several features of unintentional injury that make preventive interventions easy and several features that make such intervention difficult. In the first place, these are *unintentional* injuries, they were not sought by anyone. In the second place, we know much about injury countermeasures that can be effective in reducing the toll of unintentional injuries.[27] There is, therefore, a clear record of successes in reducing the number of unintentional injuries. As Dowswell et al explain:

> Examples of interventions that have been effective in reducing injury include: bicycle helmet legislation, area wide traffic calming measures, child safety restraint legislation, child resistant containers to prevent poisoning, and window bars to prevent falls. Interventions effective in changing behavior include bicycle helmet education and legislation, child restraint educational campaigns . . . provision of smoke detectors, and parent education on home hazard reduction. For the community based campaigns, the key to success has been the sustained use of surveillance systems, the commitment of interagency cooperation and the time needed to develop networks and implement a range of interventions.[27]

On the other hand, efforts to reduce unintentional injuries are hampered by several factors. Our data are limited, especially on the local level and especially as regards to the circumstances surrounding unintentional injuries. Certain high incidence areas, such as falls in children, have not been well studied in the literature. And the data we do have are skewed toward unintentional injury deaths (the tip of the iceberg) when public health may well have the greatest impact in reducing the much greater numbers of nonfatal injuries. Injury prevention is also hampered by the fact that the most likely victims of injury are the most vulnerable in society: the young, the old, the poor. The widespread use and abuse of alcohol—which has proven difficult to challenge—is closely tied to unintentional (as well as intentional) injury. Add to this the continuing "accidents happen" mindset, and risk—and risk taking—can be a difficult problem to deal with.

But there have been—and continue to be—important successes in reducing unintentional injuries. In reviewing childhood injuries in the United States, Rivara and Grossman note that:

> Deaths from all injuries decreased by 26.5% over the 14-year period [1978–1991], from 40.22/100,000 in 1978 to 29.58/100,000 in 1991. . . . Unintentional deaths decreased by 38.9% compared with a 47.1% increase in intentional injury deaths. The largest absolute decreases were in pedestrian (1325), occupant (1557), and drowning (615) deaths, whereas the greatest decreases in rate

of deaths were from poisoning due to gases/vapors, motorcyclist, and pedestrian injuries.[4]

---

## NOTES

1. Waller JA. *Injury Control: A Guide to the Causes and Prevention of Trauma.* Lexington, MA: Lexington Books; 1985.

2. Fingerhut LA, Warner M. Injury chartbook. In National Center for Health Statistics. *Health, United States, 1996–97 and Injury Chartbook.* Hyattsville, MD: U.S. Public Health Service; 1997.

3. Baker SP, O'Neill B, Ginsburg MJ, Li G. *The Injury Fact Book.* 2nd ed. New York: Oxford University Press; 1992.

4. Rivara FP, Grossman DC. Prevention of traumatic deaths to children in the United States: How far have we come and where do we need to go? *Pediatrics.* 1996;97: 791–797.

5. Rivara FP, Grossman DC, Cummings P. Injury prevention (Parts One and Two). *New Engl J Med.* 1997;337:543–548 and 1997;337:613–618.

6. National Highway Traffic Safety Administration. *Children and Youth Traffic Safety Data Book.* Washington, DC: U.S. Department of Transportation (DOT HS 88 385); 1996:59.

7. National Center for Statistics and Analysis, National Highway Traffic Safety Administration. *Traffic Safety Facts 1996: Pedestrians.* Washington, DC: U.S. Department of Transportation; 1997:1.

8. Stevenson MR, Sleet DA. Which prevention strategies for child pedestrian injuries? A review of the literature. *Int Q Community Health Educ.* 1996–97;16:207–217.

9. National Center for Injury Prevention and Control. Unintentional Injury Fact Sheet: Impaired Driving, at http://cdc.gov/ncipc/spotlite/factshee.htm.

10. National Center for Injury Prevention and Control. Unintentional Injury Fact Sheet: Falls and Hip Fractures in the Elderly: Injury Prevention, at http://cdc.gov/ncipc/duip/falls.htm.

11. National Center for Injury Prevention and Control. Unintentional Injury Fact Sheet: Fire-Related Injury and Death Among U.S. Residents, at http://cdc.gov/ncipc/duip/fire2.htm.

12. Runyan CW, Bangdiwala SI, Linzer MA, Sacks JJ, Butts J. Risk factors for fatal residential fires. *New Engl J Med.* 1992;327:859–863.

13. Mallonee S, Istre GR, Rosenberg M, et al. Surveillance and prevention of residential-fire injuries. *New Engl J Med.* 1996;335:27–31.

14. Katcher ML. Efforts to prevent burns from hot tap water. In: Bergman AB. *Political Approaches to Injury Control at the State Level.* Seattle: University of Washington Press; 1992:69–78.

15. McGuire A. Fires, cigarettes, and advocacy. *Law Med Health Care.* 1989;17:73–77.

16. O'Flaherty JE, Pirie PL. Prevention of pediatric drowning and near-drowning: A survey of members of the American Academy of Pediatrics. *Pediatrics.* 1997;99:169–174.

17. National Center for Injury Prevention and Control. Unintentional Injury Fact Sheet: Injury Prevention: Drowning, at http://cdc.gov/ncipc/duip/drown.htm.

18. Rimell FL, Thome A Jr, Stool S, et al. Characteristics of objects that cause choking in children. *JAMA.* 1995;274:1763–1766.

19. Baker S. Designing the death out of balloons. *JAMA.* 1995;274:1805.

20. Rauchschwalbe R, Mann NC. Pediatric window-cord strangulations in the United States, 1981–1995. *JAMA.* 1997;277:1696–1698.

21. Lescohier I, Gallagher SS. Unintentional injury. In: DiClemente RJ, Hansen W, Ponton LE. *Handbook of Adolescent Health Risk Behavior.* New York: Plenum Press; 1996: 236–237.

22. Bijur PE, Trumble M, Harel Y, Overpeck MD, Jones D, Scheidt P. Sports and recreation injuries in US children and adolescents. *Arch Pediatr Adolesc Med.* 1995;1009–1016.

23. Malek M, Chang B, Gallagher SS, Guyer B. The cost of medical care for injuries to children. *Ann Emerg Med.* 1991;20:997–1005.

24. National Institutes of Health. *Conference on Sports Injuries in Youth: Surveillance Strategies.* NIH Publication No. 93-3444; November 1992.

25. Gallagher SS. Massachusetts: A case example of how surveillance systems work. In: *Conference on Sports Injuries in Youth: Surveillance Strategies.* NIH Publication No. 93-3444; November 1992:33–38.

26. Posner M, Gallagher SS. Sports and physical education. In: *Preventing Injuries in the School Environment* (in press).

27. Dowswell T, Towner EML, Simpson G, Jarvis SN. Preventing childhood unintentional injuries—what works? A literature review. *Inj Prev.* 1996;2:140–149.

# Injury-Related Year 2000 Objectives

## UNINTENTIONAL INJURIES

**9.1** Reduce deaths caused by unintentional injuries to no more than 29.3 per 100,000 people. (Age-adjusted baseline: 34.7 per 100,000 in 1987)

**9.2** Reduce nonfatal unintentional injuries so that hospitalizations for this condition are no more than 754 per 100,000 people. (Baseline: 887 per 100,000 in 1988)

**9.3** Reduce deaths caused by motor vehicle crashes to no more than 1.5 per 100 million vehicle miles traveled (VMT) and 14.2 per 100,000 people. (Baseline: 2. 4 per 100 million vehicle miles traveled (VMT) and 19.2 per 100,000 people (age adjusted) in 1987)

**9.4** Reduce deaths from falls and fall-related injuries to no more than 2.3 per 100,000 people. (Age-adjusted baseline: 2.7 per 100,000 in 1987)

**9.5** Reduce drowning deaths to no more than 1.3 per 100,000 people. (Age-adjusted baseline: 2.1 per 100,000 in 1987)

**9.6** Reduce residential fire deaths to no more than 1.2 per 100,000 people. (Age-adjusted baseline: 1.5 per 100,000 in 1987)

**9.7** Reduce hip fractures among people aged 65 and older so that hospitalizations for this condition are no more than 607 per 100,000. (Baseline: 714 per 100,000 in 1988)

**9.8** Reduce nonfatal poisoning to no more than 88 emergency department treatments per 100,000 people. (Baseline: 108 per 100,000 in 1986)

*Source:* Reprinted from *Healthy People 2000 Midcourse Review and 1995 Revisions*, 1995, U.S. Public Health Service.

**9.9** Reduce nonfatal head injuries so that hospitalizations for this condition are no more than 106 per 100,000 people. (Baseline: 118 per 100,000 in 1988)

**9.10** Reduce nonfatal spinal cord injuries so that hospitalizations for this condition are no more than 5 per 100,000 people. (Baseline: 5.3 per 100,000 in 1988)

**9.11** Reduce by 20% the incidence of secondary conditions (i.e., pressure sores) associated with traumatic spinal cord injuries. (Baseline data unavailable)

**9.12** Increase use of safety belts and child safety seats to at least 85% of motor vehicle occupants. (Baseline: 42% in 1988)

**9.13** Increase use of helmets to at least 80% of motorcyclists and at least 50% of bicyclists. (Baseline: 60% of motorcyclists in 1988 and an estimated 8% of bicyclists in 1984)

**9.14** Extend to 50 states laws requiring safety belt and motorcycle helmet use for all ages. (Baseline: 33 states and the District of Columbia in 1989 for automobiles; 22 states, the District of Columbia, and Puerto Rico for motorcycles)

**9.15** Enact in 50 states laws requiring that new handguns be designed to minimize the likelihood of discharge by children. (Baseline: 0 states in 1989)

**9.16** Extend to 2,000 local jurisdictions the number whose codes address the installation of fire suppression sprinkler systems in those residences at highest risk for fires. (Baseline: 700 jurisdictions in 1989)

**9.17** Increase the presence of functional smoke detectors to at least one on each habitable floor of all inhabited residential dwellings. (Baseline: 81% of residential dwellings in 1989)

**9.18** Provide academic instruction on injury prevention and control, preferably as part of comprehensive school health education, in at least 50% of public school systems (grades K through 12). (Baseline data unavailable)

**9.19** Extend requirement of the use of effective head, face, eye, and mouth protection to all organizations, agencies, and institutions sponsoring sporting and recreation events that pose risks of injury. (Baseline: National Collegiate Athletic Association football, hockey, and lacrosse; high school football; amateur boxing; and amateur ice hockey in 1988)

**9.20** Increase to at least 50 the number of states that have design standards for markings, signing, and other characteristics of the roadway environment to improve the visual stimuli and protect the safety of older drivers and pedestrians. (Baseline data unavailable)

**9.21** Increase to at least 50% the proportion of primary care providers who routinely provide age-appropriate counseling on safety precautions to prevent unintentional injury. (Baseline: Percentage of pediatricians, nurse practitioners, obstetricians/gynecologists, internists, and family physicians providing this service to 81–100% of patients in 1992)

**9.22** Extend to 20 states the capability to link emergency medical services, trauma systems, and hospital data. (Baseline: 7 states in 1993)

**9.23** Reduce deaths caused by alcohol-related motor vehicle crashes to no more than 5.5 per 100,000 people. (Baseline: 9.8 per 100,000 in 1987)

**9.24** Extend to 50 states laws requiring helmets for bicycle riders. (Baseline: 9 states in 1994)

**10.1** Reduce deaths from work-related injuries to no more than 4 per 100,000 full-time workers. (Baseline: Average of 6 per 100,000 during 1983–87)

**10.2** Reduce work-related injuries resulting in medical treatment, lost time from work, or restricted work activity to no more than 6 cases per 100 full-time workers. (Baseline: 7.7 per 100 in 1987)

**10.6** Increase to at least 95% the proportion of worksites with 50 or more employees that mandate employee use of occupant protection systems, such as seatbelts, during all work-related motor vehicle travel. (Baseline: 82.4% of worksites in 1992)

**10.10** Implement occupational safety and health plans in 50 states for the identification, management, and prevention of leading work-related diseases and injuries within the state. (Baseline: 10 states in 1989)

**10.12** Increase to at least 70% the proportion of worksites with 50 or more employees that have implemented programs on worker health and safety. (Baseline: 63.8% in 1992)

**10.13** Increase to at least 50% the proportion of worksites with 50 or more employees that offer back injury prevention and rehabilitation programs. (Baseline: 28.6% offered back care activities in 1985)

**10.14** Establish in 50 states either public health or labor department programs that provide consultation and assistance to small businesses to implement safety and health programs for their employees. (Baseline: 26 states in 1991)

**10.15** Increase to at least 75% the proportion of primary care providers who routinely elicit occupational health exposures as a part of patient history and provide relevant counseling. (Baseline: 6–14% of pediatricians, nurse practitioners, obstetricians/gynecologists, internists, and family physicians reported routinely providing this service to patients in 1992)

**4.5** Increase by at least one year the average age of first use of cigarettes, alcohol, and marijuana by adolescents aged 12–17. (Baseline: Age 11.6 for cigarettes, age 13.1 for alcohol, and age 13.4 for marijuana in 1988)

**4.6** Reduce the proportion of young people who have used alcohol, marijuana, cocaine, or cigarettes in the past month.

**4.7** Reduce the proportion of high school seniors and college students engaging in recent occasions of heavy drinking of alcoholic beverages to no more than 28% of high school seniors and 32% of college students. (Baseline: 33% of high school seniors and 41.7% of college students in 1989)

**4.8** Reduce alcohol consumption by people aged 14 and older to an annual average of no more than 2 gallons of ethanol per person. (Baseline: 2.54 gallons of ethanol in 1987)

**4.9** Increase the proportion of high school seniors who perceive social disapproval of heavy use of alcohol, occasional use of marijuana, and experimentation with cocaine, or regular use of tobacco.

**4.10** Increase the proportion of high school seniors who associate physical or psychological harm with heavy use of alcohol, occasional use of marijuana, and experimentation with cocaine, or regular use of cigarettes.

**4.12** Establish and monitor in 50 states comprehensive plans to ensure access to alcohol and drug treatment programs for traditionally underserved people. (Baseline data unavailable)

**4.13** Provide to children in all school districts and private schools primary and secondary school educational programs on alcohol and other drugs, preferably as part of comprehensive school health education. (Baseline: 63% provided some instruction, 39% provided counseling, and 23% referred students for clinical assessments in 1987)

**4.14** Extend adoptions of alcohol and drug policies for the work environment to at least 60% of worksites with 50 or more employees. (Baseline: 88% of worksites had adopted alcohol policies; 89% of worksites had adopted drug policies in 1992)

**4.15** Extend to 50 states administrative driver's license suspension/revocation laws or programs of equal effectiveness for people determined to have been driving under the influence of intoxicants. (Baseline: 28 states and the District of Columbia in 1990)

**4.16** Increase to 50 the number of states that have enacted and enforce policies, beyond those in existence in 1989, to reduce access to alcoholic beverages by minors. (Baseline data unavailable)

**4.17** Increase to at least 20 the number of states that have enacted statutes to restrict promotion of alcoholic beverages that is focused principally on young audiences. (Baseline data unavailable)

**4.18** Extend to 50 states legal blood alcohol concentration (BAC) tolerance levels of .08% for motor vehicle drivers aged 21 and older and zero tolerance (.02% and lower) for those younger than age 21. (Baseline: 7 states with .08 BAC laws and 9 states with zero tolerance laws in 1993)

**4.19** Increase to at least 75% the proportion of primary care providers who screen for alcohol and other drug use problems and provide counseling and referral as needed. (Baseline: 19–63% of pediatricians, nurse practitioners, obstetricians/gynecologists, internists, and family physicians reported routinely providing services to patient in 1992)

**4.20** Increase to 30 the number of states with Hospitality Resource Panels (including representatives from state regulatory, public health, and highway safety agencies, law enforcement, insurance associations, alcohol retail and licensed beverage associations) to ensure a process of management and server training and define standards of responsible hospitality. (Baseline: 8 states in 1994)

# CHAPTER 5

# Intentional Injury

"[T]he new vision for violence prevention put forth by the public health community provides reason for optimism."

James A. Mercy, et al, *Health Affairs*, 1993

## WHAT THIS CHAPTER IS ABOUT

As intentional violence has intruded into the national psyche as a high-priority social issue, increasing attention has been directed at dealing with violence as a public health problem. What exactly does this mean? What can public health practitioners do to reduce violence? Isn't this a matter for the law enforcement, criminal justice, and mental health systems? Are there any models for a public health approach to the prevention of violence?

This chapter will review the nature of interpersonal violence in the United States, explain why many people feel that public health can offer as much as law enforcement to the prevention of intentional violence, and describe possible public health approaches to violence reduction. We will suggest ways in which health departments can play a role in dealing with this problem. As with Chapter 4, our goal is to provide an overview and an introduction, *not* a reference work. For the most up-to-date data on any aspect of intentional injury, readers should consult the most recent publications of the National Center for Health Statistics, the National Center for Injury Prevention and Control, and other sources listed in the notes at the end of this chapter, as well as the data-related World Wide Web sites included in Appendix A at the end of this book.

## INTRODUCTION

The subject of this chapter—intentional, violent injury—is not a simple classification and is difficult to define in anything other than a general sense. Not all homicides are intended; for example, death is not usually the intended consequence of shaken baby syndrome or drunk driving or boxing matches. Nor is intent the only relevant factor in preventive efforts. Prevention strategies are aimed at reducing destructive energy transfer. This is true regardless of intent. Community-based injury prevention programs may be similar for both intentional and unintentional injuries; in fact, some strategies—such as home visiting programs and product designs to make guns less accessible—can be used to reduce both types of injuries. "Violence" is itself a poor descriptor: most injury deaths can be considered the result of violent trauma. The Panel on the Understanding and Control of Violent Behavior defined violence as "behaviors by individuals that intentionally threaten, attempt, or inflict physical harm on others,"[1(p2)] yet even the panel realized the limitations of such a definition, excluding as it does self-inflicted violence, collective violence (such as war), and noncriminal corporate violence (such as the marketing of "junk guns"). At the same time, "intentional," "violent" injury does have a common sense meaning. In all so-called intentional injury deaths, the act that led to the injury (if not the actual death) was intentional. Often the death itself was intended. We will use this common sense concept of intended acts in this chapter.

The United States stands out among developed countries in terms of fatal violence; our society does not necessarily have higher levels of violent incidents than other countries, but the violence that does occur in the United States is more likely to be lethal.[2] The United States has historically demonstrated a tolerance of interpersonal violence—the myth of the "wild West," acceptance of corporal punishment and state-imposed death penalties, music videos exploiting women, acceptance of widespread firearm availability, and societal inattention to domestic violence. At the same time—or perhaps consistent with this tolerance of violence—public perceptions distort the true nature of violence in America. Violence is portrayed in the media as stranger violence (muggings and random acts), when in fact the majority of violence occurs among acquaintances and family members. Violence is popularly associated with the deviant worlds of gang warfare and drug dealing, when in fact legal alcohol use and maleness are the factors most commonly associated with interpersonal violence. Violence is seen as a special problem for youth because young people are the primary perpetrators and victims, but the critical causal factor is not youth but the socioeconomic burdens, like poverty, that particularly affect the young. And violence is often seen as an urban problem, but domestic violence and suicide, in particular, also need to be addressed— and more fully studied—in the rural areas of our country.

Violence may be "as American as apple pie,"[3] but we are not helpless against it. The fact that the United States is an outlier, with the highest homicide rate of any developed country, suggests that there is nothing natural about such high rates of interpersonal violence. Rather, violence is a learned response to interpersonal interaction and violence can be mitigated. The area of violence prevention is new for public health practitioners, but what public health has done to foster prevention of other health problems, including other injury problems, can be applied to equal avail to the problem of violence. A public health approach to violence is one that identifies risks and protective factors, evaluates intervention programs, and implements promising programs at the community level. (See Figure 1–2.)

The major categories of intentional injury will be reviewed in this chapter. These common groupings, based on the injured victim, include

- self-inflicted violence (suicide and suicide attempts)
- homicide
- nonfatal assaultive violence
- violent exploitation of women (including spousal abuse and rape or sexual assault)
- child and elder abuse

In 1995 there were 31,284 suicide deaths and 25,522 homicide deaths in the United States.[4] The toll of nonfatal intentional injuries is difficult to quantify but does seem to exceed 2.5 million injuries annually. According to Rosenberg and Mercy, "The ratio of nonfatal assaults to homicide is probably far greater than 100:1."[5(p17)] In one statewide study of children and adolescents, the ratio skyrocketed to 567:1.[6]

Although the different types of intentional injuries vary in many ways, they share certain common patterns and risk factors. These include access to firearms, alcohol abuse, maleness, certain childhood experiences (such as a personal history of abuse or violence involving a parent or caregiver), and—most important—income disparity and poverty. These common factors have clear implications for prevention, which are discussed later in the chapter.

## SELF-INFLICTED VIOLENCE (SUICIDE AND SUICIDE ATTEMPTS)

Violence is often thought of as *inter*personal, when in fact the most common type of intentionally caused death is *intra*personal. Suicide is death from intentionally self-inflicted injury. In many states—and overall, nationally—suicide is a larger problem than homicide, but it is too often a hidden problem. Suicide accounts for 30,000 deaths annually—roughly 86 deaths per day—for an annual rate of 11.9 per 100,000 population. Because the social stigma surrounding suicide often results in the mislabeling of suicide deaths, these official statistics are most likely a substantial undercount. Suicide is the cause of 21% of all injury deaths and has become the ninth leading cause of death in the United States and the fifth leading cause of premature death. Almost all suicides involve victims 15 years old or older, although recent data suggests that suicide deaths among 10 to 14 year olds are increasing. Suicide has been increasing among adolescents generally; since the late 1950s, suicide rates for young people have soared several fold. Suicide is the third leading cause of death for adolescents, after motor vehicle deaths and homicides. Males are at least four times more likely to die from suicides than are females (with the highest rates among elderly males), but females are more likely to attempt suicide than are males.[4,7,8]

By definition suicides are fatal. Suicide attempts are not, but they are clearly an important public health problem. There are an estimated 25 attempts for each completed suicide, for an annual total of 750,000 attempts. We have a rather poor understanding of what distinguishes completed from attempted suicides, other than the obvious factor of lethality of the mechanism employed (e.g., firearms being much more lethal than poisons). We do know about the means used for suicides and suicide attempts. We know that suicide among children and youth is often a very impulsive act done with little or no planning. On the other hand, suicides by those with severe or terminal illnesses can be quite carefully planned and executed. Nearly 60% of all completed suicides (and two thirds of teenage suicides) involve firearms, followed by hanging, poisoning by liquids and solids, and poisoning by carbon monoxide. Among youth, the rates for suicides using methods other than firearms has been largely stable, while the rates for suicides involving firearms has been increasing greatly. People living in households in which guns are kept have a suicide risk five times that of people living in households without guns. Almost all of the increase in the overall suicide rate between 1980 and 1994 (which for persons aged 15 to 19 was a 29% increase) can be attributed to the increase in firearm-related suicides.[9-11] When it comes to uncompleted suicide attempts, some 70% involve drug ingestion; firearms are not often involved in uncompleted suicide attempts. There is considerable variation between states and by ethnic group in preferred methods for attempting suicide.

Our epidemiological understanding of suicide is meager, particularly regarding the victim's state of mind. And we know too little about effective interventions to reduce suicide. We do know that prominent risk factors include previous suicide attempts, certain psychiatric illnesses (especially depression), personality disorders, alcohol and alcoholism, family history of suicide, divorce or separation, and firearm availability. Organizations that focus specifically on suicide prevention have not actively embraced the goal of getting firearms out of the home as a strategy especially needed in high-risk situations, such as the presence of impulsive teenagers. (In fact, means restriction—access to firearms, medications, etc.—in general is not emphasized by programs addressing suicide risk factors.) Public health practitioners need to work with these groups on this issue. Suicide prevention has tended to focus on the mental health sector rather than public health, with particular attention to individual-level intervention and treatment. But suicide is a public health problem calling for community-based prevention approaches. A decade ago a survey of state health agencies found that 85% of respondents felt that health departments have a legitimate role in the prevention of suicide.[12] A number of state health agencies are currently developing suicide prevention programs. More to the point, it is a problem that the tools of public health, if properly engaged, can help mitigate. To date, however, most of the public health community's suicide prevention efforts have focused on improving data on suicide attempts and on developing guidelines for school responses to prevent or contain suicide clusters following a youth suicide in the community.

## HOMICIDE

Homicide is death resulting from injuries inflicted by another person with the intent to injure or kill. (This definition is similar to that employed in law and law enforcement, although the law recognizes such concepts as negligent homicide and homicide by misadventure. Legal definitions get considerably more complicated in terms of how homicide is dealt with. Murder, for example, is defined legally in terms of differing levels of intent—premeditation, malice, malice aforethought—and varying "degrees" of murder are recognized. The law also recognizes a category of "voluntary" manslaughter that includes an immediate intent to injure. Moreover, legal definitions vary somewhat according to jurisdiction.) Homicide is the cause of 15% of all injury deaths. For ages 1 to 9, homicide is the fourth leading cause of death, for ages 10 to 14 it is the third, and for ages 15 to 24 it is the second. Homicide accounts for about 25% to 30% of all injury deaths among infants, teens, and young adults. Overall, homicide is the fourth leading cause of premature mortality. At the same time, however, the 1995 homicide rate of 8.6 per 100,000 population was the lowest level since 1989.[4(p17),13–17]

The number of people who die each year in the United States as the result of homicide has reached a level of 25,000 annually, 70 homicide deaths for each day of the year. For Blacks and Hispanics 15 to 24 years of age, homicide has become the leading cause of death. According to a Centers for Disease Control and Prevention (CDC) report, "Much of the disparity in the burden of death and illness experienced by blacks relative to the majority white population is attributable to rates of black homicide that are 5 to 6 times higher than those for whites."[18(p17)] When socioeconomic status is controlled for, racial difference in homicide rates become almost nonexistent. The major factor is not race but poverty. A higher percentage of Blacks live under conditions of poverty than do Whites; they are therefore more likely than Whites to live in socially disorganized communities.

It was not always so. In 1930 the U.S. homicide rate was 9 per 100,000 population (a peak that many associate with the gangster era); in 1957 it had fallen to 4 per 100,000. But by 1980 it had climbed to 11 per 100,000, and in 1988 stood at 9 per 100,000.[16(p86)] The United States has the highest homicide rate of all developed countries, and one of the highest rates among all countries that report homicide statistics to the World Health Organization.[14(p1037)] The U.S. rate is 4.4 times that for the next highest rate among industrialized nations. A large part of this difference would seem to be related to firearms, which are used in 70% of all homicides.[9]

For years homicide was viewed simply as a criminal justice problem, with emphasis on the offender and on using criminal law to deter violent acts by individual lawbreakers or to merely deal with the problem after the fact through incarceration. From this conceptual perspective, homicides appeared as unpredictable acts for which neither general nor specific deterrence really seemed to hold out much hope of significantly reducing homicide rates. But as former U.S. Surgeon General C. Everett Koop and *JAMA* Editor George Lundberg noted, "Regarding violence in our society as purely a sociologic matter, or one of law enforcement, has led to unmitigated failure."[19(pp3075-3076)]

## NONFATAL ASSAULTIVE VIOLENCE

In 1994 there were 10.9 million criminal acts of violence directed against people 12 or older, for a rate of 51 per 1,000 population. One quarter of these, or 2.7 million, resulted in injury to the victim. CDC researchers Rosenberg and Mercy define assaultive violence as "personal violence where physical force or other means is used by one person with the intent of causing harm, injury, or death to another." They note that "nonfatal assaults may constitute an even more important aspect of this public health problem than homicide"[5(p14)] (although homicide rates are a more reliable source of data). For example, in a population-based study of U.S. youth, it was found that for every homicide death there were 33 hospitalizations and 534 emergency department visits for assault. This same study found that during a three-year period 4.3% of children and adolescents treated in hospitals for assaultive violence injuries suffered from repeated violent injuries.[6]

We know much less than we would like to about the magnitude, nature, and circumstances surrounding the assaultive violence problem. Rosenberg and Mercy note that:

> Current thinking on the causes of assaultive violence suggest that biological factors (such as male sex, young age, or mental illness), psychological factors (such as history of previous abuse, history of violent behavior by parents), cultural factors (such as male belief in physical prowess and media glorification of violence), "structural" or large-scale factors (such as poverty and racial discrimination), and interactionist factors (such as alcohol and drug abuse) all may contribute to assaultive violence.[5(p15)]

The thing we know most clearly is that the distribution of violence reflects the disparities of wealth and income in the society; victimization rates decrease as family income increases. Overrepresentation of minority groups and youth as both perpetrators and victims of violence are proxy indicators for poverty.

When we think of assaults, we often think of guns; however, in one study of youth it was found that most assaults involved unarmed fights. Less than 10% of assaults involved a weapon and the most commonly used weapon was a knife.[6] This should not diminish our concern with reducing access to guns, because when guns are involved in violence the likelihood of death increases sharply; the early 1990s increases in youth deaths due to violence were largely due to gun violence, but it is clearly not enough to focus entirely on firearms in reducing nonfatal assaultive violence.

## VIOLENT EXPLOITATION OF WOMEN (INCLUDING SPOUSAL ABUSE AND RAPE OR SEXUAL ASSAULT)

Domestic violence, dating violence, battering, or abuse are usually defined as using physical force in intimate relationships. A more contemporary term for this category of violence is *intimate partner violence*, which encompasses violence perpetrated by current spouses; divorced, former, or separated spouses; current nonmarital partners (dating partners, boyfriends/girlfriends, same-sex partners); and former nonmarital partners. Abuse can take many forms: physical violence is the most extreme, but sexual violence, the threat of physical or sexual violence, and psychological attacks may also be included in such definitions. Domestic violence involving intimate partners—most often spouse abuse—can involve women or men as victims and perpetrators, but predominantly it is women who are seriously injured by abuse from men.

In any given year, 8% to 12% of all adult women in the United States experience some form of domestic violence.[20] Abuse frequently occurs during pregnancy, with estimates ranging from 6% to 17% of all pregnancies.[21] Stark and Flitcraft define spousal abuse, in terms that could be applied more generally, as "a syndrome of control and increasing entrapment . . . characterized by a history of injury, general medical complaints, isolation, stress-related psychosocial problems, and unsuccessful help-seeking."[22(pp184–185)]

Especially because of the intimate relationships involved, our information on the types of domestic abuse is very limited. Even when violence occurs between strangers or nonintimate acquaintances, victims are often hesitant to report the event to the police. This is considerably more likely to occur in intimate relationship violence. In describing spouse abuse, Stark and Flitcraft explain:

> Spouse abuse presents a challenge to epidemiology because its parameters are not well defined, its severity is highly subjective, its causes are poorly understood, and its psychosocial consequences are often linked in very complex ways to physical events. This helps explain why a problem that may affect as much as 20% of the adult female population and that results in more than three times as many injuries as auto accidents has been largely neglected by health researchers, including those specializing in injury.[22(pp123,125)]

Cohen and Swift suggest that while

> violence against women, in particular spouse and partner battering and sexual assault, is increasing, it is still paid less attention than violence directed at men for three reasons:
>
> 1. *Under-reporting.* Often victims do not file reports because of the shame and fear of retribution that generally accompany these types of assaults. The frequent insensitivity of law enforcement and court personnel also discourage reporting.
>
> 2. *Statistical undercount.* Because rape and sexual assault injuries are not always captured by hospitalization and death statistics, their frequency and severity can be underestimated.
>
> 3. *Extent of injury underplayed.* Because the medical and criminal justice systems are still largely administered by men, there may be times when the true scope of pain and injury caused by such assaults are not fully understood and can be down-played.[23]

Along with spousal abuse, women in the United States are the victims of the highest rate of sexual assault of any industrialized nation. A national study of college students found that 27.5% of the women surveyed said they had suffered rape or attempted rape at least once since age 14.[24,25] An estimated 500,000 to 700,000 rapes occur each year in the United States, nearly half of which are committed by friends or acquaintances of the victim. The majority of rapes involve minors as victims.[25,26] Rape is unfortunately a common occurrence within intimate relationships. Abuse is also common in dating relationships; the average prevalence rate for nonsexual dating violence is 22% among male and female high school students and 32% among college students.[25,27]

Many factors contribute to violence toward women, but it is clear that underlying the problem is the low social status and objectification of women. It has taken a long time for society to realize that sexism, not the behavior of victims, is the obstacle that needs to be addressed if violent exploitation of women is to be reduced.

## CHILD AND ELDER ABUSE

There are between 250,000 and 350,000 cases of physical abuse of U.S. children annually.[4(p45),28(p101),29] Based on reports from all but three states, in 1994 there were 1,011,628 cases of "substantiated" or "indicated" child abuse and neglect affecting children 18 and younger (out of close to 3 million children involved in reports to child protective services agencies). One half of these cases involved neglect, one quarter involved physical abuse, and 14% involved sexual abuse. It is estimated that 27% of the cases involved children under 4 years of age. For the 43 states that provided data on child abuse deaths, there were 1,111 children known to have died as the result of abuse or neglect.[4(p48)] Child abuse affects children of all ages; it affects boys slightly more than girls. Close to 80% of the maltreatment of children is at the hands of birth parents (in contrast to sexual abuse of children, half of which seems to involve perpetrators other than parents or parental figures).

The number of substantiated and probable victims of child abuse has increased over the last decade; this may be the result of greater public willingness to report child maltreatment. A 1995 national survey by the National Committee to Prevent Child Abuse found a 39% increase in confirmed child abuse fatalities (and a 49% increase in the total number of child abuse reports) from 1985 to 1995, an increase the committee attributed to increases in poverty and substance abuse.[30] Estimates of the involvement of alcohol abuse in child maltreatment range up to 80% of substantiated cases, suggesting substance abuse treatment is a promising avenue for prevention of child abuse. Although child abuse cuts across all socioeconomic boundaries, it is clear that family stress—especially economic stress—is a leading determinant of abuse. It is also clear that adults who were abused as children are most likely to become abusive parents themselves. There is also some evidence that being abused as a child increases the victim's likelihood of subsequently committing a violent crime.

Child sexual abuse is a problem for which data is very scant. But although the prevalence of the problem is unclear, it is certainly widespread enough to be a significant social concern.

Elder abuse is a rather recently recognized problem for which we have even less data than for child and spousal abuse. Victims seem to be especially the "old old," i.e., those 75 and over. Most often the victims reside with the abuser. As with child and spousal abuse, elder abuse can include neglect and psychological abuse as well as physical violence.[31] As the elderly population in the United States grows, the rate of elder abuse is also increasing.

Stark and Flitcraft note that "of the four components of prevention—shelter, law enforcement, legislation, and health care—the health response remains the least developed."[22] Mandatory reporting laws are most developed for child abuse, but even here there is controversy over the potential effectiveness of such systems. If necessary, the state can intervene to remove children from the custody of abusive caregivers. The same situation does not exist for adult victims of abuse.

An approach used at the state level to analyze the most serious cases of child abuse more accurately is the child death review team, an approach also being tried with other types of domestic violence. These multidisciplinary teams allow for in-depth study of suspicious and confirmed intentional deaths, providing a clearer picture of what is going on and how we can best prevent it. (See Chapter 10 for more information.) The Year 2000 Health Objectives included implementation of such teams in 45 states by the year 2000.[32]

## EPIDEMIOLOGY

A standard way of dealing with public health problems is to identify specific risk factors and then intervene in ways tailored to dealing with these factors. A variety of factors seem to be associated with the epidemic of violence in the United States. The most notable factors are poverty and unemployment, racism and sexism, alcohol and drug use, firearm availability, social disorganization, family dysfunction, and media emphasis on violence. Other risk factors include male sex, adolescence, mental illness, history of previous physical and psychological abuse, history of violent behavior by parents and the witnessing of violence, and a male belief in physical prowess.[33,34] An important risk factor is the relationship between homicide victim and perpetrator. Federal Bureau of Investigation figures for 1986 show 40% of reported homicides involved friends and acquaintances, 15.1% family members, and 12.5% strangers. Rosenberg and Mercy speculate that much of the remaining 32.4% "unknown relationship" homicides may involve strangers.[14(p1035)] These differences underscore the fact that most homicides are committed by friends and relations, rather than by strangers involved in criminal activities, suggesting that interventions and prevention strategies may need to vary according to the relationship between homicide victim and perpetrator.

In *The Injury Fact Book,* Baker et al note that homicide rates are highest for males, especially those 25 to 29 years old, and are two-and-one-half times as high in low-income areas as in high-income areas for all races combined—with this becoming a ten-fold disparity in central cities. "When socioeconomic status is controlled for, racial differences in homicide rates decrease markedly. . . . The inverse correlation between homicide rates and income is most pronounced for firearm homicides."[16(p83)] Such correlations are reminders that (1) increased homicide risk is yet another disadvantage of poverty and (2) stereotypes based on race are as unhelpful as they are wrong. For example, a social disorganization study by Sampson et al found that social cohesion among neighbors combined with their willingness to intervene on behalf of the common good, is linked to reduced violence. Black neighborhoods with adequate social cohesion—even when poor—had violence rates similar to those of White, middle-class communities.[35]

Another study reports a similar point regarding recent hysteria over "youth violence." Males points out that:

> The official/media-generated crisis of "children killing children" (and innocent adults) collapses in one simple calculation. Divide the arrest rate for murder or violent crime (which includes murder, rape, robbery, and aggravated assault) for each age group by the number of persons in that age group living in poverty. The result: The fact that teenagers are more likely to live in poverty than adults in their 20s and 30s fully explains the higher rates of murder and violent crime among teenagers . . . . Teenagers do not respond to poverty more or less violently than do grownups—teenagers just experience more poverty. Once the poverty factor is removed, "teen violence" disappears.[28(pp107–108)]

Alcohol and drug use have been associated with all categories of homicide except child homicide, although the relationship is not completely clear. Researchers continue to debate whether the disinhibiting effect of alcohol may be more psychological than physiological. We do know that alcohol is often present in both the perpetrators *and* the victims of violence. Drugs can affect behavior in the same way as alcohol, lowering inhibitions, dulling senses, impairing reasoning, and increasing vulnerability. In addition, drugs play a critical role in homicide because of their illegal nature; criminal activities mean high monetary stakes combined with a violent private enforcement system. "It has been estimated . . . that a minimum of 10% of homicides nationwide are related to illicit drug use."[36,37,38] This figure is much lower than the standard portrayals by the news and entertainment media imply.

Finally, firearms play a key role in homicides. Rosenberg and Mercy reported that in 1986, three fifths of all homicides were committed with firearms; three quarters of the victims were killed with handguns.[14] A more recent CDC report puts the percentage of homicides committed with a firearm at more than 70%.[9] This increase has been even sharper among 15 to 24 year olds, rising from 67% in 1985 to 87% in 1994.[39] Firearm-associated family and intimate assaults are three times more likely to result in death than those involving knives or other cutting instruments and 23.4 times more likely to result in death than those involving other weapons or the use of bodily force.[40,41] The greater lethality of firearms is exacerbated by the fact that firearms have become more plentiful and more readily available throughout the United States since the early 1960s. The dramatic increase in gun ownership seems to be related to fear of crime and civil disorder and a mistaken belief that guns provide self-defense advantages and heightened safety.[42] The Position Paper on Violence Prevention prepared for the federal government's Third National Injury Control Conference, noting that firearms—especially handguns—are much less accessible in other countries, stated: "Trends in our overall rates of violent death are largely determined by firearm violence. . . . Most developed countries report near-negligible numbers of firearm deaths, and their rates of overall violence are far lower than ours."[43(pI-15)]

This represents a dramatic escalation of gun violence in the United States. Baker et al note that: "between 1960 and 1980 the death rate from firearm homicide increased by 160% (from 2.6 to 6.8 per 100,000), while the rate for all other homicides increased by 100% (from 1.9 to 3.8)."[16(p86)]

As a dramatic symbol of the change that has been occurring, by the early 1990s seven states and the District of Columbia shared the distinction of having more firearm deaths than motor vehicle deaths.[44,45]

A problem in the epidemiology of homicide is that complete data is hard to collect (although it is much easier to acquire homicide data than data on nonfatal assaultive violence). Sources of national data include the Federal Bureau of Investigation Uniform Crime Report, the National Crime Victimization Survey, the National Center for Health Statistics Mortality Data, and other such data sources. Unfortunately, all of these systems have serious limitations; dependable data on weapon employed, circumstances, and relationship of perpetrator and victim are often incomplete, especially as to weapon type.[46,47]

Violence prevention interventions have been initiated based on political perspectives, the fear of crime, or a community agency agenda, rather than on sound prevention practices incorporating an understanding of risk factors and population characteristics. On the state and federal levels, "three-strikes" laws and sentencing guidelines that require incarceration of nonviolent drug users provide prime examples of the former. Many local initiatives are narrowly focused on school-based violence prevention interventions rather than taking a comprehensive approach. For example, the use of metal detectors in schools is a popular "prevention" approach, one that is expensive but which does nothing to change the at-risk behaviors of students. It is public health's role to ensure that interventions are epidemiologically informed.

## APPROACHES TO SOLUTIONS

The public health community began to take note of the problem of violence with the 1985 Surgeon General's report on Violence as a Public Health Problem, in which a violence prevention role for public health agencies was delineated.[48] The concern was with fostering a primary prevention approach to the problem, rather than just case identification and risk avoidance. The Surgeon General's report outlined a five-part approach:

1. Provide the constituency to get violence prevention into the mainstream of public health.
2. Define the problem carefully, using the tools of public health.

3. Provide information and education for *policy makers* to assist them in developing new public policy approaches, to *children* through the development of violence prevention curricula, and to the *general public* through media focus on violence prevention.
4. Develop intervention strategies and systems to evaluate their impact.
5. Provide a stabilizing input into this process in order to sustain it and keep it from being merely a temporary fad.

A previous Surgeon General—Antonia Novello—warned that "violence in the United States is a public health emergency."[49(p3007)] Most violent injuries are not the result of organized criminal activity and are closely tied to social ills, ranging from poverty and racism to alcohol abuse and family dysfunction. Both the magnitude and nature of the problem make it sensible for homicide and other types of intentional violence to be approached as public health problems having large impacts on health and productive years of life lost. Most often victims know their assailants, who are family members, friends, or acquaintances. Most violent injuries are not random, but in fact are predictable; they are amenable to public health techniques for surveillance, epidemiological analysis, and interdisciplinary primary prevention. This approach is one that recognizes multicausal explanations and which emphasizes environmental factors while eschewing concentration on victim fault.

Criminal justice professionals might argue that violence *prevention* is not a new idea, that they have long been concerned with prevention as well as enforcement, but much of the focus of past efforts was on general and specific deterrence, incapacitation, and rehabilitation to prevent further violence. What public health offers that goes beyond this is an approach that looks at etiology in detail, discovering that violence is multicausal, with many discrete points at which to intervene for prevention. Public health also offers the concept of "contagion," a powerful analytic approach to better define the problem of the spread of violence, breaking the problem up into manageable prevention steps.

Where does this leave us regarding our understanding of violence? We can identify three root risk factors for violence—economics, oppression, and mental health—and six community risk factors—guns, media, alcohol and other drugs, incarceration, witnessing acts of violence, and community deterioration.[50] We know that interventions must include individual factors and social factors. And we know that the application of limited strategies in isolation from an overall approach to violence prevention yields small benefits and questionable permanence of results.

How are public health practitioners to work with this knowledge? The public health approach to violence prevention can begin with surveillance and assessment, lead to universal prevention approaches, and move on to selective prevention for high-risk populations. Public health practitioners need to get the message out that most violence in the United States is between family members and friends, often involves alcohol, is particularly inflicted on the young, and most often is self-inflicted. Public health practitioners can't reduce poverty or end unemployment, but they can help direct communities away from unhelpful approaches and toward helpful ones. They can help communities go beyond single strategies like school-based curricula to the development of comprehensive prevention approaches that include environmental and enforcement strategies such as tracking weapons confiscated from young people and identifying (and shutting down) dealers who illegally sell firearms to minors. And they can help foster collaboration and coalitions involving local law enforcement, education, social services, and public health to build on the strengths each discipline has to offer.

Before undertaking a violence prevention initiative in a community, you need to accurately determine the true nature of the violence problem. An anecdote-based perception of the problem may be distorted. Are firearms the critical problem for this community, or do knives and physical fighting cause more injuries? Are illegal drugs a significant factor? Public health has the tools to help the community do an assessment of the true nature of their injury problem.

Violence is a complex problem, which means it requires multifaceted solutions. Public health practitioners can help communities understand what works and what doesn't when it comes to the problem of violence. Approaches to solution include both *violence prevention interventions,* specific, targeted activities for preventing violence that can either stand alone or comprise part of a program, and *violence prevention programs*, multifaceted prevention efforts, consisting of a combination of two or more interventions designed to prevent or reduce violence.

There are a variety of specific violence prevention interventions available. Unfortunately, many intervention efforts focus on changing just one risk factor and usually focus on changing only the individual rather than social or environmental characteristics. Such narrow interventions may be necessary but insufficient to reduce violence in a meaningful way. We need to be more comprehensive.

Despite limitations in available data, it is relatively clear which preventive approaches are most likely to reduce homicide rates. Four critical interventions would be

1. increases in social support spending
2. limitations on alcohol consumption
3. restrictions on the access to and lethality of firearms and ammunition
4. reductions in access to media violence

We know that interpersonal violence is exacerbated by the media portrayals of violence with which the public is continually bombarded.[51] Media violence via news and entertainment programming continues at horrific levels. Although the percentage of television shows containing guns did drop from 25% to 23% between the 1994–1995 and 1995–1996 television seasons, during that same period programs containing violence rose from 58% to 61% and there was a 10% increase in the number of children's programs that portrayed violence in a humorous context.[52]

Although no adequate case-control studies of the phenomena can be performed (given that virtually the entire population is exposed) the American Psychological Association has reported that "since 1955, about 1,000 studies, reports, and commentaries concerning the impact of television violence have been published. The accumulated research clearly demonstrates a correlation between viewing violence and aggressive behavior."[53] This harmful effect results from media portrayals of violence that (1) model aggressive attitudes and behaviors, (2) produce emotional desensitization toward real world violence, and (3) increase the fear and mistrust associated with violence.

There is a great need for injury prevention professionals to advocate for the responsible treatment of violence in the media. Mediascope, an organization dedicated to promoting responsible depictions of health and social issues in the media, urges filmmakers to realize the effects of violence on viewers and to portray the pain and suffering that violence causes without glamorizing and romanticizing it. Research shows that realistic portrayals of violence can be an effective tool in preventing violence. What is needed, before viewers become completely desensitized to violence, is constructive dialog and cooperation amongst parents, children, public health and education experts, the television industry, local stations, and the Federal Communications Commission.

A related concern is the media's coverage of suicides, particularly teenage suicides. News reports of actual suicides can induce "copycat" suicides. Often, suicide deaths of the famous or of fellow students are treated in ways that enhance idolization of them and their deaths. Media portrayals of suicide should be handled with care and responsibility.[54,55]

Extensive and detailed recommendations for reducing homicide and other types of assaultive violence were developed for the 1985 Surgeon General's Workshop on Violence and Public Health.[56] Similar recommendations are included in a 1992 review article by Rosenberg and Mercy.[14] These recommendations for intervention include (1) social and cultural changes, such as decreasing the cultural acceptance of violence, reducing racial discrimination, reducing gender inequality, and reducing the consumption of alcohol and other drugs; (2) health and related social service changes, such as developing education programs to teach conflict resolution skills and increasing education for family life, family planning, and child rearing (such as violence prevention messages within home health visits or domestic violence screening at family planning clinics); and (3) environmental and other changes such as developing strategies to reduce injuries associated with firearms.[14,57]

How can state and local health departments begin to implement these types of violence prevention recommendations? There are several useful models that can be pointed to. For example, in Contra Costa County, California, located in the San Francisco Bay area, the County Health Services Prevention Program is an interdisciplinary public health program that focuses on the prevention of violence, childhood injuries, and chronic disease. Rather than create new, stand-alone programs, the Contra Costa Prevention Program coordinates, cultivates, and links existing community resources in a systems approach. A *Countywide Action Plan* delineating 25 critical recommendations for reducing violence was developed by the Health Department and placed on the November 1994 election ballot by the county board of supervisors. The recommendations dealt with six themes: safe homes, safe schools, safe neighborhoods, safe workplaces, government service, and policy initiatives. The focus was primarily on assault, homicide, sexual assault, and battering. The recommendations served as organizing principles around which each community in the county could develop a specific violence prevention action plan for implementation[50]; 78% of the voters supported this action plan.

The Contra Costa Prevention Program is organized around a six-part "spectrum of prevention," which includes

1. strengthening individual knowledge and skills
2. educating the community
3. training providers
4. building coalitions
5. changing organizations' practices
6. influencing policy and legislation[23]

In Washington State, the State Department of Health convened an Advisory Council on Youth Suicide Prevention to develop a state *Youth Suicide Prevention Plan*. Prevention strategies were identified, evaluated, and prioritized. Focus groups were held throughout the state to gather the perspectives of multiple high-risk groups of youth. This plan recommended three promising preventive approaches. The first was *universal communitywide* youth suicide prevention approaches, such as a statewide public education campaign, a high school– and college-based education campaign, an effort to reduce access to firearms and other lethal means for suicide, and a program to educate the media and health professionals in an effort to decrease suicide "contagion" effects. The second encompassed *selective* youth suicide prevention approaches for high-risk populations, such as screening programs to identify and assess high-risk youth and a "gatekeeper" program to train adults working with high-risk populations. The third was *indicated* youth suicide prevention approaches for high-risk individuals such as high school– and college-based support and skill-building groups and family support training.

Where intervention programs do exist for suicide prevention—as in Washington State—they usually work with teenage youth rather than with young adults and the elderly. In *Youth Suicide Prevention Programs: A Resource Guide*, the CDC noted two conceptual categories in suicide prevention programs for adolescents and young adults: (1) strategies to identify and refer suicidal adolescents and young adults for mental health care and (2) strategies to address known or suspected risk factors for suicide among adolescents and young adults. The CDC recommended that suicide prevention programs be linked as closely as possible with professional mental health resources in the community, that reliance on a single prevention strategy be avoided, that suicide prevention effort be expanded for young adults, and that evaluation efforts be incorporated into suicide prevention programs.[58]

In New Mexico, the state Department of Health and Environment established a coordinated state network of knowledgeable professionals and community members committed to working on violence prevention. The goal was to foster primary prevention activities and programs at the local and state level to prevent a range of violent behavior including homicide, suicide, child abuse, domestic violence, and rape. They funded violence prevention programs in the schools and developed firearm violence curricula.[59] In New Hampshire, a promising cooperative effort by the state Department of Public Health and state Department of Mental Health has been directed at reducing suicide. And Massachusetts was the first state to develop a weapons injury surveillance system for hospital emergency departments.

A variety of state and local programs and strategies to prevent injury and violence among children and youth were highlighted in *Building Safe Communities*, a publication distributed by the Maternal and Child Health Bureau of the U.S. Department of Health and Human Services.[59] These programs included

- the Ohio Department of Health's protocol on sexual assault
- the Massachusetts Department of Public Health's protocol to detect and treat battered adult and adolescent women
- the Colorado Health Department's adolescent suicide prevention program
- the Contra Costa County, California, Health Services Department's Firearm Injury Reporting, Surveillance, and Tracking (FIRST) System
- the Monterey County, California, Health Department's Gun Storage Education and Trigger Lock Coupon Program

The CDC has published a manual intended to provide a framework for community action to reduce the number of injuries and deaths produced by violence. The manual:

includes a menu of specific activities for communities to undertake plus a framework for putting those activities effectively into place. The manual is based on the principles of effective, community-based health promotion programs that have been success-fully used to address a variety of chronic diseases as well as prob-lems of youth, such as sexually transmitted diseases and teenage pregnancy.[60]

The manual reviews what is known about youth violence through scientific research and what has been learned through community efforts. It discusses information gathering and analysis, setting goals and objectives, locating resources, organizing the community, and monitoring program progress.[60]

Unfortunately, few evaluation studies have been done on violence prevention programs. Many popular community approaches focus on only a narrow aspect of the violence problem (e.g., school-based violence) and are of unproven value. These include metal detectors and locker searches in schools, along with school dress codes to discourage gang identification; community curfews; and neighborhood crime watch associations. Perhaps most widespread have been programs to introduce conflict resolution curricula into the schools, where implementation far outstripped evaluation. One of the first randomized controlled trials of this approach, which found "a modest positive effect," was not published until after a decade of experience with such violence prevention curricula.[61] Another popular public health approach to violence prevention has been the development of community programs, such as building community programs to increase awareness of violence, change community norms, and provide alternative activities for adolescents. Evaluation is needed here also. The same applies to suicide prevention hotlines, where evidence of effectiveness is unclear. In fact, there has been some concern that existing school-based suicide prevention programs may have *adverse* consequences for students. The fact is that many suicide prevention interventions are maintained in the absence of careful evaluation of their impact. This includes, for example, such apparently promising approaches as peer support programs for those who attempt suicide and high-risk youth, the strengthening of ties between suicide prevention programs and existing mental health resources, training to enhance recognition and referral of suicidal youth, and strategies aimed at specific risk factors.

Public health practitioners need to stress evaluation, because there is a big gap between the most commonly used programs and the most frequently evaluated ones. And it is unclear what programs work for what types of violence and for which groups of high-risk victims of violence. This includes evaluating injury prevention laws,[62] an important area of study that includes questions such as whether restricting access to guns—especially in the home—will reduce gun injuries[14(p1037)] and whether restraining orders are effective in providing protection against domestic violence.

One review of juvenile violence prevention initiatives was completed in late 1997 by the Center for the Study and Prevention of Violence. Center Director Delbert Elliott noted that: "After reviewing over 400 violence prevention programs, we have identified 10 programs that meet the highest scientific standards for demonstrating that they can successfully prevent or reduce levels of violence." Handbooks describing each of these successful programs will be developed by the center. The 10 specific prevention programs identified by this evaluation study met three criteria of effectiveness: "the programs demonstrated reductions in violence, deviance or substance use with a careful experimental study; showed sustained impact for at least one year after participants left the program; and had been successfully replicated at multiple sites with diverse populations." The 10 "Blueprints for Violence Prevention" programs were

1. prenatal and infancy home visitation by nurses
2. bullying prevention program
3. promoting alternative thinking strategies
4. Big Brothers Big Sisters of America
5. Quantum Opportunities Program
6. multisystemic therapy
7. functional family therapy
8. Midwestern Prevention Project
9. life skills training
10. multidimensional treatment foster care[63]

Another important area for evaluation and training involves the role of health care practitioners in dealing with interpersonal violence. Practitioners must know what needs to be reported to legal authorities, where and how to refer both victims and perpetrators of violence, and how to provide anticipatory guidance regarding such matters as firearms in the home and youth suicide. These can be complicated issues. For example, referral requires knowing what resources are available and what their limitations are—for example, do they accept unemancipated minors? It is helpful to have standard protocols for use in addressing suspected episodes of violence in patients, including guidance on how to question these patients and what to document in the medical record. Practitioners also need to know how to deal with special needs such as battering during pregnancy. Much of what is done in this area, including reporting, referral, and guidance, has been incompletely evaluated.

There are several injury prevention resources that can be helpful to you and the communities you work with. These include the Children's Safety Network's National Injury and Violence Prevention Resource Center, the National Network of Violence Prevention Practitioners, the CDC's National Center for Injury Prevention and Control (which offers CDC Community Guidelines), and the Center for the Study and Prevention of Violence. World Wide Web sites for these organizations appear in Appendix A at the end of the book.

## CONCLUSION

Despite the magnitude of the suicide and homicide problem in the United States and the identification of promising interventions by the research and public health communities, policy makers have followed an almost opposite course. They have underfunded social support and early intervention programs while heavily funding crime fighting and after-the-fact incarceration, thus all but guaranteeing increased social crises, including increased homicide. And they have not been at all interested in the careful scientific evaluation of what works and what doesn't.

Instead, during the 1980s in particular, politicians embraced an ideology of selfishness, urging individuals to get what they could for themselves without regard for their neighbor. Similarly, governmental and extra-governmental attitudes about the inferiority of minority citizens, especially African Americans and Hispanics, magnified the homicide problem in the United States. Rather than deal with the central problem of poverty, the U.S. political system has overseen a dramatic increase in the gap between rich and poor in our country.

Most tragically, a large number of politicians have resisted efforts to reduce firearm injuries. In the United States, firearms are readily available with few restrictions and they are expressly omitted from regulation as consumer products by any federal agency.[64-66] This ease of access and lack of safety standards has made the United States one of the most "gun violent" countries in the world. Particularly tragic is that suicide has not been part of the firearms debate despite the fact that nearly 60% of completed suicides (and two thirds of teen suicides) are carried out with firearms. The political leadership of the nation has facilitated suicide and homicide even as public health and medical communities have geared up to reduce intentional violence. Politicians have avoided offending a powerful gun lobby by hiding behind a mythical individual "right" to guns.

They have played out this deceit even though the U.S. Supreme Court has made it clear that the Second Amendment to the Constitution has no significant limiting impact on efforts by government to control (and even ban) firearms. Two Supreme Court decisions defining the meaning of the Second Amendment have made it clear that there is no Constitutional right to possess firearms.[67–69] Politicians have bent to gun industry pressures regularly enough that federal agencies have become fearful of even funding research that might help us better understand the problem of firearm deaths. Because of a specific congressional directive, the CDC includes in its grant funding awards a "Prohibition on Use of CDC Funds for Certain Gun Control Activities," stating that "CDC's funds may not be spent on political action **or other** activities designed to affect the passage of specific Federal, State, or local legislation **intended** to restrict or control the purchase or use of firearms."[70]

In the face of such misdirected social policy, public health efforts to reduce violence may seem like swimming upstream against a strong current. But the fact that misguided, counterproductive policies are being pursued is all the more reason that public health practitioners must seek to have an impact on violence. Public health practitioners can share their prevention insights, can evaluate current violence reduction efforts, and can highlight those things that seem to work best. They can work toward strengthening health-based data systems that can provide a different perspective on the problem of violence. And they can encourage coordination of approaches amongst the criminal justice, law enforcement, mental health, and public health communities.

Violence is an important public health issue, not only in terms of direct injury impact (mortality and morbidity) but also in terms of the indirect impact of its long-term effect on survivors, families, and friends.[71] The Year 2000 Health Objectives include numerous health status, risk reduction, and services and protection objectives related to intentional injury (see Appendix 5–A).

This is a new area for public health. Public health can bring important skills and insights to violence prevention. Rosenberg and Mercy point to four aspects of the public health epidemiological approach that can be usefully applied to violence reduction

1. public health surveillance
2. risk group identification
3. risk factor identification
4. program development, implementation, and evaluation[5]

The follow-up to these steps should be dissemination of evaluation results, leading to replication elsewhere. Public health can bring an interdisciplinary approach to dealing with the problem of intentional violence. In introducing a collection of studies on *Violence in America: A Public Health Approach*, former CDC Director William Foege noted that:

> Health departments should be seen as crucial but not sufficient. This is a lesson learned in many areas, even in what is regarded as standard public health. Health departments are simply not strong enough, sufficiently influential, or rich enough to carry out programs by themselves. . . .
>
> With violence, it is even more important to involve the largest diversity of professional and volunteer groups possible if a significant impact is to be realized.
>
> What, then, should be the role of health departments? (1) Health departments could assist to get violence into the mainstream of public health. (2) Health departments could be involved in problem definition, an area of considerable experience and expertise. (3) Health departments could be involved in the education of politicians and those who could change what is now done, education of children through the development of appropriate curricula, and education of the public by providing information to the media. (4) Health departments should develop intervention strategies and evaluate their impact. (5) Health departments must work to keep this interest from being a fad. They must develop the stabilizing interest to sustain a search for answers into the future.[72(pix–x)]

Surveillance, identification of risk factors, developing interventions, empowering communities, training, and evaluation are hallmarks of the public health approach and can be usefully directed at better understanding and dealing with violence in the United States. It is an approach that has played an important role in reducing unintentional injuries. Those successes should provide inspiration and direction as public health practitioners tackle the violence problem.

---

## NOTES

1. Reiss AJ, Jr, Roth JA. *Understanding and Preventing Violence.* Washington, DC: National Academy Press; 1993.

2. Zimring FE, Hawkins G. *Crime Is Not the Problem: Lethal Violence in America* (Studies in Crime and Public Policy). New York: Oxford University Press; 1997.

3. An observation first credited to H. Rap Brown of the Student Nonviolent Coordinating Committee during the 1960s civil rights movement.

4. Fingerhut LA, Warner M. Injury chartbook. In: National Center for Health Statistics. *Health, United States, 1996–97 and Injury Chartbook.* Hyattsville, MD: U.S. Public Health Service; 1997.

5. Rosenberg ML, Mercy JA. Assaultive violence. In: Rosenberg ML, Fenley MA. *Violence in America: A Public Health Approach.* New York: Oxford University Press: 1991.

6. Guyer B, Lescohier I, Gallagher SS, et al. Intentional injuries among children and adolescents in Massachusetts. *New Engl J Med.* 1989;321:1584–1589.

7. *Suicide Rates Among U.S. Males, by Method: Ages 10–14, 1980 and 1981.* U.S. Centers for Disease Control and Prevention, LP 188.

8. Kachur SP, Potter LD, Powell KE, et al. Suicide: Epidemiology, prevention, treatment. *Adolesc Med.* 1995;6:171–182.

9. National Center for Injury Prevention and Control. *National Summary of Injury Mortality Data, 1987–1994.* Atlanta, GA: U.S. Centers for Disease Control; 1996.

10. Kellerman AL, Rivara FP, Somes G, et al. Suicide in the home in relation to gun ownership. *New Engl J Med.* 1992;327:467–472.

11. Children's Safety Network. *A Data Book of Child and Adolescent Injury.* Washington, DC: NCEMCH; 1991.

12. Harrington C, Gallagher SS, Burgess LL, Guyer B. *Injury Prevention Programs in State Health Departments: A National Survey.* Boston, MA: Childhood Injury Prevention Resource Center, Harvard School of Public Health; 1988.

13. National Center for Injury Prevention and Control. *Violence: Division of Violence Prevention*, at http://www.cdc.gov/ncipc/dvp/dvp.htm.

14. Rosenberg ML, Mercy JA. Assaultive violence. In: Last JM, Wallace RB. *Maxcy-Rosenau-Last: Public Health and Preventive Medicine.* 13th ed. Norwalk, CT: Appleton & Lange; 1992:1035–1039.

15. Fingerhut LA, Kleinman JC. International and interstate comparisons of homicides among young males. *JAMA.* 1990;263:3292–3295.

16. Baker SP, O'Neill B, Ginsburg MJ, Li G. *The Injury Fact Book,* 2nd ed. New York: Oxford University Press; 1991.

17. Priority Area 7: Violent and Abusive Behavior. In: National Center for Health Statistics. *Healthy People 2000 Review, 1997.* Hyattsville, MD: U.S. Public Health Service; 1997:78–84.

18. Division of Injury Epidemiology and Control. *Draft Report of the Interagency Workgroup, Year 2000 Health Objectives for the Nation: Reduce Violent and Abusive Behavior.* Atlanta, GA: U.S. Centers for Disease Control; 1989.

19. Koop CE, Lundberg GD. Violence in America: A public health emergency. *JAMA.* 1992;267:3075–3076.

20. Wilt S, Olson S. Prevalence of domestic violence in the United States. *JAMA.* 1996;275:77–82.

21. Guard A. *Violence and Teen Pregnancy: A Resource Guide for Maternal and Child Health Practitioners.* Newton, MA: Children's Safety Network, Education Development Center; 1997.

22. Stark E, Flitcraft AE. Spouse abuse. In: Rosenberg ML, Fenley MA. *Violence in America: A Public Health Approach.* New York: Oxford University Press, 1991.

23. Cohen L, Swift S. A public health approach to the violence epidemic in the United States. *Environ Urbanization.* 1993;15:50–66.

24. Koss MP, Gidycz CA, Wisniewski N. The scope of rape: Incidence and prevalence of sexual aggression and victimization in a national sample of higher education students. *J Consult Clin Psychol.* 1987;55:162–170.

25. National Center for Injury Prevention and Control. *Violence: Fact Sheet on Dating Violence.* http://www.cdc.gov/ncipc/dvp/datviol.htm.

26. Bachman R, Saltzman LE. *Violence against Women: Estimates from the Redesigned Survey.* Washington, DC: Bureau of Justice Statistics, Special Report, U.S. Department of Justice; 1995.

27. Sugarman DB, Hotaling GT. Dating violence: Prevalence, context and risk markers. In: Pirog-Good MA, Stets JE. *Violence in Dating Relationships.* New York: Praeger; 1989: 3–32.

28. Males MA. *The Scapegoat Generation: America's War on Adolescents.* Monroe, ME: Common Courage Press; 1996.

29. National abuse and neglect data system. *Child Maltreatment 1993 (April 1995).* In: *Statistical Abstract of the United States, 1995.* Washington, DC: U.S. Department of Commerce; Table 346.

30. National Committee to Prevent Child Abuse. *Prevention of Child Abuse and Neglect Fatalities.* http://www.childabuse.org/fs9.html.

31. Pillemer K, Frankel S. Domestic violence against the elderly. In: Rosenberg ML, Fenley MA. *Violence in America: A Public Health Approach.* New York: Oxford University Press; 1991:158–183.

32. Maternal and Child Health Bureau, Health Resources and Services Administration. *Recommendations of the Child Fatality Review Advisory Workgroup.* Washington, DC: Public Health Service, U.S. Department of Health and Human Services; 1993.

33. Rosenberg ML, Mercy JA. *Homicide and Assaultive Violence: Background Paper Prepared for the Surgeon General's Workshop on Violence and Public Health.* Atlanta, GA: U.S. Centers for Disease Control; 1985: H2.

34. Hawkins D. Intentional injury: Are there no solutions? *Law Med Health Care.* 1989;17:32–41.

35. Sampson RJ, Raudenbush SW, Earls F. Neighborhoods and violent crime: A multilevel study of collective efficacy. *Science.* 1977;277:918–924.

36. Division of Injury Epidemiology and Control. *Draft Report of the Interagency Workgroup, Year 2000 Health Objectives for the Nation: Reduce Violent and Abusive Behavior.* Atlanta, GA: U.S. Centers for Disease Control; 1989.

37. Goldstein PJ, Brownstein HH, Ryan PJ, Bellucci PA. Crack and homicide in New York City, 1988: A conceptually based event analysis. *Contemp Drug Problems.* 1989:16:651–687.

38. Goldstein PJ. Drugs and violent crime. In: *Pathways to Criminal Violence.* Beverly Hills, CA: Sage Publications; 1990:16–48.

39. Trends in rates of homicide—United States, 1985–1994. *MMWR.* 1996;45:460–464.

40. Saltzman LE, Mercy JA, O'Carroll PW, Rosenberg ML, Rhodes PH. Weapon involvement and injury outcomes in family and intimate assaults. *JAMA.* 1992;267:3043–3047.

41. Kellermann A. The epidemiologic basis for the prevention of firearm injuries. *Annu Rev Public Health.* 1991;12:17–40.

42. Kellermann AL, Rivara FP, Rushford NB, et al. Gun ownership as a risk factor for homicide in the home. *New Engl J Med.* 1993;329:1084–1091.

43. Panel on Violence Prevention. *Draft Position Paper on Violence Prevention.* Atlanta, GA: U.S. Centers for Disease Control; 1991: I-15.

44. The states were California, Louisiana, Maryland, Nevada, New York, Texas, and Virginia. See Deaths resulting from firearm and motor vehicle related injuries, US, 1968–1991. *MMWR.* 1994;43(3):37–42.

45. Lewin T. 1990 gun deaths top auto fatalities in Texas. *New York Times* (National Edition), November 9, 1991, page Y7.

46. Ryan PJ, Goldstein PJ, Brownstein HH, Bellucci PA. Who's right: Different outcomes when police and scientists view the same set of homicide events, New York City, 1988. In: NIDA Research Monograph 103. *Drugs and Violence: Causes, Correlates, and Consequences.* Rockville, MD: National Institute on Drug Abuse; 1990:239–264.

47. Rokaw WM, Mercy JA, Smith JC. Comparing death certificate data with FBI crime reporting statistics on U.S. homicides. *Public Health Rep.* 1987;105:447–455.

48. Department of Human Services, Department of Justice. Surgeon General's Workshop on Violence and Public Health: Report, Leesburg, Virginia, October 27–28, 1985. Washington, DC: Health Resources and Services Administration, 1986. (DHHS Pub. no. HRS-D-MC86 1).

49. Novello AC, Shosky J, Froehlke R. From the Surgeon General, U.S. Public Health Service: A medical response to violence. *JAMA.* 1992;267:3007.

50. Contra Costa Health Services Department Prevention Program. *Preventing Violence in Contra Costa County: A Countywide Action Plan.* Pleasant Hill, CA: Contra Costa Health Services Department; 1994.

51. Centerwall BS. Television and violence: The scale of the problem and where to go from here. *JAMA.* 1992;267:3059–3063.

52. Mediascope. *National Television Violence Study Scientific Papers.* Studio City, CA: Mediascope; 1996.

53. Quoted in Conflict in the media, *Children's Advocate.* January–February 1997.

54. Programs for the prevention of suicide among adolescents and young adults. *MMWR.* 1994;43:RR–6.

55. Suicide contagion and reporting of suicide: Recommendations from a national workshop. *MMWR.* 1994;43:13–18.

56. *Surgeon General's Workshop on Violence and Public Health, Recommendations from the Working Groups.* Leesburg, VA: October 27–29, 1985

57. Hawkins DF. Inequality, culture, and interpersonal violence. *Health Aff.* 1993;12:80–95.

58. National Center for Injury Prevention and Control. *Youth Suicide Prevention Programs: A Resource Guide.* Atlanta, GA: CDC; 1992.

59. Children's Safety Network. *Building Safe Communities: State and Local Strategies for Preventing Injury and Violence.* Arlington, VA: National Center for Education in Maternal and Child Health; 1993:V27–31.

60. National Center for Injury Prevention and Control. *The Prevention of Youth Violence: A Framework for Community Action.* Atlanta, GA: Centers for Disease Control and Prevention; 1993.

61. Grossman DC, Neckerman HJ, Koepsell TD, et al. Effectiveness of a violence prevention curriculum among children in elementary school: A randomized controlled trial. *JAMA.* 1997;277:1605–1611.

62. Christoffel T, Teret SP. *Protecting the Public: Legal Issues in Injury Prevention.* New York: Oxford University Press; 1993.

63. "Blueprints" for violence prevention presented by University of Colorado. Boulder, CO: Office of Public Relations, University of Colorado at Boulder; December 10, 1997.

64. Children's Safety Network. *A Consumer Protection Approach to Firearms Safety.* Boston: Education Development Center; 1997.

65. *A Model Handgun Safety Standard Act.* Baltimore, MD: Johns Hopkins Center for Handgun Policy; 1996.

66. Karlson T, Hargarten S. *Reducing Firearm Injury and Death: A Public Health Sourcebook on Guns.* New Brunswick, NJ: Rutgers University Press; 1997.

67. *Presser v. Illinois.* 116 U. S. 252 (1886).

68. *United States v. Miller.* 307 U. S. 174 (1939).

69. Henigan DA, Nicholson EB, Hemenway D. *Guns and the Constitution: The Myth of Second Amendment Protection for Firearms in America.* Northhampton, MA: Aletheia Press; 1995.

70. CDC grant award requirement based on the agency's interpretation of the gun control prohibition contained in The Department of Labor, Health and Human Services, and Education, and Related Agencies Appropriations Act, 1997 (emphasis in original).

71. Rosenberg ML, O'Carroll PW, Powell KE. Let's be clear: Violence is a public health problem. *JAMA.* 1992;267:3071–3072.

72. Foege W. In: Rosenberg ML, Fenley MA. *Violence in America: A Public Health Approach.* New York: Oxford University Press; 1991: ix–x.

# Injury-Related Year 2000 Objectives

## PREVENTION OF VIOLENCE AND INJURIES DUE TO VIOLENCE

**6.1** Reduce suicides to no more than 10.5 per 100,000 people. (Age-adjusted baseline: 11.7 per 100,000 in 1987)

**6.2** Reduce to 1.8% the incidence of injurious suicide attempts among adolescents aged 14–17. (Baseline: 2.1% in 1990)

**6.10** Increase to 50 the number of states with officially established protocols that engage mental health, alcohol and drug, and public health authorities with corrections authorities to facilitate identification and appropriate intervention to prevent suicide by jail inmates. (Baseline: 3 states in 1992)

**7.1** Reduce homicides to no more than 7.2 per 100,000 people. (Age-adjusted baseline: 8.5 per 100,000 in 1987)

**7.3** Reduce firearm-related deaths to no more than 11.6 per 100,000 people from major causes. (Baseline: 14.6 firearm-related deaths in 1990)

**7.4** Reverse to less than 22.6 per 1,000 children the rising incidence of maltreatment of children younger than age 18. (Baseline: 22.6 per 1,000 in 1986)

**7.5** Reduce physical abuse directed at women by male partners to no more than 27 per 1,000 couples. (Baseline: 30 per 1,000 in 1985)

*Source:* Reprinted with permission from *Healthy People 2000 Midcourse Review and 1995 Revisions*, 1995, U.S. Public Health Service.

**7.6** Reduce assault injuries among people aged 12 and older to no more than 8.7 per 1,000 people. (Baseline: 9.7 per 1,000 in 1986)

**7.7** Reduce rape and attempted rape of women aged 12 and older to no more than 108 per 100,000 women. (Baseline: 120 per 100,000 in 1986)

**7.9** Reduce to 110 per 1,000 the incidence of physical fighting among adolescents aged 14–17. (Baseline: 137 incidents per 1,000 high school students per month in 1991)

**7.10** Reduce to 86 per 1,000 the incidence of weapon carrying by adolescents aged 14–17. (Baseline: 107 incidents per 1,000 high school students per month in 1991)

**7.11** Reduce by 20% the proportion of people who possess weapons that are inappropriately stored and therefore dangerously available. (Baseline data unavailable)

**7.12** Extend protocols for routinely identifying, treating, and properly referring suicide attempters, victims of sexual assault, and victims of spouse, elder, and child abuse to at least 90% of hospital emergency departments. (Baseline data unavailable)

**7.13** Extend to at least 45 states implementation of unexplained child death review systems. (Baseline: 33 states in 1991)

**7.14** Increase to at least 30 the number of states in which at least 50% of children identified as neglected or physically or sexually abused receive physical and mental evaluation with appropriate follow-up as a means of breaking the intergenerational cycle of abuse. (Baseline data unavailable)

**7.15** Reduce to less than 10% the proportion of battered women and their children turned away from emergency housing due to lack of space. (Baseline: 40% in 1987)

**7.16** Increase to at least 50% the proportion of elementary and secondary schools that teach nonviolent conflict resolution skills, preferably as a part of comprehensive school health education. (Baseline data unavailable)

**7.17** Extend coordinated, comprehensive violence prevention programs to at least 80% of local jurisdictions with populations over 100,000. (Baseline data unavailable)

**7.19** Enact in 50 states and the District of Columbia laws requiring that firearms be properly stored to minimize access and the likelihood of discharge by minors. (Baseline: Zero states in 1993)

**10.16** Reduce deaths from work-related homicides to no more than 0.5 per 100,000 full-time workers (Baseline: Average of 0.7 per 100,000 during 1980–1989)

**4.5** Increase by at least 1 year the average age of first use of cigarettes, alcohol, and marijuana by adolescents aged 12–17. (Baseline: Age 11.6 for cigarettes, age 13.1 for alcohol, and age 13.4 for marijuana in 1988)

**4.6** Reduce the proportion of young people who have used alcohol, marijuana, cocaine, or cigarettes in the past month.

**4.7** Reduce the proportion of high school seniors and college students engaging in recent occasions of heavy drinking of alcoholic beverages to no more than 28% of high school seniors and 32% of college students. (Baseline: 33% of high school seniors and 41.7% of college students in 1989)

**4.8** Reduce alcohol consumption by people aged 14 and older to an annual average of no more than 2 gallons of ethanol per person. (Baseline: 2.54 gallons of ethanol in 1987)

**4.9** Increase the proportion of high school seniors who perceive social disapproval of heavy use of alcohol, occasional use of marijuana, and experimentation with cocaine, or regular use of tobacco.

**4.10** Increase the proportion of high school seniors who associate physical or psychological harm with heavy use of alcohol, occasional use of marijuana, and experimentation with cocaine, or regular use of cigarettes.

**4.12** Establish and monitor in 50 states comprehensive plans to ensure access to alcohol and drug treatment programs for traditionally underserved people. (Baseline data unavailable)

**4.13** Provide to children in all school districts and private schools primary and secondary school educational programs on alcohol and other drugs, preferably as part of comprehensive school health education. (Baseline: 63% provided some instruction, 39% provided counseling, and 23% referred students for clinical assessments in 1987)

**4.14** Extend adoptions of alcohol and drug policies for the work environment to at least 60% of worksites with 50 or more employees. (Baseline: 88% of worksites had adopted alcohol policies; 89% of worksites had adopted drug policies in 1992)

**4.15** Extend to 50 states administrative driver's license suspension/revocation laws or programs of equal effectiveness for people determined to have been driving under the influence of intoxicants. (Baseline: 28 states and the District of Columbia in 1990)

**4.16** Increase to 50 the number of states that have enacted and enforce policies, beyond those in existence in 1989, to reduce access to alcohol beverages by minors. (Baseline data unavailable)

**4.17** Increase to at least 20 the number of states that have enacted statutes to restrict promotion of alcoholic beverages that is focused principally on young audiences. (Baseline data unavailable)

**4.18** Extend to 50 states legal blood alcohol concentration (BAC) tolerance levels of .08% for motor vehicle drivers aged 21 and older and zero tolerance (.02% and lower) for those younger than age 21. (Baseline: 7 states with .08 BAC laws and 9 states with zero tolerance laws in 1993)

**4.19** Increase to at least 75% the proportion of primary care providers who screen for alcohol and other drug use problems and provide counseling and referral as needed. (Baseline: 19–63% of pediatricians, nurse practitioners, obstetricians/gynecologists, internists, and family physicians reported routinely providing services to patient in 1992)

**4.20** Increase to 30 the number of states with Hospitality Resource Panels (including representatives from state regulatory, public health, and highway safety agencies, law enforcement, insurance associations, alcohol retail and licensed beverage associations) to ensure a process of management and server training and define standards of responsible hospitality. (Baseline: 8 states in 1994)

# PART II

# Basic Concepts of Injury Prevention

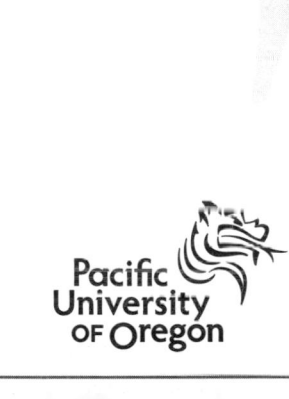

# CHAPTER 6

# Injury Prevention: General Principles

"The fundamental tasks in injury control are (a) to prevent the agents from reaching people in amounts or at rates that exceed injury thresholds, and (b) to minimize the consequences of injury."

William Haddon, Jr., and Susan P. Baker,
in *Preventive and Community Medicine*, 1981

## WHAT THIS CHAPTER IS ABOUT

We have seen that injuries—both unintentional and intentional—are a major problem for the nation. We have reviewed the magnitude, cost, and nature of these injuries, as well as the conceptual, historical, and epidemiological background of the injury problem. But where does that leave us? Can society do anything to reduce the number of injuries and the severity of those that do occur? The answer is yes. The chapters in Part II review ways in which this can be done.

Public health is grounded in prevention, the firm belief that it is much better to prevent problems from happening in the first place than to labor to ameliorate problems after they occur; this certainly applies to injury. Although injuries were long thought of as unpredictable, uncontrollable events, we now understand that we can anticipate and reduce the occurrence of injuries. We can do so using the time-honored approaches of public health. We have significant successes to build on.

This chapter will explain the how and why of injury prevention. (Arguments can be made regarding the aptness of prevention versus control or reduction, or for combining terms—as the Centers for Disease Control and Prevention [CDC] now does with its institutional name. We will follow the more traditional use of prevention.) What can be done to prevent injuries?

What has been done? What remains to be done? After laying out the basics of injury prevention in this chapter, we will use the following three chapters to summarize the three major approaches to injury prevention: educational, environmental, and legal interventions.

## INTRODUCTION

The public health approach to prevention is one based on measuring the occurrence of a disease or injury problem (surveillance), identifying relevant risk factors (epidemiologic analysis), ascertaining the natural history of the problem, intervening to reduce the number or severity of cases, and evaluating the results. (See Figure 1–2.) As injury prevention researchers from the CDC have explained it:

> The public health approach consists of health-event surveillance, epidemiologic analysis, and intervention design and evaluation, focused unwaveringly on a single, clear outcome—the prevention of a particular illness or injury. This approach was originally developed to combat infectious diseases, when such diseases were the leading causes of death. It has been successfully applied, however, to many causes of premature death and preventable physical illness including lung cancer, coronary heart disease, and, more recently, motor vehicle crashes.[1(p3071)]

Interventions may focus on eliminating the general conditions and factors that lead to injury, as when efforts are undertaken to separate vehicular and pedestrian traffic to prevent pedestrian injury. Or they may focus on identifying and intervening to protect persons at particular risk, such as women who have experienced ongoing abuse.

Injury prevention efforts can be categorized in three general approaches: (1) use the tools of persuasion and *education* to promote behavior changes so that individuals are cautious and avoid risk (and so that policy makers produce more enlightened decisions); (2) use the tools of *environmental modification* to create safer surroundings; and/or (3) use the tools of *legal requirements and prohibitions* to reduce risk. These three approaches have been referred to as the "three Es" of injury prevention: education, engineering, and enforcement.

The public health approach to prevention is interdisciplinary in nature, which means not working in isolation but rather working with government agencies, the private sector, and communities to develop multifaceted approaches to injury problems. Public health can take credit for focusing new and effective strategies on injury problems, but public health cannot take credit for the resulting successes, for these have truly been interdisciplinary in nature, drawing on the efforts of engineering, law, psychology, law enforcement, social marketing, medicine, and other fields.

Baker et al note that:

> Throughout most of this century, the death rate from injuries has declined. Most of this decline has occurred in the general category of unintentional injury deaths not related to motor vehicle crashes. . . . Although the non-motor-vehicle injury per capita death rate declined by 76% between 1910 and 1986, the death rate from motor vehicle crashes increased approximately tenfold between 1910 and 1930 and has decreased by about 25% since that time.[2(p33)]

More recent trends are reported in the injury chartbook in *Health, United States, 1996–97*,[3] where it is reported that from 1985 to 1994 the age-adjusted motor vehicle traffic death rate declined 14%, suffocation declined 9%, fall deaths declined 11%, and drownings declined 31%. Poisoning deaths remained fairly stable, and firearm deaths increased 18%.

What has brought about these reductions in injury rates and the increased safety for our citizens? Let's look at the critical prevention principles involved, beginning with the conceptual advances made by William Haddon, Jr., who, as a physician, engineer, and public health leader, personally encapsulated the interdisciplinary approach to injury prevention.

## GENERAL PRINCIPLES OF INJURY PREVENTION

In what has become known as the "Haddon Matrix," William Haddon, Jr., assessed injury prevention interventions by the phase in time at which intervention was attempted (preinjury-event phase, injury-event phase, or postinjury-event phase) and by the contributing factors that might be altered (human, agent or vehicle, physical environment, and social environment). The physical environment is the physical context within which the injury event occurs, while the social environment includes the socioeconomic, political, and cultural context surrounding the injury event (e.g., attitudes toward drinking and driving). The Haddon Matrix is graphically presented in Chapter 2 as Exhibit 2–1.

Breaking down the injury event according to time phases and contributing factors can make it easier to discern that there are multiple points for intervention for each type of injury and, in turn, allows for interventions that can be more carefully tailored and complementary of one another than would be a general, nondifferentiated approach to prevention. Table 6–1 provides examples of the intervention points for each cell of the matrix as applied to motor vehicle injury.

Haddon, working with Susan Baker, highlighted the considerations involved in selecting strategies for injury prevention:

> The choice of countermeasures should *not* be determined by the relative importance of causal or contributing factors or by their earliness in the sequence of events. The behaviors that exposed

**Table 6–1** Haddon Matrix Example

| Phases | Human Factors | Agent or Vehicle | Physical Environment | Sociocultural Environment |
|---|---|---|---|---|
| Pre-event | Driver ability/ driver training | Maintenance of brakes, tires, etc./ vehicle inspection programs | Adequate roadway markings and lighting | Public attitudes on drinking and driving, speeding, etc. |
| Event | Spread out energy in time and space with airbag and/ or seatbelt | Crashworthiness ("crush space," forgiving windshield, no dash protrusions) | Presence of fixed objects near roadway | Enforcement of mandatory seatbelt use laws |
| Postevent | Crash victim's general health status (including sobriety) | Gas tanks designed to minimize likelihood of postcrash fires | Availability of effective trauma response system | Public support for trauma care and rehabilitation |

people to polio viruses, although important, were not relevant to the eventual solution of the polio problem; similarly, while psychological factors may be important in the initiation of motor vehicle crashes, it does not follow that psychological screening of drivers would be fruitful. Rather, priority and emphasis should be given to measures that will *most effectively* reduce injury losses. As a result of failure to understand this point, emphasis on human error as the cause of most injuries has resulted in undue emphasis on changing behavior, rather than on using more effective measures to reduce injuries and their results.[4]

These experts, and their disciples, have urged that a mixed strategy of injury prevention should be used, one which addresses each of the three temporal phases of injury (preinjury, injury, postinjury). For example, efforts to reduce swimming deaths among toddlers have included required fencing around home swimming pools, monitoring and alarm systems for such pools, and teaching lifesaving and cardiopulmonary resuscitation techniques. Also, whenever possible passive or automatic approaches should be employed, ones that do not require individual compliance to be effective (such as the automatic brake now standard on all power lawnmowers). Product and environmental design may hold the greatest potential for effective injury prevention intervention, although laws may often be needed to bring about such design modifications. In turn, it is difficult to get laws enacted without first generating support by educating policy makers and the public about injury prevention. Injury prevention measures must also be carefully and continually evaluated as to effectiveness and cost to prevent misallocation, and possible waste, of scarce injury prevention resources (political as well as financial).

Although there are many things that can be done to reduce injury frequency and severity, specific injury prevention countermeasures all fall into certain patterns. As discussed more fully in Chapter 2, Haddon noted that once we move beyond education and persuasion, all such countermeasures fall into one or another of 10 basic conceptual approaches to intervention. These approaches, the Haddon Ten, are:

1. Prevent the creation of the hazard.
2. Reduce the amount of the hazard.
3. Prevent the release of a hazard that already exists.
4. Modify the rate or spatial distribution of the hazard.

5. Separate, in time or space, the hazard from that which is to be protected.
6. Separate the hazard from that which is to be protected by a material
   barrier.
7. Modify relevant basic qualities of the hazard.
8. Make what is to be protected more resistant to damage from the hazard.
9. Begin to counter the damage already done by the hazard.
10. Stabilize, repair, and rehabilitate the object of the damage.

Each of these 10 countermeasures is conceptually distinct. They are also
all inclusive; no eleventh approach has been added. Most importantly,
these generic countermeasures provide a broad armamentarium for dealing
with injury. If a particular approach, such as preventing the creation of the
hazard, is simply not feasible, no effort need be wasted trying to implement that type of intervention. Instead, other countermeasure approaches
can be used to protect the public. Exhibit 6–1 presents the National Center
for Injury Prevention and Control's summary of the public health approach
to injury prevention.

## IMPLEMENTATION

There are a variety of approaches that can be taken to reduce injury. And
they are being undertaken, on the local, state, and federal levels. It should
be noted that Haddon's countermeasures one through seven all involve
product or environmental design approaches and that all but countermeasure eight often involve governmental action. In *Injury in America*, the
Committee on Trauma Research used the terms "persuade," "require," and
"provide automatic protection" to refer to education, enforcement, and engineering approaches to injury prevention, noting that such efforts can be
directed so as to[5]:

- *Persuade* people at risk of injury to alter their behavior for increased
  self-protection—for example, to use seatbelts or install smoke detectors.
- *Require* individual behavior change by law or administrative rule—
  for example, by laws requiring seatbelt use or requiring installation of
  smoke detectors in all new buildings.
- *Provide automatic protection* by product and environmental design—
  for example, by the installation of seatbelts that automatically encom-

**Exhibit 6–1** Prevention: The Public Health Approach

- Injury is a serious public health problem because of its impact on the health of Americans, including premature death, disability, and the burden on our health care system.

- Like diseases, injuries do not occur at random and are preventable. National Center for Injury Prevention and Control is using the same scientific methods to prevent injuries that have been used in preventing disease: carefully describing the problem through surveillance, studying what puts people at risk for injury, and designing and evaluating intervention strategies that target these risk factors.

- The public health community has the experience as well as the public and private partners necessary to research, develop, and communicate effective methods to prevent injury.

- Injury prevention strategies focus primarily on environmental design (e.g., road construction that permits optimum visibility), product design, human behavior, education, and legislative and regulatory requirements that support environmental and behavioral change.

- Public health efforts to prevent injuries have been highly successful. For example, 240,000 lives were saved between 1966 and 1990 because of improved motor vehicle and highway design, increased use of safety belts and motorcycle helmets, and enforcement of laws regarding drinking and driving and speeding. Similar results are possible with other types of injuries.

*Source:* Reprinted from http://www.cdc.gov/ncipc/about/about.htm, National Center for Injury Prevention and Control.

pass occupants of motor vehicles or built-in sprinkler systems that automatically extinguish fires.

The committee went on to observe that:

Each of these general strategies has a role in any comprehensive injury-control program; however, a basic finding from research is that the second strategy—requiring behavior change—will generally be more effective than the first, and that the third—providing automatic protection—will be the most effective.[5(p7)]

In fact, however, none of these approaches should be used in isolation. Each has a role to play in injury prevention and each is needed in a combined way to be truly effective. Moreover, the persuasion approach is important in mobilizing the community to make the demands for the other two strategies.

What does this mean for local public health agencies, especially those with little history of injury prevention activity? Governmental injury prevention efforts in public health agencies are often focused on public education, but local agencies can do more; legal sanctions and service delivery are not necessarily outside of their purview. Public health agencies often have more authority and potential for carrying out injury prevention interventions than may at first be apparent. For example, day care licensing can provide an opportunity to focus on safety issues in a context that affords authority to inspect facilities and impose legal sanctions. Another example is provided by state sanitary codes, which are often promulgated by a state health agency with statutory authority for enforcement given to local or county boards of health. These codes may include requirements related to household hazards and injury prevention in the home. For example, in Massachusetts, the State Sanitary Code provides that:

- The owner of a dwelling that is required by law to be equipped with smoke detectors must maintain them in compliance with regulations of the State Board of Fire Prevention. If a violation of these regulations is observed during an inspection of a dwelling, the board of health must notify the proper fire official. . . .
- The owner of a dwelling is responsible for maintaining all means of egress in a safe, operable condition at all times. . . .
- The temperature of the hot water [provided by hot water heaters] is not to exceed 130° Fahrenheit. . . .
- A safe handrail must be provided for every stairway used for or intended for use by the occupants. . . .
- Every opening exterior window of a dwelling must be . . . fitted with a functioning locking device. . . .
- No wiring shall lie under any floor cover nor shall it extend through a doorway, window or any other opening. . . .
- No lead paint may be used in painting any surface on the premises.[6]

Other types of safety-related measures that may be found in state sanitary codes include requirements for safety glass in glass doors and lighting in stairwells, as well as bans on the use of space heaters and standards for the safe installation of wood stoves.

In most states the sanitary code has the force of law including criminal penalties for failure to comply. A study assessing the feasibility of local health departments carrying out injury prevention activities as part of their responsibility for inspecting dwellings on a regular basis or on complaint found that normal housing code procedures combined with education and installation of safety devices were effective in significantly reducing hazards in the home.[7]

Service delivery is another important part of the public health system that provides an opportunity for incorporating attention to injury prevention. In most states, contracts are awarded at the local or state level for provision of prenatal care; women, infants, and children nutrition programs (WIC); adolescent health services; early intervention for developmentally delayed children; home visiting for mothers of newborns; and immunizations. Very often such service delivery is targeted at populations that are at high risk for injury and violence. It makes sense to include prevention of injury and violence developmentally appropriate to the target audience, incorporating educational and environmental injury prevention strategies into routine service delivery through anticipatory guidance, referrals to other agencies (such as those offering low-cost or giveaway child safety seat programs), and information on legal requirements (such as mandated smoke detectors in rental housing). A goal for injury prevention practitioners should be the integration of the general principles of injury prevention into the existing base of routine service delivery of public health agencies. In fact, injury prevention efforts need to be integrated into all levels of ongoing state programming (e.g., social workers transporting very young foster children should have toddler car safety seats and booster seats available and should receive training on their proper use and installation).

Public health agencies are not limited to any single injury prevention approach; they can engage in a wide-ranging effort to reduce injury. First, public health agencies are crucial to the surveillance and epidemiologic analyses that are prerequisites to injury prevention intervention. Second, it is through public health agencies that effective injury prevention efforts can be coordinated and evaluated—as described in Part III of this book. The authors of *Injury Prevention: Meeting the Challenge* argued that:

> In addition to their data collection and analysis capabilities, public health agencies can offer practical experience in the successful management of communitywide health problems through the de-

sign, implementation, and evaluation of community-based prevention programs. And, in its recognition that health problems have multiple causes and are therefore multidisciplinary by nature, public health understands the need to coordinate and participate in fashioning multidisciplinary solutions.[8(p9)]

This will not be easy, not because we don't know what we could and should do as a society but because the professions involved—public health, medicine, public policy—still do not fully embrace the fact that something can be done to prevent "accidents." As the National Conference on Injury Control explained:

> [T]he prevention of injuries has received scant attention from the scientific community and from federal, state and local governments. As a result, there is a gross imbalance between the significance of the health problem resulting from injuries and the degree to which efforts to prevent them are represented in most public health and medical school curricula, health department programs and governmental budgets.[9]

Exhibit 6–2 lays out a National Plan for Action on injury control, the recommendations of which were distilled by staff of the National Center for Injury Prevention and Control from input provided by the injury prevention community. An agenda is only useful, however, if it suggests priorities, which must be tailored according to local data, resources, and support. To prioritize and decide which injury problem to tackle first, it may be useful to consider the following questions:

1. Frequency: How often do such injuries occur?
2. Severity: Are these mostly deaths, hospitalizations, emergency department visits? Do severe disabilities result?
3. Cost: What are the costs of health care? What other costs do these injuries impose upon society?
4. Strategies available: Is there a proven or promising prevention strategy available?
5. Resources: What resources will be required for implementation?
6. Acceptability: Would implementation (*and enforcement*) of this strategy be acceptable to the community in general?
7. Political feasibility: Would there be significant opposition to implementation by specific and important actors?

**Exhibit 6–2** Injury Control in the 1990s: A National Plan for Action

**Recommendation 1:** Establish and support a center for injury control within CDC to emphasize the importance of injuries as a public health issue and to lead a national program of effective action to address the problem.

**Recommendation 2:** Increase the recognition, awareness, and support of injury control at all levels of the public and private sectors. This education and communication campaign should include prevention of injuries, and acute care and rehabilitation of persons with injuries.

**Recommendation 3:** Mandate the inclusion of codes to identify external causes of injury (E codes) in hospital discharge data whenever an injury is the principal diagnosis. Federal and private health insurance systems should require E codes for reimbursement.

**Recommendation 4:** Develop, implement, and evaluate a uniform system to collect etiologic data on injury fatalities not related to motor vehicles similar to the system for motor vehicle traffic fatalities sponsored by the National Highway Traffic Safety Administration.

**Recommendation 5:** Link traffic and medical records to provide statewide surveillance systems for nonfatal motor vehicle injuries.

**Recommendation 6:** Improve data on occupational injuries and worker populations. Promote standardized reporting of work-related injury fatalities on death certificates and improve coding of occupation and industry on death certificates.

**Recommendation 7:** Develop, implement, and evaluate national uniform data sets for trauma care and for rehabilitation.

**Recommendation 8:** Conduct biomechanics, behavioral science, and other research on a range of injury issues covering vehicle and road design and driver or pedestrian behavior. Research should address prevention and the reduction of severity of injury.

**Recommendation 9:** Delineate more precisely the risks and benefits of ready access to handguns and other firearms.

**Recommendation 10:** Determine the potential impact of improving and enforcing building codes and other safety codes to prevent injuries in the home and residential facilities.

*continues*

**Exhibit 6–2** continued

**Recommendation 11:** Conduct research to identify occupational hazards and high-risk workers. Evaluate the effectiveness of new and existing worker protection strategies, including engineering control, standards, inspection strategies, training, and education.

**Recommendation 12:** Evaluate the effectiveness of an inclusive trauma care system.

**Recommendation 13:** Conduct research on optimal acute care interventions and monitoring.

**Recommendation 14:** Conduct research on the health care system and rehabilitation services, such as access and payment, cost-benefit analyses, employment training, incentives to work, traditional and nontraditional services, therapeutic methods, and quality of life.

**Recommendation 15:** Continue implementation of and strengthen programs for reducing impaired driving and improving occupant protection (safety belt use, child safety seats, airbag use); motorcycle, pedestrian, and bicycle safety; and speed limit enforcement to prevent motor vehicle injuries.

**Recommendation 16:** Develop, implement, and evaluate programs to reduce injuries related to violence. Areas of emphasis are injuries from firearms, injuries associated with alcohol and other drug use, early childhood experiences that affect the risk of future violent behavior or victimization, and mental and addictive disorders associated with suicide for which there are effective treatments.

**Recommendation 17:** Develop, implement, and evaluate programs to reduce injuries related to home and leisure activities.

**Recommendation 18:** Develop, implement, and evaluate programs to prevent and control occupational injuries.

**Recommendation 19:** Develop, implement, and evaluate an inclusive trauma care system.

**Recommendation 20:** Formulate objective treatment guidelines for use by medical providers in the emergency phase of care.

**Recommendation 21:** Develop systems of care to increase capacity for delivering rehabilitation services for all people with injuries that produce sig-

*continues*

**Exhibit 6–2** continued

nificant limitations in function and evaluate the effectiveness of these systems. The goal of these systems should be focused toward independent living.

**Recommendation 22:** Enhance the training of professionals (practitioners and researchers) at all levels of prevention, acute care, and rehabilitation. Develop and implement a strategic plan for national training based on national injury control priorities and on sound education technology.

*Source:* Reprinted from *Injury Control in the 1990s: A National Plan for Action*, 1993, National Center for Injury Prevention and Control, Centers for Disease Control and Prevention.

An injury prevention agenda by state and local agencies must also address (1) common difficulties in the implementation and evaluation of programs (e.g., developing the appropriate tools and materials to integrate injury prevention within existing service delivery routes) and (2) gaps in current approaches (such as developing effective interventions for recent immigrants and non–English-speaking cultures).

## CONCLUSION

The challenges are multiple, but the need, the potential, and the models for emulation are many. What remains to be done is fairly clear. Intentional injuries stand out as a high priority, particularly deaths related to firearms. Motor vehicle deaths could be reduced further. Our entire system for dealing with the injury problem could be greatly enhanced. Based on figures for 1995, as a nation we still endure 147,891 injury deaths each year, accompanied by 2,591,000 hospital discharges, 36,981,000 emergency department visits, and a total of 59,127,000 annual episodes of reported injuries.[3]

The injury problem will continue to be an important one. We will need to build on our successes with hard work if we are to reduce the impact of injury on our society. This will involve time, cooperation, resources, and dedication. The success stories of the past (including the work of individuals such as William Haddon, Jr.) required years of effort. But as a result of past successes—and failures—we know what works, we know what can be effective, and we know that there can be successes. We need to build on them using the "three Es" of injury prevention: *education, engineering, and enforcement.*

---

## NOTES

1. Rosenberg ML, O'Carroll PW, Powell KE. Let's be clear: Violence is a public health problem. *JAMA* 1992;267:3071–3072.
2. Baker SP, O'Neill B, Ginsburg MJ, Li G. *The Injury Fact Book.* 2nd ed. New York: Oxford University Press; 1992.
3. Fingerhut LA, Warner M. Injury chartbook. In: National Center for Health Statistics. *Health, United States, 1996–97 and Injury Chartbook.* Hyattsville, MD: U.S. Public Health Service; 1997.
4. Haddon WJ, Jr, Baker SP. Injury control. In: Clark D, MacMahon B. *Preventive and Community Medicine.* Boston: Little, Brown & Company; 1981:109–140.
5. Committee on Trauma Research, Commission on Life Sciences, National Research Council and Institute of Medicine. *Injury in America: A Continuing Public Health Problem.* Washington, DC: National Academy Press; 1985.
6. *Safe & Sanitary Housing for Massachusetts Residents: Highlights of Chapter II of the State Sanitary Code.* Boston: Office of the Secretary of State, undated.
7. Gallagher SS, Hunter P, Guyer B. A home injury prevention program for children. *Pediatr Clin North Am.* 1985;32:95–112.
8. National Committee for Injury Prevention and Control. *Injury Prevention: Meeting the Challenge.* New York: Oxford University Press (Published as a supplement to the *Am J Prev Med.* 1989;5:9).
9. Johns Hopkins School of Hygiene and Public Health. *Report of the National Conference on Injury Control.* Atlanta, GA: U.S. Centers for Disease Control; 1981.

# CHAPTER 7

# Injury Prevention: Educational Strategies

"A basic cultural theme in the United States, perhaps as widely shared as any in a diverse society, is that sufficient education will resolve almost any problem."

Leon Robertson, *Injuries: Causes, Control Strategies and Public Policy*, 1983

## WHAT THIS CHAPTER IS ABOUT

Educational approaches to injury prevention assume that injury is often the result of inadequate knowledge, skill, or attitudes. Educational strategies are intended to increase individual knowledge and alter individual attitudes, fostering safer behaviors and reducing risky behaviors. Often the educational messages are directed at <u>parents</u> to alert them to supervision issues or how to best protect their children from common but underappreciated dangers, such as the danger of tap water scalds, riding a bicycle without a helmet, or teen driving without accumulating more hours behind the wheel. Many messages conveyed in public information campaigns, such as not to drink and drive, are used to remind people of known risks and to encourage safety precautions.

Educational interventions have long been a mainstay of public health practice, and for a long time education was the dominant approach to injury prevention, an approach viewed as the most logical way to induce safer behaviors. More recently many critics have argued that the educational approach is a diversion from the much more effective uses of passive environmental protections and legislation. Is there any middle ground between these diametrically opposed views? If so, what is it? What do we mean when we talk about injury prevention education? And how—if at

139

all—should education be integrated into a comprehensive injury prevention program? These are the questions that underlie this chapter. It reviews the role of education in injury prevention and provides a view of education as a potentially effective part of an overall injury prevention strategy.

## INTRODUCTION

Education has been a longstanding tool in the field of public health. It has been the first "E" of injury prevention: education, engineering, and enforcement. Injury prevention education is generally viewed as a process having three sequential goals. First, educational strategies seek to *provide information* regarding injury risks and how to avoid them. Many risks are quite obvious; it is apparent to most adults that scaling steep cliffs or driving at high speeds requires caution, but it is not intuitively evident that baby walkers are hazardous or that some BB guns have a higher muzzle velocity than some powder firearms. Moreover, the best way to reduce perceived hazards is not always manifest; the proven value of bicycle helmets, smoke detectors, or window guards is valuable information that must be imparted to people if they are to be convinced to use these protective devices. And critical skills, such as safe driving, may best be enhanced through extended behind-the-wheel training programs, a type of education.

But as noted in *Injury in America*, "Many injuries (including highway injuries) result less from lack of knowledge than from failure to apply what is known."[1(p38)] Information is only helpful if it affects how people view the world around them. The second goal of injury prevention education is to *change attitudes* toward risk and safety. For example, family traditions, core values, and work ethics sometimes compromise the safety of children on farms and override parents' perspective of actual risk. In other areas, parents—even safety-conscious parents—may feel that their own children are exceptional and therefore less likely to be injured than their peers; somehow the warning on a toy that it is "not safe for children under three" does not apply to their 2 year old.

This still is not enough, however. The third goal of injury prevention education is to *alter behaviors*. It is not enough for people to simply learn that seatbelts save lives. They must also believe that it is important to buckle up and to make the decision to do so. Yet even that falls short of the overall goal, which is to get people to actually wear their seatbelts on a routine basis, to adopt the behavior that is the goal of the educational intervention. Behavior change is the goal, change that is sustained over time and which results in reduced injury rates. Without this type of documented result, the effort is unsuccessful and could even be counterproductive.

## CONCEPTUAL PRINCIPLES

Because the goal is behavior change, it might be more appropriate to use the term "persuasion" rather than "education." More important, some conceptual model of what is being attempted should be articulated. How do we define what is usually referred to as health education? Pless and Arsenault interpret the term quite broadly when they suggest that health education is intended:

> first, to encompass programs that are strictly educational in nature, whether the message is delivered verbally, visually, or by written material. It also includes educational programs that have a behavioral or social learning component, and those that combine information with other forms of persuasion, such as legislation. Implicit in the definition, or in assessing the success of the process, is the question of what health education is intended to accomplish. At one extreme there is the view that the goal is to assure that, within a given group, a certain percentage of persons attain a certain minimal level of knowledge—a measure of breadth, or diffusion, or a concept. . . . At the other is the assumption that the only meaningful objective is a change in the targeted event, in this case actual injuries. . . . Within the gamut of strategies employed by those in health education, two further divisions may be recognized. The first involves programs focused on those at greatest risk; the second includes those that are generally unselective. Extreme examples of the latter are programs that distribute literature to parents of children of all ages, with the intention of preventing all or most injuries. Such a "shotgun" approach has little chance of success, but at least gives the appearance of being economical. On the other hand, interventions focused on high-risk groups are more likely to be successful but equally likely to be more expensive.[2]

Leon Robertson notes that for "education to change behavior that leads to injury or to induce increased protection, its assumptions must be valid.

Following are four assumptions that are included, either explicitly or implicitly, in educational efforts to reduce injury:

1. Persons informed of risk will retain the information and take recommended action to reduce the risk.
2. Persons skilled in a given hazardous endeavor are less likely to be injured than those less skilled.
3. The educator has the means available to teach information or skills, and to cause behavior change related to emotions, attitudes, and values.
4. The training of people to perform a hazardous activity will not result in an increase in the activity to the point that any injury-reducing effect of the training is more than offset by increased injuries resulting from use of the new skill.[3(pp91–92)]

How does behavior change take place? The work of James Prochaska has received considerable attention in recent years from health agencies dealing with substance abuse and other destructive behaviors. Prochaska and his colleagues have described a research-based model for intentional behavior change—both self-initiated and professionally facilitated—that consists of the following six-stage process within which shifts in an individual's attitudes, intentions, and behaviors occur[4]:

1. *Precontemplation*: no intention to change behavior; unaware or underaware of their problems.
2. *Contemplation:* aware that a problem exists and seriously thinking about overcoming it, but have not yet made a commitment to take action; weigh the pros and cons of the problem and the solution to the problem; can remain stuck here for long periods.
3. *Preparation:* intend to take action soon; have made some small behavior changes.
4. *Action:* modify behavior, experiences, and/or environment in order to overcome the problems.
5. *Maintenance:* prevent relapse and consolidate gains attained during action.
6. *Termination*: maintaining change is effortless.

Prochaska et al argue that "Each of these . . . is a predictable, well-defined stage; it takes place in a period of time and entails a series of tasks that need to be completed before progressing to the next stage. Each stage does not inevitably lead to the next—it is possible to become stuck at one stage or another."[4] Without an appreciation of these discrete stages, it is much harder to understand, inspire, guide, and achieve behavior changes.

Early injury prevention education was not attuned to this change process. Such early efforts also failed to specifically target messages in ways that were developmentally appropriate and that accounted for individual differences. There are variations in the pace and manner of child and adult learning, variations rooted in families, learning styles, culture, and socioeconomic status. One size does not necessarily fit all. Child development and learning styles must be considered when developing educational approaches. Current behavioral theory and developmental theory identifies four aspects of child development: physical, cognitive, emotional, and social. All four must be considered in order to create effective educational strategies.[5] Often, focus group studies are needed to determine the effectiveness of approaches and materials.

## TECHNIQUES FOR EDUCATING AND PERSUADING

We should definitely approach injury prevention education as having the potential to be something more than simply providing information. Injury prevention education can be

- anticipatory guidance by health care professionals who counsel their patients about what they can do to avoid injury
- coordinated efforts to use education to enhance environmental approaches to injury prevention—for example, demonstrating proper vehicle restraint use
- community education campaigns, such as that which transformed the concept of "designated driver" into a common practice
- long-term efforts to alter the public's perception of risk to change social norms, such as the social acceptability of drinking and driving
- the creation of demand for a safer environment, safer products, and effective injury prevention laws
- education to make enforcement of laws acceptable and a high priority

What are the standard approaches and techniques? Lawrence Green defines basic health education as "any combination of learning experiences designed to predispose, enable, and reinforce voluntary adaptations of individual or collective behavior conducive to health."[6] Green's conceptualization of health education is a broad one; he suggests that:

Health education occurs thorough the mass media and in various settings: worksites (occupational health and safety, employee health promotion), medical (patient education, health education in primary care settings and hospitals), community agencies (voluntary health organizations, health fairs, health promotion events), and schools.[6(p789)]

Alan Andreasen lists technologies that seek to induce behavior change: health education, health communications, health promotion, mass communications, media advocacy, public advertising, public communications, social advertising, and social mobilization. He groups these technologies into four general approaches:

**The Education Approach:** The education approach begins with the primary assumption that individuals will do the right thing if only they understand why they need to do what is being advocated and know how to carry it out. The educator's task is to bring the facts to the target audience in the most lucid and compelling fashion possible. It is the approach that underlies the Health Belief Model (HBM) used extensively in the health care field. . . . In the early versions of this model, behavior was seen as driven by four sets of key beliefs.

- perceived susceptibility to a given health problem
- perceived severity of the problem
- perceived benefits from acting
- perceived barriers to taking the action

Although some authors caution that the HBM "does not presuppose or imply a strategy for change,". . . most practitioners conclude that any behavior-change strategy must focus on directly modifying these beliefs. In such strategies, careful attention is paid to using the right channels of communications and the right spokespeople. Messages are carefully assessed for readability to, and understanding by, the target audience. . . .

**The Persuasion Approach:** This approach recognizes a number of deficiencies of the education approach and takes it one step further. Adherents to this approach have a fundamental belief that actions take place only if people are sufficiently motivated. Thus, the goal of the persuasionist is to discover the careful arguments and motivational hot buttons that will get the educated consumer to "get off the dime." It is an approach that underlies . . . social advertising . . . causes and ideas such as the "Just Say No" anti-drug campaign.

The problem is that the persuasion approach is one of getting the consumer to adopt the persuasionist's view of the world. This group knows what is good for consumers and attempts to push this view of the world on them.

**The Behavioral Modification Approach:** This approach tends to minimize the influence of thoughts and feelings on individual behavior. It stresses very simple principles of learning theory that argue that people do what they do because they (a) learn the techniques necessary for the action and (b) find the outcomes rewarding. Behaviorists emphasize training and modeling of desired behavior and then give careful attention to rewarding the behavior when it occurs. . . . A basic problem with this approach is that it is very costly. Whereas education and persuasion can be aimed at the masses as well as at individual customers, the behavioral modification approach almost always has to be at the individual level.

**The Social Influence Approach:** [A]dvocates of this approach argue that campaigns directed at influencing community norms and collective behavior are the most cost-effective way to reach and change individuals and families. . . . Thus, they see changing social norms . . . as the best way to convince individuals that they must act in the prescribed way or risk social isolation. However, the approach may be limited to situations in which:

- Social issues and norms are well understood and accepted . . .
- The pressures to conform are extremely strong . . .
- The behavior to be influenced is socially important and visible.[7(pp9–12)]

Andreasen recommends a fifth approach, *social marketing,* which has features in common with each of the above four approaches. He defines social marketing as:

the application of commercial marketing technologies to the analysis, planning, execution, and evaluation of programs designed to influence the voluntary behavior of target audiences in order to improve their personal welfare and that of their society.[7(p7)]

Social marketing has been coming increasingly into vogue in public health. The Centers for Disease Control and Prevention has been emphasizing social marketing approaches. A national conference on social marketing in public health has been held annually since 1991.[8] Andreasen attributes successes in establishing the practice of designated drivers to social marketing approaches.

## WHO ARE WE EDUCATING?

Aside from the question of which techniques may be most successful in inducing behavior change, there is also the question of which target audiences these techniques should be used on. It would be a mistake to assume that the focus is only on the day-to-day behaviors of the general public. Towner notes that the frequent criticisms of health education tend to:

relate specifically to the traditional "preventive" model, in which people are persuaded to adopt healthy lifestyles. But, in addition to individual decision making, education can also be directed at professionals, at lobbying and advocacy, at changing the political agenda, and at general awareness. . . . The *preventive* model is an individually focused and medically dominated form of health education. . . . It provides people with information on which they are expected to act, assuming individual responsibility for their own health. This model seeks approved behavioral outcomes and has been criticized because of its tendency to blame the victim. . . . The *radical* model, in contrast, is more collectivist in outlook. It is an environmental "upstream" model that challenges the view that the individual is to blame for his/her own health. . . . Within *empowerment* models, process is more important than outcomes. . . . It enhances self esteem and a willingness to take control.[9]

Although the main focus of health education and behavior change has been aimed, as Towner notes, on people (i.e., the population whose possible injury we wish to prevent), there are several other populations that need to be the focus of education and persuasion about injury risks and prevention. These include health care professionals, media, policy makers, the business community, law enforcement, and public health agency staff—each of whom have an important impact on the injury risks and the injury avoidance behaviors of the general public.

## Health Professionals

Health professionals provide injury prevention counseling in primary care settings, especially for children and their parents. This is often referred to as anticipatory guidance, which alerts parents to safety hazards facing their children and suggests preventive measures to reduce risk. This method was long assumed to be a self-evident good, although the amount of time pediatricians devoted to discussing such issues has been minimal.[10] As Abraham Bergman stated in a 1982 article in the *Pediatric Clinics of North America*, anticipatory guidance "is a cornerstone of pediatric practice. Clinicians who spend time in health education activities are assured of a seat in heaven. And given the magnitude of the injury problem in children . . . a goodly proportion of that time would be spent on injury prevention."[11] But Bergman went on to throw some cold water on this angelic enterprise. Simply imparting information is "worthless in terms of reducing mortality and morbidity." And as for more sophisticated educational strategies, wrote Bergman, the relatively few studies that had been done "cast doubt on the efficacy of educational efforts directed toward the prevention of childhood injuries." On the other hand, "none of the studies showed harm, but rather demonstrated that success was not as dramatic as hoped." Bergman advised physicians to continue injury prevention counseling while better tools were developed to evaluate and direct such counseling. And, in fact, soon thereafter the American Academy of Pediatrics created The Injury Prevention Program (TIPP), which includes specific injury prevention advice, suggested counseling schedules from birth to 12 years of age, a series of safety surveys for parents, and related educational materials.

The critical point is that to contribute effectively to injury prevention, health professionals must themselves be well educated and well prepared. An educational goal for the injury prevention community must be to impart knowledge and skills to health care providers so they can be effective in counseling patients regarding injury. An example is the area of domestic violence, where health professionals can play an important role in screening and counseling. Yet to do so, they must understand the nature of the domestic violence problem and how to recognize that problem, the need for appropriate interventions, how to properly question patients, and how and where to refer both victims and perpetrators of violence. They need to know how to deal with special needs, such as battering during pregnancy. Health professionals also need to be able to provide anticipatory guidance regarding matters such as firearms in the home. They can often learn these things through their own professional organizations. It is also important that health professionals be involved in all local and statewide injury prevention coalitions.

Recommended guidelines for counseling on injury prevention appear in a number of documents produced by expert panels,[12] professional associations,[13] and federal agencies.[14] Although the expectations have grown for physicians to perform such counseling, there is still a need to find incentives for them to include counseling in their practices and for residency programs to include training in this area. A 1997 study of an urban pediatric clinic serving low-income families indicates that only 47% of pediatric well-child visits with children younger than 5 years of age included injury prevention counseling. An average of only 1.08 minutes was spent on injury prevention counseling during which time 1.96 injury topics were discussed. This study indicates a need for pediatricians to prioritize their injury prevention counseling so that the most important injury problems and most effective prevention strategies are covered in the limited time available.[15] Another recent study estimated that if all young children received all of the recommended American Academy of Pediatrics injury prevention counseling, the annual savings in medical spending due to decreased injuries would be $230 million, with total injury costs to society reduced by $3.4 billion.[16]

## The Media

Print and broadcast media play a critical role in forming public attitudes regarding what is acceptable and unacceptable in our society (e.g., regarding drinking and driving, where the media has played a mixed role) and what is achievable in terms of reducing injury levels (e.g., gun violence, where the media has played a negative role). One problem is that few people working in the media understand injury issues; rather, they accept and pass on the idea of random, unpredictable accidents that cannot be avoided. Thus educating those who work in print and broadcast journalism should be a high priority for injury prevention education.[17]

## Policy Makers and the Business Community

The same point can and should be made regarding policy makers and the business community. An aspect of education that has been neglected by the injury prevention community is introducing policy makers to the issues surrounding injury prevention. These are the people who make the decisions that can lead to needed legislative, regulatory, and engineering changes. With them, as with other audiences, education should be an ongoing process rather than isolated and sporadic events occurring only when critical policy measures are being debated. Education directed at policy makers, whether they are public officials or corporate leaders, should focus on background information, data, and effective, proven initiatives. (Policy-related education is also necessary to build grassroots support for injury prevention.)

## Law Enforcement Officials

Law enforcement officials, especially those involved in enforcing motor vehicle laws, are well aware of injury problems and are familiar with the enforcement end of prevention. It is important to incorporate them into educational efforts, for some of the greatest successes in injury prevention—e.g., effective use of child car seats—seem to have come from a combination of education and enforcement.

## Public Health Agency Staff

Regardless of whether or not they work directly on injury issues, public health agency staff need to know about the nature of the injury problem and about which preventive measures work and which do not. Thus one aspect of injury prevention education involves educating your colleagues—and yourself.

## WHEN AND HOW TO USE EDUCATIONAL STRATEGIES: A BALANCED APPROACH

Despite the criticisms and limited documentation of effectiveness, there are certain circumstances in which education is particularly useful. This would include areas of new knowledge, such as the hazard presented by most—but not all—airbags to out-of-position, small individuals. It would also include situations where there is no other preventive approach. Neither legislation nor passive protections can be used to prevent bathtub drownings or toddlers choking on peanuts, popcorn, or grapes, for example. Most important, many environmental and legislative strategies would never come into being were the public not educated to demand such changes of manufacturers or legislators not educated to understand the true impact of their support or lack thereof for injury prevention laws. To be effective, health education should not be used in isolation; rather, it should be part of a balanced approach.

Education can be particularly useful in reducing injury in four areas.

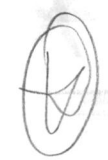

1. Teaching young children basic safety behaviors and skills that stay with them later in life. Examples might include what to do when a smoke detector sounds an alarm (e.g., crawl under the smoke), calling 911 for help in an emergency, or fastening seatbelts.
2. For certain types and causes of injury and certain age groups, educating may be the only strategy available. For example, in the case of infants and toddlers choking on carrots, peanuts, and other foods, redesigning the shape of the food or taking it off the supermarket shelves may not be feasible.
3. Altering the public's perception of risk and acceptable risk to change social norms and attitudes. This is what happened regarding drinking and driving and what is occurring now with wearing helmets when bike riding.
4. Promoting policy change and educating consumers to demand safer products. Health education can be used to marshal widespread support to bring about systematic implementation of what we know works.

Much of the criticism of the educational approach to injury prevention has been directed at the narrowness of the approach, either those that rely on information transmittal without integration into an overall strategy or those that are directed at an undifferentiated population. Roadside signs advising drivers to drive safely would be an example of the former; ads in newspapers would be an example of the latter. One reason that primary care–based counseling to prevent unintentional childhood injuries may have some positive effect is that it is integrated into a one-on-one visit with a respected professional, provides an opportunity for two-way discussion, and is usually accompanied by take-home written materials. Behavioral compliance may increase when tangible objects—for example, a thermometer to test home hot water temperatures or a smoke detector for early warning—are made available and made part of the educational effort.[18]

Education used in isolation may have limited impact, but when the same approaches are combined with other methods can have positive results.  Enforcement combined with publicity has provided an important and feasible method for increasing compliance with seatbelt use laws.[19] In one study, police enforcement at "Click It or Ticket" checkpoints combined with publicity (i.e., posters, pamphlets) and education (i.e., proper restraint demonstrations for parents and direct education with children) resulted in short-term gains in proper restraint use.[20] Education plus legislative efforts have been a successful combination in promoting bicycle helmet use, with  one study documenting a 47% increase in use one year after legislation enactment plus implementation of an education program. This is compared to an increased use of 19% and 4% in control communities with legislation only.[21,22] Another study analyzed 43 studies of seatbelt use campaigns according to intervention approach—i.e., law enforcement (state-specific laws, policies, and enforcement practices, such as warnings and fines), education (presentations, films, and discussions that provided information directly in a formal setting), incentives (immediate and delayed rewards, such as raffle tickets, merchandise coupons, and prizes for individuals or groups), monitoring (information provided along with notice that seatbelt use would be monitored), and prompts (posters, dashboard stickers, payroll stuffers). The maximum increase in safety belt use occurred with a program that combined incentives and law enforcement approaches.[23]

Perhaps the question should not be what health education *is* but rather what health education *does*. Are there key components of any promising injury prevention educational strategy? Larry Cohen, formerly with the Contra Costa County Health Services Prevention Program, California, suggests a *spectrum of prevention*, a six-part strategy that can provide a more integrated response to the problem of injury. It uses health education activities for both individual and environmental change. The spectrum includes[24]

1. Strengthening individual knowledge and skills, an approach best exemplified by one-on-one counseling, which is the traditional method health practitioners use to encourage changes in behavior and reinforce positive health practices. This can be undertaken as anticipatory guidance or as follow-up to an injury event.

2. Promoting community education to raise awareness through traditional, albeit often ineffective in isolation, approaches such as billboards with a health education message, brochures, dissemination of literature, media publicity, and media portrayal of safe practices such as wearing a helmut when riding a bicycle.

3. Educating providers of community services, a training-of-trainers approach to reinforcing injury prevention messages in a variety of settings or to developing advocates with more skills in prevention. For example, physicians need to understand their role in injury prevention vis-à-vis clinical practice, community education, and public policy and receive specific training on dealing with suspected cases of domestic violence or screening all patients for domestic violence. In a more unusual example, California radio traffic reporters participated in an invitational luncheon conference that focused on changes in seatbelt and bicycle helmet laws. This was a very effective method to get them to include health education messages and law changes in their "sky high" reporting.

4. Fostering coalitions and networks, a more coordinated approach where groups of community people work together to identify common goals, mobilize resources, and develop and implement solutions to injury problems.[25] At the state level, these often occur as task forces working on a particular injury problem. But the idea is to garner a broader base of support. For example, this would include bicycle helmet manufacturers and bike shop owners if a helmet initiative were being developed.

5. Changing organizational practices to improve health and the environment in public agencies and private industry. For example, in the United States young adolescents often ride bicycles to deliver local newspapers. The employing agency provides orientation on keeping papers dry, collecting money on a weekly basis, and dealing with stray dogs, while safe bicycling practices are overlooked. The deaths

of two local carriers finally made one newspaper chain consider including such orientation and making bicycle helmets and a balanced load standard practices. Similarly, to facilitate safer transportation to school, schools should provide lockers to store bicycle helmets during the school day.

6. Influencing policy and legislation, especially among regulatory agencies. Although this approach takes longer to establish, it can have the greatest impact. Examples might include passing zoning restrictions on selling alcoholic beverages at gas stations or near schools or influencing medical education by demanding more education and training on injury control. Determining how to gain the support of those in a position to influence policy is seldom easy (see Chapter 14).

Our health education efforts need to evolve from focusing on the first three parts of this spectrum to making a commitment to parts four through six, which seem to present the greatest opportunities for injury prevention. Used together, the combined spectrum allows for interaction, reinforcement, and complementary practices. The spectrum of prevention is a tool for programmatic integration, one that can be enhanced by following Bergman's recommendations and drawing on Rosenstock, that whatever approach is used, it build on the individual's perception of susceptibility, seriousness, benefits of taking action, and barriers to action.[26]

In addition to the educational approaches, mediums, and methods mentioned so far, two other avenues of health education should be mentioned. The first is *home visitation,* which is a proven intervention for reducing child abuse and the lifetime chain of violence it can precipitate. Education during such visits can improve parenting skills, which may also lead to a reduction in unintentional injuries. Home safety and safety equipment checks—which have worked well in Philadelphia—could also be made an integral part of any home visitation program.[27,28] For example, social marketing concepts and tools provide a means to enhance the effectiveness of educational strategies by involving injury prevention professionals and the community in an "exchange" process rather than a "word from on high" approach. (This is akin to the empowerment model mentioned earlier.)

The second method is through the *school system.* Schools, however, may provide a problematic setting for injury prevention education. There would seem to be a role for the schools in reducing both unintentional and intentional injuries. As Green points out, "there appears to be some disappointment with the [intervention] outcomes."[6] School-based efforts aimed at reducing teenage pregnancies, drug and alcohol abuse, and overall injury rates have not succeeded. Moreover, drivers' education has been shown to actually be counterproductive when it facilitates licensing of drivers at a younger age.[29] On the other hand, recent efforts to integrate conflict resolution and "No Bullying" curricula have met with some success (see Chapter 5).[30]

Academic instruction about injury prevention is supported by the *Healthy People 2000* national health objectives and the National Health Education Standards. The latter provide that "students will demonstrate the ability to practice health-enforcing behaviors and reduce health risks." School-based curricula devoted to injury and violence prevention are evident throughout our nation's schools. A recent study found that 61% of all U.S. school districts require conflict resolution/violence prevention be taught in required courses, that 74% of school districts require injury prevention and safety be taught in required courses, and that 67% of districts require suicide prevention be taught in required courses.[31] Yet, while we know that these topics are required to be taught, we do not have adequate information about the quality of existing curricula, the types of materials used, the frequency in which these topics are taught, or the proportion of students reached. The quality, comprehensiveness, and effectiveness of injury and violence prevention curricula have just not been well studied. A recent task force report from the American School Health Association recommends that "existing curricula should be compiled, reviewed by experts and consumers, evaluated and revised to ensure that they utilize current health education theoretical models and are consistent with the National Health Education Standards and the goals of *Healthy People 2000*."[32] The report also suggests that components of a model injury prevention curriculum should be defined.

Green argues that to be effective, school-based health education programs must be focused on end points (i.e., health outcomes) that address the primary function of schools, education.[6] This may explain why some of the violence prevention efforts have had some success, as schools struggle to reduce violence as an impediment to education. For example, a recent review by an expert panel has identified nine critical elements of a promising violence prevention program. Promising programs begin in the primary grades and are reinforced across grade levels, are developmentally tailored, cover appropriate content, and provide teacher training.[33]

But the fact remains that few school-based health education efforts have been adequately evaluated. Such evaluation is necessary to identify and replicate those approaches that truly do work to reduce injury. And we need to remember that curricula need not be the only component of school-based injury prevention, and that the model that the school system sets in dealing with the risk of injury can have a profound effect on students.

Whatever method, medium, or strategy used, injury prevention education must take into account ethnic, cultural, geographic, and class differences. Julian Waller notes, for example, that families in the lower socioeconomic levels may be:

> immune to middle-class modes of communication, such as pamphlets, community campaigns, group discussions, and school-oriented check lists, which have been conceived and developed by middle-class professionals who make ethnocentric assumptions about the information sources of people at other socioeconomic levels.[34(p288)]

Partnerships with community-based support services and organizations, youth centers, street outreach programs, churches, and neighborhood businesses may be vital to development of a successful education strategy.

## EVALUATING RESULTS

Education has gotten something of a bad name in the injury prevention field because of its earlier use in isolation from other prevention strategies, its sole focus on media-based information campaigns, and its application in poorly designed intervention programs that were bound to fail. Rather than view education, passive environmental protections, and legislation as being complementary to one another, many in the injury prevention field came to view educational strategies as ineffective diversions. As a result, there emerged what Michael Roberts refers to as "interdisciplinary antagonism." Roberts notes that "not all people in the field of public health adamantly hold to the passive structural position, nor do psychologists blindly assert that their contributions to health and safety are the only viable ones, but the potential for professional antagonism remains."[35] It is critical that the public health community rise above such antagonism and promote education as an essential component of injury prevention and an important complement to other prevention strategies.

In recent years many of the assumptions underlying educational strategies to reduce injuries have been put to the test of evaluation studies. The assessment that has emerged is a mixed one: some strategies have shown a positive effect, many have not, and a few have actually been shown to increase injury rates.[36] As one discussion of the issue put it: "To educate or not to educate: Is that the question?"[37]

Towner, in the course of advocating a broader view of injury prevention education, quotes several critics,[9] including Stone, who has suggested that:

> an inverse proportion law operates, with preventive activities receiving official support in inverse proportion to their effectiveness. "Socio-environmental change is costly, radical and unpredictable" and is consequently unattractive to politicians, in contrast to health education, which is, "cheap, generally uncontroversial and safe." Roberts *et al* support this viewpoint: "It is unclear what part, if any, educational health promotion messages have played in the reduction of accidents", as does Sibert: "The evidence that these [educational campaigns] are effective is unconvincing" and in most cases, effective solutions "involve environmental changes."[38(pp890–891),39,40]

Efforts to scientifically evaluate the results of office-based counseling have improved. By 1993 it was possible for a panel representing the American Academy of Pediatrics (AAP) to conclude, based on a critical review of the scientific literature, that in the appropriate circumstances primary care–based counseling to prevent childhood unintentional injuries can be effective. The panel observed that:

> Injury prevention efforts such as legislation that provides automatic, passive protections are most effective and are essential to public health efforts to reduce injuries. However, legislation and passive devices often need educational reinforcement. For some injuries, passive strategies are not available and behavioral change through pediatric counseling is the only practical approach.[41]

Studies demonstrating a positive effect of counseling on childhood injury prevention behaviors are now available for a number of hazards, including car seat use, smoke detector purchase, tap water temperature reduction, fall reduction, syrup of ipecac availability, safe home environment knowledge, and poison prevention strategies. Car seats provide a good example of how the "three Es" are complementary. Mandatory child restraint laws will be of limited value unless parents are persuaded that restraint systems make sense. And compliance with these laws needs to be appropriate compliance. Technology has developed better and better infant safety restraints, but the current technology requires education for correct installation and use. Currently the rates of usage are high, but misuse is also high, more than 50%.

## CONCLUSION

What is the current view of educational approaches to injury prevention? At the risk of overgeneralizing, several observations can be made. Once the dominant approach to injury prevention, health education lost favor. Now the pendulum seems to have settled at a middle ground. While legislative and passive approaches may be viewed as being the most effective ways to reduce injury, educational strategies are also seen as playing an important role, particularly in laying the foundation for all injury prevention approaches. Thus, injury prevention laws will not be enacted unless a base of popular support has been developed for them, nor will they be enforced without the support of police and other authorities (see Chapters 9 and 14). And injury prevention laws will not work if their requirements are too dissonant from popular norms and beliefs.[3(p133)]

Clearly more needs to be done to evaluate the impact of educational strategies, but in the meantime we cannot afford to abandon any approaches to reducing injury unless clearly counterproductive. The AAP panel "identified some positive outcomes in most of the published studies. A plausible theoretical mechanism, which supports these positive findings [is that] given the strong motivation that parents have to protect their children from hazards, pertinent education for parents concerned about protecting their children can be expected to have a positive effect on outcomes."[41(p549)]

The debate over the value of injury prevention educational strategies will continue, which is in itself a helpful thing. By evaluating the effectiveness of past educational programs, integrating newer techniques—such as social marketing  into future programs, and integrating all educational efforts into a comprehensive approach to injury prevention, the role of education in injury prevention can only be strengthened.

## NOTES

1. Committee on Trauma Research, Commission on Life Sciences, National Research Council and Institute of Medicine. *Injury in America: A Continuing Public Health Problem.* Washington, DC: National Academy Press; 1985.

2. Pless IB, Arsenault L. The role of health education in the prevention of injuries to children. *J Soc Issues.* 1987;43:87–103.

3. Robertson LS. *Injuries: Causes, Control Strategies, and Public Policy.* Lexington, MA: Lexington Books; 1983.

4. Prochaska JO, Norcross JC, DiClemente CC. *Changing for Good.* New York: William Morrow; 1994.

5. S. Bredekamp C. Copple, eds. *Developmentally Appropriate Practice in Early Childhood Programs.* Washington, DC: National Association for the Education of Young Children; 1997.

6. Green LW. Prevention and health education. In: Last JM, Wallace RB. *Maxcy-Rosenau-Last: Public Health and Preventive Medicine.* 13th ed. Norwalk, CT: Appleton & Lange; 1992: 787–802.

7. Andreasen, AR. *Marketing Social Change: Changing Behavior To Promote Health, Social Development, and the Environment.* San Francisco: Josssey-Bass; 1995.

8. Health Canada maintains a social marketing Web site at http://www.hc-sc.gc.ca/socialmarketing.

9. Towner EML. The role of health education in childhood injury prevention. *Inj Prev.* 1995;1:53–58.

10. Reisinger KS, Bires BA. Anticipatory guidance in pediatric practice. *Pediatrics.* 1980;66:889–892.

11. Bergman AB. Use of education in preventing injuries. *Pediatr Clin North Am.* 1982:29:331–338.

12. U.S. Preventive Services Task Force. *Guide to Clinical Preventive Services.* Baltimore, MD: Williams & Wilkins; 1989.

13. American Medical Association, Department of Adolescent Health. *Guidelines for Adolescent Preventive Services.* Chicago: American Medical Association; 1992.

14. National Center for Education in Maternal and Child Health. *Bright Futures: National Guidelines for Health Supervision of Infants, Children, and Adolescents.* Arlington, VA: Maternal and Child Health Bureau; 1993.

15. Gelen AC, McDonald EM, Forrest CB, et al. Injury prevention counseling in an urban pediatric clinic. *Arch Pediatr Adolesc Med.* 1997;151:146–151.

16. Miller TR, Galbraith M. Injury prevention counseling by pediatricians: A benefit-cost comparison. *Pediatrics.* 1995;96:1–4.

17. *Publicity and Advocacy for Injury Prevention.* Newton, MA: Education Development Center; 1988.

18. Katcher ML. Efforts to prevent burns from hot tap water. In: Bergman AB. *Political Approaches to Injury Control at the State Level.* Seattle: University of Washington Press; 1992:72.

19. Williams AF, Lund AK, Preusser D, Blomberg RD. Results of a seat belt use law enforcement and publicity campaign in Elmira, New York. *Accident Analysis Prev.* 1987;19:243–249.

20. William AF, Wells JK, Ferguson SA. Development and evaluation of programs to increase proper child restraint use. *J Safety Res.* 1997;28:197–202.

21. Cote TR, Sacks JJ, Lambert-Hubert DA, et al. Bicycle helmet use among Maryland children: Effect of legislation and education. *Pediatrics.* 1992;89:1216–1220.

22. MacKnin M, VangerBrieg S. Association between bicycle helmet legislation, bicycle safety education, and use of bicycle helmets in children. *Arch Pediatr Adolesc Med.* 1994;148:255–259.

23. Johnston JJ, Hendricks SA, Fike JM. Effectiveness of behavioral safety belt interventions. *Accident Analysis Prev.* 1994;26:315–323.

24. Gallagher, S. Health Education—Beyond Brochures, Injury Prevention: What Works Conference, London, 1995.

25. Hingson R, McGovern T, Howland J, Heeren T, Winter M, Zakocs R. Reducing alcohol-impaired driving in Massachusetts: The Saving Lives Program. *Am J Public Health.* 1996;86:791–797.

26. Rosenstock, IM. Why people use health services. *Milbank Memorial Fund Q.* 1966;44(Part 2):94.

27. *Home Visiting: A Promising Early Intervention Strategy for At-Risk Families.* Washington, DC: U.S. General Accounting Office; 1990.

28. Olds D, Henderson C, Chamberlin R, and Tatelbaum R. Preventing child abuse and neglect: A randomized trial of nurse home visitation. *Pediatrics.* 1986;78:65–78.

29. Robertson LS, Zador PL. Driver education and crash involvement of teenaged drivers. *Am J Public Health.* 1978;68:959–965.

30. Grossman DC, Neckerman HJ, Koepsell TD, et al. Effectiveness of a violence prevention curriculum among children in elementary school: A randomized controlled trial. *JAMA.* 1997;277:1605–1611.

31. Collins JL, Small ML, Kann L, Pateman BC, Gold RS, Kolbe LJ. School health education. *J Sch Health.* 1995;65:302–311.

32. Injury Prevention Task Force of the American School Health Association. *Report of the National Injury Prevention Task Force.* Kent, OH: American School Health Association; 1998.

33. Dusenbury L, Falco M, Lake A, Brannigan R, Bosworth K. Nine critical elements of promising violence prevention programs. *J Sch Health.* 1997;67:409–414.

34. Waller JA. *Injury Control: A Guide to the Causes and Prevention of Trauma.* Lexington, MA: Lexington Books; 1985.

35. Roberts MC. Public health and health psychology: Two cats of Kilkenny? *Professional Psychol Res Pract.* 1987;18:145–149.

36. Robertson LS. *Injury Epidemiology.* New York: Oxford University Press: 1992: 112–119.

37. Green LW. To educate or not to educate: Is that the question? *Am J Public Health.* 1980;70:625–626.

38. Stone D. Upside down prevention. *Health Serv J.* 1989;99:890–891.

39. Roberts H, Smith S, Bryce C. Prevention is better. . . . *Sociol Health Illness.* 1993;15:447–463.

40. Sibert JR. Accidents to children: The doctor's role. Education or environmental change. *Arch Dis Child.* 1991;66:890–893.

41. Bass JL, Christoffel KK, Widome M, et al. Childhood injury prevention counseling in primary care settings: A critical review of the literature. *Pediatrics.* 1993;92:544–550.

# CHAPTER 8

# Injury Prevention: Environmental Modification

"Poverty, unemployment, dangerous working conditions, bad housing, overcrowding, and a poor environment all make [injuries] more likely."

Allison Quick, *Unequal Risks*, 1991

## WHAT THIS CHAPTER IS ABOUT

Educating the public about risks and how to avoid them—the subject of the previous chapter—is a time-honored public health approach. "Practice safe sex." "Don't smoke." "Don't share needles." "Buckle your seatbelt." These are important public health messages, but they have their limits. It is difficult to change attitudes and behaviors, particularly among high-risk groups; therefore, public health attempts other approaches to reducing risk as well. One such approach is to enact laws. Another—the subject of this chapter—is to modify the environment to make behavior change easier or, better yet, to make behavior change unnecessary by providing automatic or passive protections.

This chapter will look at how changes in physical surroundings and product designs can reduce injury risk. This is a critical part of injury prevention (*Injury in America*[1] identified it as the "most effective" approach) but it may seem somewhat remote to a public health audience. After all, what role can public health professionals play in re-engineering the environment? The answer is that they can play an important role, and this chapter will conclude with a discussion of that role.

## INTRODUCTION

Injury avoidance behaviors can be demanding on the individual. For example, parents must be convinced that car restraints are important to the well-being of their child. They must acquire a child safety seat. They must use the child safety seat. They must use the child safety seat correctly. And they must do so every time they transport the child, over and over again, regardless of complaints, difficulties, and need to make haste. That this happens at all may seem a wonder. That it happens with some frequency is in large part a tribute to the public health and safety community.

The primary limit on health behavior education is that success depends on effort and action by the target audience. The more effort required on the part of the individual, the less successful the educational (or legal) approach is likely to be. The authors of *Injury in America* proposed that: "Injuries can be prevented with a variety of strategies. The effectiveness of these strategies varies inversely with the extra effort required to keep people from being harmed and the degree to which people must change their usual behavior patterns."[1(p7)]

Thus educational efforts alone would seem to have their limits. Both educational and legal approaches to modifying human behavior take an injurious environment as a given and seek to accommodate human actions to that injurious environment. But focusing on education tends to unduly stress the human component of injury and the pre-event phase of the injury occurrence. Environmental modification provides an entirely different, but complementary, approach to injury prevention.

What do we mean by "environmental modification?" Environment is used here in the broadest sense, to include physical surroundings (such as highway layout and construction) as well as specific mechanisms for injury (such as automobile design features) and, finally, the social environment (such as attitudes toward drinking and driving). Environmental modification rather than engineering is used to encompass the broad range of possible interventions, ranging from product design to social attitudes.

Environmental modifications are premised on the assumption that humans can alter and control their surroundings to make them less hazardous. This is hardly a startling insight, although it is too frequently ignored (as, for example, in the case of firearm design and accessibility). It is especially nonstartling given that most of the injury risk we encounter has been created by humans in the first place. As Leon Robertson notes, "The vast majority of injurious human contact with energy . . . is the result of human use and alteration of that energy, usually in ways that increase its concentration at points where it is likely to do harm in contact with human beings."[2(p139)] Motor vehicles, firearms, occupational settings, poisonous chemicals, stairs, house fires, infant furniture, and playground equipment all are factors in major categories of injury and all involve human creations. And what humans create they can re-create.

## MODIFYING THE ENVIRONMENT

"On the Escape of Tigers" is the title of a now-classic 1970 essay on injury prevention by William Haddon, Jr. As Haddon explained, human injuries result from the dangerous, uncontrolled transfer of energy in such ways and amounts, and at such rapid rates, that inanimate or animate structures are damaged. Haddon pointed out that an escaped tiger can be viewed as a dangerous, uncontrolled accumulation of energy, energy that can cause severe harm—including death—to any living creature unfortunate enough to come in contact with the beast. It is this high potential for sudden, uncontrolled, and destructive energy release that leads society to take extreme care to keep people separated from tigers: either by not having them around at all or else by keeping them securely confined. Our injury prevention approach is not one of educating the public on how to safely deal with escaped tigers.

Unfortunately the same logic is not always applied to more common injury risks. Controlling the physical and social environments to control injury risk should be the starting point for thinking about injury prevention. But as Robertson notes:

> Too often these factors are neglected. For example, early studies of injuries from all-terrain vehicles focused primarily on variations in user characteristics—age, sex, height, weight, alcohol use, use of helmets, gloves, goggles, or boots—and certain circumstances such as number of riders, setting, terrain, estimated speed, maneuver, and type of crash (hit object, overturned, etc.). Variations in potential effects of stability of the vehicles, maximum speed capability, exposed moving parts, and seating allowing passengers were not examined.[3(p169-170)]

The same logic of tiger control should apply to all other types of injury: the best injury prevention approach is for society to take extreme care to keep people separated from destructive energy release and to minimize whatever unwanted energy release does occur. A good example is the concept of automobile "crashworthiness." Safety advocates argued for decades that automobiles could and should be built to afford occupants optimal conditions for withstanding a crash. And yet the conventional wisdom well into the 1960s was that automobiles were designed to transport people, that a crash was the result of driver error having nothing to do with automobile design, and that if a crash occurred injury was inevitable. (Following this logic it would be acceptable for automobile manufacturers to market automobiles made out of glass as long as they handled well.) Today the situation is dramatically different. Not only do federal laws require various "crashworthy" design features (such as nonshattering windshields), but failure to design for crash survivability can be negligence on the part of the manufacturer. Exhibit 8–1 describes the potential in this approach.

The concern for a more safety-friendly environment extends well beyond crashworthy vehicles. No longer do we accept as given that swimming pools must be "attractive nuisances" beckoning to toddlers, that factories must mean "enter-at-your-own-risk" peril, or that homes must contain an assortment of injury-producing booby-traps. The Committee on Trauma Research concluded that:

> The most successful injury-prevention approaches have involved improved product designs and changes in the man-made environment that will protect everyone. Such built-in or automatic protection, now taken for granted in insulated electric hand tools and household fuses, is gradually gaining acceptance in other realms, because of its great potential for preventing deaths and injuries.[1(p40)]

There has been a growing recognition that the developmental factors that limit a child's ability to deal with the injury environment are a reason for modifying that environment rather than a cause for blaming the child's (or the parents') injury-avoiding inadequacies.[4] And "[s]ome product and environmental changes achieve important changes in behavior. For example, experimental equipping of fleets of vehicles with high-mounted brake lights substantially reduced the incidence of rear-end crashes."[1(p41)]

## EXAMPLES

It is possible to envision an environment with fewer hazards and one with more forgiving injury points. All that is required is the ability to see

**Exhibit 8–1** The Story of the Research Safety Vehicle

During the 1970s the U.S. Department of Transportation funded the development of a prototype automobile known as the "Research Safety Vehicle." Using "off-the-shelf" technology, a compact-sized passenger vehicle was built incorporating all the then-current safety technology, such as airbags, padded dashboards, reinforced side doors, considerable "crush space" between the front of the vehicle and the passenger compartment, and the latest in crash-avoidance technology. The resulting vehicle was one in which occupants had a high chance of surviving a 50-mile-per-hour crash with minimal or no injury. It was a vehicle that provided the styling and comfort preferred by the public. And it was a vehicle that the Department estimated could, if mass produced, be priced competitively with other compact cars then on the market. The Research Safety Vehicle toured the country and began to generate some public interest. But with the advent of the Reagan administration in 1981, the project was put in limbo and no manufacturer ever chose to emulate the vehicle.

the status quo as unacceptable and the creativity to visualize a better state of affairs. It then becomes possible to contemplate ways in which a less hazardous environment can be created. The fact is that—to modify an old saying of public health—a society can have any level of safety it is willing to pay for. The Haddon Ten countermeasures, which were discussed in Chapters 2 and 6, emphasize the primacy of environmental approaches to injury prevention in working towards such a goal. The number of ways in which these injury prevention countermeasures can be applied to re-engineer the environment for greater safety is virtually infinite. Exhibit 8–2 outlines ways in which these potential environmental modifications can be categorized. Robertson notes that:

Manufacturers of products and builders of roads, housing, and other structures, have the opportunity to modify their products to reduce the incidence and severity of injurious energy exchanges. The vast majority of serious injuries originate with use of the products of industry and builders in everyday or frequent use: among them, motor vehicles, road characteristics, guns, agricultural and industrial machines, stairs, cigarettes, matches, propane lighters, stoves and space heaters, clothing, bedding, swimming pools, and watercraft.[3(p167)]

**Exhibit 8–2**  Modifying the Physical and Social Environments

- Minimize or eliminate the need for the potential hazard
- Design safer physical surroundings
- Design safer consumer products
- Redesign operating protocols and practices
- Change social attitudes

One approach to a safer environment is to minimize or eliminate the need for risk-producing surroundings or conditions. An example would be to encourage the use of mass transit so that motor vehicle use and its attendant greater hazards are reduced. Environmental modifications such as bicycle racks at subway stations and bicycle carriers on buses would also help encourage mass transit use. Another example of this approach would be reducing residential fires by greatly curtailing smoking through heavy taxes on cigarettes. *These measures are not dependent on actions by those being protected; they simply remove or lower the injury risk from the environment.*

Another environmental approach to injury prevention is to design safer physical surroundings, so that injury events will not occur, and, when injury events do occur, the consequences are not as severe. Roadways can be designed not only to minimize the occurrence of crashes by simplifying the driving task, but also to reduce the severity of crashes that do occur by minimizing roadside hazards such as rigid signposts and bridge abutments; it should not and need not be the case that when a vehicle veers off the roadway—even at high speeds—that injury is an inevitable result. Motor vehicle traffic can be separated from bicycle and pedestrian traffic by means of bike paths and lanes, pedestrian walkways, and overpasses and underpasses—and from oncoming motor vehicles with medians.

Fencing around all four sides of swimming pool areas, with locked access points, can keep young children from falling or jumping into swimming pools. Antislip surfaces and adequate hand supports can reduce the number of bathtub falls. Improved stairway lighting can reduce the incidence of falls, as can improved stair tread design. The installation of window guards in high-rise buildings has greatly reduced fall deaths by young children. Impact-absorbing playground surfaces and detachable, break-away baseball bases create more forgiving environments for children at play. Airbags can be installed in motor vehicles to redistribute the energy release of crashes in time and space. *All of these are injury reduction measures that are not dependent on actions by those being protected; they do not require behavior changes, they do not require constant vigilance, they are passive, automatic, and constant in their protective effects.*

Another design approach to injury prevention focuses specifically on consumer products, which also can be designed with injury reduction in mind. In recent years lawnmowers, chain saws, hair dryers, and many other consumer items have been redesigned to reduce what had been classic injuries associated with each. For example, "deadman" brakes on lawnmower blades have made it almost impossible for operators to lose feet and hands while operating the mower, a goal that education and common sense had not been able to achieve. Childproof caps on pharmaceuticals and child-resistant packaging on other toxic household products have greatly reduced childhood poisonings. Closely placed slats on cribs have virtually eliminated strangulation deaths of youngsters whose heads would get caught in wider slat openings. Special flame-resistant sleepwear for children, automatic shut-offs on space heaters that tip over, and child-resistant cigarette lighters have eliminated significant sources of tragic fire injuries. The addition of safety straps on products such as changing tables, high chairs, and shopping carts have contributed to a reduction in falls by infants and toddlers. And universal application of anti-scald plumbing fixtures has the potential to greatly reduce scald burns from tap water.

Three technically feasible product design features with great potential to reduce injuries have so far not been adopted by the industries involved

- "personalized" handguns that can only be fired by their legal owner (see Exhibit 8–3)
- "fire-safe" cigarettes that will not ignite furniture if left unattended
- sports utility vehicles, pickup trucks, and mini-vans redesigned to reduce their overall weight and height to make them less hazardous to the occupants of other vehicles.

*Again, these are injury reduction measures that are not dependent on actions by those being protected; they do not require behavior changes, they do not require constant vigilance, they are passive, automatic, and constant in their protective effects.*

Another way in which environmental factors can be modified to minimize injury is to redesign the way in which things are done by implement-

**Exhibit 8–3**  The "Personalized" Handgun

> A personalized handgun is designed so it can be fired only by an authorized user. The gun uses radio frequency technology, with the authorized user wearing a tiny transponder (often located in a finger ring) that communicates with an antenna in the gun's grip to authorize operation. Without the transponder in close proximity to the gun, it will not fire. The technology making personalized guns possible has existed for several years, with the first patents granted in 1976. Costs of such guns would not be prohibitive.
>
> Obviously this design feature will not end all gun violence. But—provided the transponder ring is not kept with the gun—it would be important in keeping children from firing guns they discover in the home, would eliminate the danger of a gun being grabbed and used against its authorized user, and would make a stolen gun inoperable. Most important, it would do these things without requiring that the gun owner take any action; it would not require behavior changes and constant vigilance. The personalized handgun provides a safety feature that is passive, automatic, and constant in its protective effects.
>
> So why aren't such guns flooding the market? It is hoped that at least some manufacturers—such as Colt—will soon be marketing them.

ing operating protocols and practices for various systems. Traffic patterns can be improved. This could include "traffic-calming" initiatives[5] such as speed bumps and roundabouts. Traffic patterns can also be modified to provide longer walk-light timing at crossings where elderly pedestrians are common or longer amber-light timing to reduce vehicle crashes; right-turn-on-red can be eliminated in high-pedestrian or bicycle use areas. Hot water heaters can be set at lower temperatures as they leave the factory. Work rules can be changed so that the pace or manner of factory or other job sites operation does not make it impossible to observe safety precautions. Well-lit streets and areas may provide some increased protection from sexual and other physical assaults, as may better placement of bus stops, ATMs, and the like. The adoption of universal child restraint attachment systems (thereby bypassing the adult restraint systems, which vary by auto manufacturer) could reduce incorrect restraint usage. *Yet again, all of these are injury reduction measures that are not dependent on actions by those being protected; they do not require behavior changes, they do not require constant vigilance, they are passive, automatic, and constant in their protective effects.*

Another way in which environmental factors can be modified is to change aspects of the social environment that contribute to the likelihood of injury. The social acceptability of drunk driving, of drive-through liquor purchases, of intimate partner violence, or of exceeding the speed limit, all provide an environment within which it is relatively easier for persons to engage in those practices. But norms of social acceptability can be changed. For example, by no longer making alcohol an acceptable part of office parties, sports events, or college campus fraternities, an environment is created that makes it harder for those who would overindulge in such settings to do so. Conversely, the current social attitudes toward gun availability and toward television violence provide a social context that makes it easier for those who would commit gun violence to do so. Changing the social environment is often an important part of the introduction of new injury prevention technology and equipment. For example, the development of sport safety gear such as helmets, elbow and knee pads, protective eyewear, or personal flotation devices will lead to reductions in injury only if those items are used. A task for injury prevention professionals is to help make people aware of such protective equipment and to help change the social environment to make use both acceptable and routine. (Exhibit 8–4 offers an example of one such area in which product design and social environmental factors need to work hand in hand.) *Even this area of social environmental factors involves injury reduction measures that are not dependent on actions by those being protected; they do not require changes in individual attitudes, they do not require constant individual vigilance, they are passive, automatic, and constant in their protective effects.* Although they can be circumvented by those determined to do so, they make it harder for anyone to do so.

Do these environmental modifications actually work to reduce injuries? Many of the interventions to reduce injury have been evaluated and many have been shown to be effective, which is why there is such strong support within the injury prevention community for this approach.[1,6] But despite the documented successes, there is need for much more evaluation to determine what works and what doesn't. Robertson argues that:

> Well-designed epidemiological studies can reveal the injuries associated with the characteristics of products and environments.

**Exhibit 8–4** Reducing Baseball Injuries

Baseball, softball, and tee-ball are among the most popular sports for youth. In a population-based study of injuries to children and youth, baseball accounted for 9% of all sports-related injuries requiring emergency room treatment or hospital admission. The most common body parts injured were lower limb (29.7%), finger (26.2%), upper limb (13.6%), face (10.4%), head (2%), and chest (1.4%). More than a third of these injuries were associated with a product such as a baseball, bat, base, or fence. Among the 862 cases identified, 3.5% required hospital admission (i.e., one out of every 29 children with a baseball injury was hospitalized.[a]) An analysis of 88 baseball-related deaths to children ages 5–14 showed that ball impact to the chest was the most frequent cause of death (43%) followed by ball impact to the head (24%). Another 15% died from being hit by a bat. The same study also indicated an estimated 404,364 baseball-related injuries were treated in hospital emergency departments during 1994.[b]

There are many different types of safety equipment on the market to prevent injuries in baseball. None are mandatory. These include reduced injury factor baseballs with a softer than standard core (price comparable to standard balls), face guards for batting helmets (about $10 each), chest protector vests, and safety release bases that leave no holes in the ground or parts of the base sticking up in order to reduce sliding injuries ($300 to $595 compared with $150 for a standard set of bases, but they tend to outlast regular bases and are portable rather than permanent).

In 1996 the Consumer Product Safety Commission commissioned an independent expert review panel to analyze the published scientific literature on protective sports equipment. This study found that the use of softer than standard baseballs, age- and sex-graded safety bases, and batting helmet face guards could reduce the number and severity of more than one third of baseball-related injuries to children each year. Only the effectiveness of chest protectors in reducing injuries could not be determined.[b] The American Academy of Pediatrics has also developed environmental injury prevention recommendations for ball sports. They include elimination of the on-deck circle, protective fencing of dugouts and benches, protective equipment that is sized appropriately, and the use of polycarbonate eye protectors on batting helmets.[c]

The critical issue here is getting the routine use of protective equipment and other environmental strategies put in place. This is where public health professionals can make a difference, working with parents, coaches, youth

*continues*

**Exhibit 8–4**  continued

organizations, and youth themselves to make them aware of such options and to change the social environment to make it acceptable to use such protective equipment. Insurers should also be drawn into the process.

ᵃSchuster M, Gallagher SS. Baseball related injuries among children. Boston: Massachusetts Department of Public Health, 1991, unpublished.
ᵇKyle SB, Adler P, Monticone RC. Reducing youth baseball injuries with protective equipment. *Consumer Product Safety Review.* 1996; 1:1–5.
ᶜCommittee on Sports Medicine and Fitness, American Academy of Pediatrics. Risk of injury from baseball and softball in children 5–14 years of age. *Pediatrics.* 1994: 93(4):690–692.

They can also aid in the evaluation of the effectiveness of modifications of products, protective equipment, and environments in injury control.[3(p167)]

Kraus and Robertson also note that using epidemiological studies to evaluate environmental interventions can help set priorities by concentrating attention on those interventions that are most cost-effective.[6(p1031)]

## THE ROLE OF PUBLIC HEALTH PROFESSIONALS

From a public health perspective, an environmental approach to injury prevention has clear advantages. First, it is an approach aimed at protecting everyone. Rather than having to reach potential victims with injury prevention messages, the risk itself is targeted. Second, the environmental approach results in built-in, or "automatic," protection. People do not have to take action in order to reduce injury risk.

Much of the work involved in creating safer environments involves engineers and planners, architects and builders. Can public health professionals also play a role in re-engineering the environment? The answer is that they can indeed, and an important role at that. Public health practitioners and the agencies in which they work can educate architects, designers, industry, retailers, the media, and other entities that can affect the safety environment. They can develop and circulate voluntary standards and protocols. They can identify environmental hazards and risks and share this information widely. They can assist in the development of community coalitions to create and advocate for environmental modifications. They can develop information and programs aimed at particular injury factors such as alcohol and firearms. And they can assist other agencies of government to recognize the injury implications of the work they do.

There are a variety of local, state, and federal agencies—along with nongovernmental agencies—involved in whole or part in efforts to make the environment less a source of injury hazards. On the local level this includes zoning boards, police and fire departments, sanitarians, alcohol control agencies, school health programs, traffic engineers, and the like. At the state level this includes highway safety and law enforcement, departments of motor vehicles, occupational safety and health agencies, day care licensing agencies, and the like. (Exhibit 8–5 provides a discussion of the potential role of public health professionals in encouraging safer out-of-home child care environments.)

At the federal level, agencies involved in environmental approaches to injury prevention include the National Highway Traffic Safety Administration, the Consumer Product Safety Commission, the Federal Aviation Administration, the Occupational Safety and Health Administration, and the Centers for Disease Control and Prevention. In most cases these agencies enforce laws enacted to reduce environmental injury hazards (the subject of the next chapter). Exhibit 8–6 lists some examples of the injury prevention statutes enforced by these agencies. In other cases, these agencies develop guidelines (or provide funding for professional organizations to develop guidelines) that can foster decreases in environmental injury hazards. For example, the Maternal and Child Health Bureau is playing a lead role in the development of health, safety, and mental health guidelines for schools. The Division of Adolescent and School Health of the Centers for Disease Control and Prevention is currently developing guidelines for injury and violence prevention within a comprehensive program of health education. And in some cases, these agencies work with industry to develop voluntary product standards. (See Exhibit 8–7.)

The role of local and state health departments should be to work with these other agencies, educating, informing, guiding, and assisting—providing data, ideas, and evaluation results.

Other entities, be they other units of government or a particular industry, have their own agendas and goals. It is obviously not a matter of telling them that you know how to do their jobs better than they do, but rather of providing useful information and perspectives to help in dealing with the

**Exhibit 8–5** Out-of-Home Child Care Standards

There are no federal regulations for out-of-home child care. Each state formulates its own regulations and criteria. Responsibility for inspecting and monitoring child care facilities varies by state. Most state agency regulatory and inspection staff will not have a public health orientation or special knowledge of children's safety and injury prevention.

The factors that contribute to injuries in child care centers may include[a]

- playground equipment: 13%
- another child involved (e.g., pushing, throwing): 12.8%
- furniture (e.g., bookshelves, chairs): 11.5%
- part of the building (e.g., radiators, glass doors): 10.7%
- vegetation (e.g., berries, trees): 8.4%
- toys: 5.2%
- fixed outdoor equipment (e.g., fence, gate): 3.1%
- bicycle: 2.5%
- sled: 2.5%
- other and unspecified: 30.5%

A 1991 national assessment of state agencies indicates that there are wide variations and gaps in the content of regulations related to safety for out of home child care.[b] Only 5 of 36 safety criteria were met by at least half of the states. Fifteen criteria were not mentioned by half of the states. For 24 of 36 criteria, more than half the states' regulations were below the criteria or failed to mention the safety topic. Given that playgrounds are the most frequent site of injuries in day care centers, it is significant that 96% of states' regulations did not mention playground surfacing. Also, 38% did not mention tap water temperature, a frequent cause of burns in young children. These figures indicate a need for attention to the development, content, and monitoring of safety regulations for child care settings. This assessment suggested that oversight of day care safety is diffuse and there is little input from injury prevention specialists.

Public health professionals can proactively contact relevant agencies to

- determine what inspection processes are used for out-of-home child care
- ascertain which environmental hazards are part of the inspection protocol
- suggest additional items to improve safety
- learn of opportunities to provide training for licensing staff

*continues*

**Exhibit 8–5** continued

- provide written safety materials for staff to give to centers
- furnish such tools as voluntary playground standards developed by the Consumer Product Safety Commission

State agency and regulatory staff also need to understand that environmental changes will be more effective than changes engendered solely through education or enforcement of regulations. Some state agencies require reporting of injuries that occur in day care settings for legal purposes, but regulatory staff seldom examine such data for prevention. Public health professionals can compile such data to look for risk patterns and feed this information back to the agency staff for their use.

National guidelines for health and safety in child care programs were jointly developed by the American Public Health Association and the American Academy of Pediatrics in 1992.[c] Public health professionals can compare their state regulations to the nationally recommended standards and then work with agencies to develop out-of-home child care standards that meet recommended practices.

[a]Sellstrom E, Bremberg S, Chang A. Injuries in Swedish day care centers. *Pediatrics* 1994; 94:1033-1036.

[b]Runyan CW, Gray DE, Kotch JB, Kreuter MW. Analysis of U.S. child care safety regulations. *Am J Public Health.* 1991; 81: 981–985.

[c]American Public Health Association and American Academy of Pediatrics. *Caring for Our Children—National Health and Safety Performance Standards: Guidelines for Out-of-Home Child Care Programs.* Washington, DC and Elk Grove Village, IL: American Public Health Association and American Academy of Pediatrics, 1992.

continuing injury problem. For example, in England a nongovernmental organization, the Childhood Injury Prevention Trust, produced materials that could assist architects in designing homes that were safer for young children, an area often neglected because it had not previously been emphasized in the training of architects. These materials were made available to architectural organizations, which could share them with their members. This kind of win-win collaboration forwarded the interests and goals of all involved. In New York State, a county health department identified the instability of commercial refuse bins as a cause of injury and death for children. The department petitioned the federal Consumer Product Safety

**Exhibit 8–6** Examples of Injury Prevention Statutes Enforced by Federal Agencies

---

- The National Highway Traffic Safety Administration, part of the U.S. Department of Transportation, promulgates motor vehicle safety standards under the authority of the National Traffic and Motor Vehicle Safety Act.
- The Occupational Safety and Health Administration, part of the U.S. Department of Labor, has authority to develop and enforce workplace safety rules under the authority of the Occupational Safety and Health Act.
- The Consumer Product Safety Commission has authority to develop and enforce standards under the Consumer Product Safety Act, the Flammable Fabrics Act, the Hazardous Substances Act, and the Poison Prevention Packaging Act.
- The Mine Safety and Health Administration administers the Federal Mine Safety and Health Act.
- The Bureau of Alcohol, Tobacco, and Firearms within the Treasury Department has some authority over the interstate commerce in firearms under the Gun Control Act of 1968 and the Handgun Violence Prevention Act (the Brady Bill).

---

Commission for a study of the problem; this ultimately resulted in design changes. The department also identified home tent fires as a source of several deaths in children and discovered that voluntary flame-retardant standards were available for tents, but were not in use in New York State. Several of the flammable tents were burned in televised demonstrations, leading to a flame-retardant tent regulation.[7]

Of course this type of collaborative effort requires effort and finesse. It will be politically more difficult to enact environmental injury prevention measures than it is to implement educational injury prevention measures because the former are likely to step on the toes of those with power (they may force action on corporations) while the latter are less intrusive of powerful interests (they usually recommend voluntary actions by individuals). As Kraus and Robertson put it, "when manufacturers resist change or continue to introduce unnecessarily hazardous products, skill in dealing with political, social, and economic issues is often required for implementation."[6(p1030)]

**Exhibit 8–7** Developing Voluntary Standards for Safer Product Design

Through its medical examiners and coroners alert system, its National Electronic Injury Surveillance System and consumer complaints, the Consumer Product Safety Commission (CPSC) identified drawstrings on children's clothing as responsible for 17 deaths and 42 nonfatal incidents. Strangulations from drawstring entanglements occurred primarily on playground slides, but also occurred from catching in school bus doors, cribs, an escalator, a fence, a farm grinder, a turn signal lever, a ski chair lift, and a tricycle.

CPSC first worked with manufacturers to try to remove catch points on playground slides and other products. Consumer alerts were issued and publicized. In 1994, CPSC later brought together representatives from manufacturers of children's clothing and provided them with the data showing that drawstrings could kill children. The industry agreed to remove drawstrings from the necks and hoods of jackets, coats, and sweatshirts, replacing them with snaps and Velcro. Through voluntary cooperation a safer product for consumers appeared in stores with the 1995 fall clothing line.

CPSC also issued voluntary guidelines advising clothing manufacturers to replace drawstrings with safer alternatives and advising parents to remove drawstrings from hoods and necks and shorten drawstrings on bottoms of clothes.

Successful redesign of products in such a short period of time and on a voluntary basis with full participation of industry is the ideal situation. Engaging manufacturers in discussions to address serious hazards is critical as is the availability of inexpensive alternatives.

When additional research and the development of new technology is needed, as was the case for building electrocution protection into handheld hair dryers, standards are delayed. Electrocutions due to hair dryer immersions have been reduced from an average of 18 per year in 1980 to 2 deaths in 1992. But the process evolved from CPSC recommendations to improve the Underwriters Laboratories standard for hair dryers, to a requirement of a pictorial warning in use and care instructions, to a label permanently attached to the cord (1980), to a requirement for a polarized attachment plug, to consumer literature to install ground fault circuit interrupters (1985), to installation of an inexpensive component to build in electrocution protection when products are immersed with the switch "off" (1987), to a requirement for similar protection in both the "on" and "off" positions (1991).

*Source:* Reprinted from *Saving Lives through Smart Government—Success Stories*, 1996, U.S. Government Product Safety Commission.

In her analysis of injury risk, Allison Quick points out that:

> Poverty, unemployment, dangerous working conditions, bad housing, overcrowding, and a poor environment all make [injuries] more likely. The risk of [injury] is one of the clearest instances of health inequality in our society.[8]

Changing these factors for the better would obviously be the most meaningful environmental intervention to reduce injury risk. Equally obvious is the fact that public health practitioners are extremely limited in the extent to which they can have any impact on these broad social factors; however, limited social policy interventions may be feasible.

Drawing on the Safe Communities effort in Sweden and elsewhere, the World Health Organization's *Manifesto for Safe Communities* suggests that:

> Governments should create environments supportive of injury prevention by reducing the hazards associated with modern amenities, such as motorized transport and manufactured products. In other words, safety should be a normal component of policies and programs for sustainable development.[9]

Under "Create Supportive Environments" the WHO Manifesto states:

> People live and work in environments that can pose unnecessary risks of accidents and injury. People use products that can be unnecessarily and often unexpectedly hazardous. . . . People who develop efforts to safeguard humans from the injurious effects of mechanical, chemical, and electrical energy must recognize that people like extremely diverse environments because this diversity enriches their lives.

> A balance must be found between the hazards and benefits of modern amenities such as motorized transportation. Those committed to safe communities must develop an approach that emphasizes consultation, negotiation, and coalition building. Strong advocates are needed to put safety and injury control high on the policy makers' agenda. Non-governmental organizations must be encouraged to endorse safety activities. The news media must assist in the public's education and in interpreting complex policy issues on safety and injury control.[9]

## CONCLUSION

We design and build most of our environment, from lawnmowers and pickup trucks to high-rise buildings and traffic interchanges. Most injury involves man-made factors: motor vehicles, highways, firearms, poisonous chemicals, swimming pools, factories, various consumer products, and the like. The environment that injures us is one that we have created. And what we have created we should be able to redesign for greater safety.

Unfortunately, it is not always quite as self-evident and straightforward as that. There are many subquestions involved in the concept of designing the environment for greater safety: Who is to be responsible? Are their actions to be voluntary or required? Can the economic marketplace play a role? What is the role for engineers, architects, and other technical experts? How widely can the concept of "crashworthiness" be applied to engineering our environment? Why is there so much opposition to safer designs for safer environments? What, if anything, can health departments do about environmental design?

Discourse in this critical area *must* involve public health practitioners. We cannot abandon the field and risk the loss of the preventive perspective. This means that public health practitioners must do more than collect and disseminate data on injury. They must network with those who will have an impact on how our physical environment affects our safety. They must show how environmental modifications are important and feasible. And they must evaluate the impact of such changes to ensure that they truly achieve their intended effect.

---

### NOTES

1. Committee on Trauma Research, Commission on Life Sciences, National Research Council and Institute of Medicine. *Injury in America: A Continuing Public Health Problem*. Washington, DC: National Academy Press; 1985.
2. Robertson LS. *Injuries: Causes, Control Strategies, and Public Policy*. Lexington, MA: Lexington Books; 1983.
3. Robertson LS. *Injury Epidemiology: Research and Control Strategies*. 2nd ed. New York: Oxford University Press; 1998.
4. See, for example, Kane DN. *Environmental Hazards to Young Children*. Phoenix: Oryx Press; 1985.

5. Stevenson MR, Sleet DA. Which prevention strategies for child pedestrian injuries? A review of the literature. *Int J Community Health Education.* 1996–1997;16:207–217.

6. See references in Kraus JF, Robertson LS. Injuries and the public health. In: Last JM, Wallace RB. *Maxcy-Rosenau-Last: Public Health and Preventive Medicine.* 13th ed. Norwalk, CT: Appleton & Lange; 1992:1021–1034.

7. Fisher L. Childhood injuries—Causes, preventive theories, and case studies. *J Environ Health.* 1988; 50:355–360.

8. Quick A. *Unequal Risks: Accidents and Social Policy.* London: Socialist Health Association; 1991.

9. World Health Organization. *Manifesto for Safe Communities. Safety—A Universal Concern and Responsibility for All.* Adopted in Stockholm, Sweden, 1989, at the first World Conference on Accident and Injury Prevention. Geneva: World Health Organization; 1989.

# CHAPTER 9

# Injury Prevention: The Role of Law

"The reach of public health law is as broad as the reach of public health itself."

Frank P. Grad, *The Public Health Law Manual*, 1990

## WHAT THIS CHAPTER IS ABOUT

Public health traditionally has relied on the law to enforce standards and promote behavior change. Injury prevention laws exist at the federal, state, and local level. What do these laws do? What gives government the authority to require safety precautions or to prohibit risky behaviors and conditions? And, most important, what role can the nonlawyer public health practitioner play in developing and applying injury prevention laws? This chapter will look at these questions to help the reader better understand law as a tool, not a barrier, in injury prevention practice.

## INTRODUCTION

Injury is a major public health problem. Law is one way to deal with this problem. The nation's courts have been consistent and strong in their support for public health laws of all types. Injury prevention laws have been no exception.

In dealing with any public health problem, governments can fund programs or enact new laws (i.e., statutory controls). Funded public health programs include screening efforts, health education, and a variety of preventive services. In each case, government provides public services that can be voluntarily accepted or rejected. Statutory controls, on the other hand, take the form of either specific statutory requirements—such as mandatory school immunization laws, seatbelt use laws, or zoning ordinances requiring the installation of fire sprinklers—or of broad regulatory programs, such as those created by the federal Consumer Product Safety Act, the National Traffic and Motor Vehicle Safety Act, and the Occupational Safety and Health Act.

Statutory and regulatory controls are usually not voluntary in nature. Public health traditionally has possessed an extensive legal armamentarium, including legal authority to isolate or quarantine, to abate nuisances and obtain other injunctive relief, to impose penal sanctions, to establish permit and license requirements, and to seize, embargo, modify, or ban dangerous items.

Courts have been quite willing to uphold compulsory public health measures, not only with respect to communicable disease but also for noncontagious health problems, such as the mandating of fluoride in public drinking water or requiring vision and hearing tests for school children. Where clear risk of disease or injury has been identified and where the proposed response is supported by relevant public health expertise, government has been afforded extensive authority to intervene in order to protect public health.

## THE NUMBER AND VARIETY OF INJURY PREVENTION LAWS

The number and variety of injury prevention laws are considerable. For example, Massachusetts alone has 124 statutes relating to the prevention of unintentional injuries to children, the majority dealing with motor vehicle, burn, and poisoning injuries. These laws are intended to do the following:

- Regulate the maximum speed capability, color, seat practices, and safety equipment in school buses (lights, mirror, markings, driver seatbelt, flares, etc.).
- License the manufacturing, ban private possession and use of, and regulate the authorized use of fireworks.
- Limit temperatures of residential hot water heaters.
- Authorize the State Burn Registry.
- Require child abuse reporting.
- Specify speed limits.
- Require that hazardous substances be packaged in containers designed to foil the attempts of small children to open them.
- Require schools to provide driver education courses.

- Regulate the design of bicycles (strength, stopping distance, markings, etc.) and "rules of the road" for bikes.
- Require swimming pools to be fenced, inaccessible to unauthorized children, drained when not in use, and inspected.
- Regulate, inspect, and require reporting of injuries on amusement park equipment, ski lifts, recreational vehicles, and camps.
- Ban the sale of air rifles to minors.
- Require all children up to 5 years of age to be restrained in a properly adjusted car seat or seatbelt while riding in a motor vehicle.
- Require that bicycle operators display specific reflective devices visible to 500 feet to the front and 600 feet to the rear when approached by a vehicle with lawful low beam headlamps.[1]

Although Massachusetts may be one of the states with the most injury prevention laws—the data is not readily available—the laws just listed typify some of the hundreds of different injury prevention laws that could be found in one or another of the 50 states. In addition, most municipalities have their own extensive array of injury prevention laws, including the important area of building codes. And the federal government has created several regulatory agencies charged with implementing injury prevention statutes, most notably those dealing with motor vehicles, consumer products, food and drugs, and occupational injury hazards. Exhibit 9–1 lists some notable milestones in the history of injury prevention law.

Thus injury prevention laws are numerous, they are ubiquitous, and they are far reaching. Many, such as regulations regarding the storage of explosives, have been on the books for decades or centuries. Others, such as smoke detector and motor vehicle occupant restraint requirements, are relatively new governmental approaches. In fact, one problem with these laws is that they have been enacted over time in such an unplanned and uncoordinated fashion that the result is generally an unsystematic array of laws, without a rational codification or classification. Tellingly, states do not compile their injury prevention laws into a single chapter or code.

## STATE POLICE POWER

The greatest number of injury prevention laws are found at the state level, since the states traditionally have exercised the most clearly established public health powers. State governments (and, by delegation, their various subdivisions) possess the authority to enact and enforce injury pre-

**Exhibit 9–1** Some Milestones in Injury Prevention Law

| | |
|---|---|
| 1966 | National Highway Safety Bureau (later the National Highway Traffic Safety Administration) established as part of the U.S. Department of Transportation. |
| 1970 | Occupational Safety and Health Act enacted by Congress. |
| 1972 | Consumer Product Safety Act, Flammable Fabrics Act, Hazardous Substances Act, and Poison Prevention Packaging Act passed by Congress. |
| 1973 | Congress enacts Emergency Medical Services Systems Act. |
| 1974 | Congress passes Child Abuse and Prevention and Treatment Act. |
| 1978 | Tennessee becomes the first state to enact a child passenger safety law. |
| 1987 | California enacts first legislation requiring helmets for child bicycle passengers 4 years old and under. |
| 1988 | Congress enacts Child Abuse Prevention, Adoption and Family Services Act. |
| 1989 | All states have enacted occupant protection laws covering children under 4 years old. |
| 1990 | Howard County, Maryland, adopts law requiring children 16 years and under to wear helmets while riding as either passengers or operators of bicycles. |
| 1993 | Congress passes the Handgun Violence Prevention Act (the Brady Bill). |
| 1997 | E coding mandated in 23 states. Using consumer protection authority, Massachusetts becomes the first state to mandate child-resistant safety mechanisms on all handguns manufactured in the state. |

*Note:* See Appendix 2–A for additional timeline information.

vention and other public health laws under what is known as "police power," a broad concept encompassing the functions historically undertaken by governments in regulating society.

Police power has been used to uphold actions by the states, many quite broad in their reach and impact. Generally such laws will be upheld if it can be shown they are reasonable attempts to protect and promote the public's health, safety, and general welfare, and that the laws are not arbitrary or capricious attempts to accomplish such an end. State authority in this area has been sustained not only regarding laws aimed at protecting the public's health and safety in general, but also for laws aimed at protecting individuals, even when such laws restrict property rights and individual autonomy.

The U.S. Supreme Court has noted that, "The police power is one of the least limitable of governmental powers." The observation was made in *Queeenside Hills Co. v. Saxl*,[2] a decision that deals with a typical injury prevention law issue; namely, how far can government go in controlling individual autonomy and private property in the name of protecting public safety? The short answer, as we will see, is that government can go quite far as long as it can demonstrate a rational need and basis for the injury prevention law. In *Queeenside Hills* a commercial building owner had objected to a new municipal ordinance requiring the installation of automatic fire sprinkler systems, arguing that the sprinklers were not needed, were too costly, and that the law was not being fairly applied. The Supreme Court rejected all of these arguments in the face of the city's need and authority to protect the safety of its citizens. (See Exhibit 9–2.)

## FEDERAL AUTHORITY

The federal government does not have police power authority. The Constitution enumerates those things the federal government is empowered to do, but does not mention the protection of public health and safety. The Constitution has been interpreted broadly by the Supreme Court as authorizing the federal government to do those things necessary to advance its enumerated powers. Two enumerated powers—the power to regulate interstate commerce and spending—have been broadly construed to provide a constitutional rationale for the wide range of federal public health efforts, including injury prevention. Thus, for example, the Consumer Product Safety Act and the Occupational Safety and Health Act are constitutionally based on the federal government's interstate commerce authority (see Exhibit 9–3). Other federal safety provisions, such as the 55-mile-per-hour speed limit and the 21-year-old drinking age, are based on the spending power—if states wish to qualify for federal funds they must institute such safety-related laws.

## THE NATURE OF INJURY PREVENTION LAWS

In enacting statutory laws, legislative bodies can pursue several different conceptual approaches. Statutory commands can either require or prohibit and they can be directed at individual behavior (people), at products (things), or at environmental conditions (places). Examples of injury pre-

**Exhibit 9–2** *Queenside Hills v. Saxl*

Protection of the safety of persons is one of the traditional uses of the police power of the States. Experts may differ as to the most appropriate way of dealing with fire hazards in lodging houses. Appellant, indeed, says that its building, far from being a fire-trap, is largely fireproof; and to the extent that any fire hazards exist, they are adequately safeguarded by a fire alarm system, constant watchman service, and other safety arrangements. But the legislature may choose not to take the chance that human life will be lost in lodging house fires and adopt the most conservative course which science and engineering offer. . . . The question of validity turns on the power of the legislature to deal with the prescribed class. That power plainly exists here.

*Source:* Reprinted from *Queenside Hills Realty Co., Inc., v. Saxl, Commissioner of Housing and Buildings of the City of New York*, 328 U.S. 80, (1946).

vention laws directed at people that require particular behaviors are mandatory seatbelt, child restraint, and helmet use laws. Examples of laws that prohibit individual behaviors are drunk driving laws, speed limits, and making assaultive behavior a crime. Although research on the subject is limited, we assume that fear of enforcement leads most people to tailor their behavior to comply with laws (i.e., that there is some deterrent effect). In addition, the fact that "it's the law" will lead many people to comply with legal requirements simply out of citizenship obligations and communicates social expectations and provides a model of moral authority that can influence behavior. In effect, it helps establish the social environment. Robertson notes that compliance with laws is most likely if a high propensity to conform exists independent of the law, if detection is easy, and if few exceptions to compliance are permitted.[3(p133)] Legal requirements that apply to "things" include design and performance standards, such as the federal Motor Vehicle Safety Standards and the standards promulgated by the Consumer Product Safety Commission (e.g., a mandatory standard making cigarette lighters child resistant). Prohibitions applying to "things" include restrictions on machine guns, dangerous animals, and flammable fabrics. Legal requirements applied to "places" include the installation of breakaway signposts along highways and fencing around swimming pools. Prohibitions applied to "places" include the outlawing of rigid structures alongside highways and firearms in airport terminals.

**Exhibit 9–3** Federal Injury Prevention Laws and Interstate Commerce

Congress finds that personal injuries and illnesses arising out of work situations impose a substantial burden upon, and are a hindrance to, interstate commerce in terms of lost production, wage loss, medical expenses, and disability compensation payments. . . . Congress declares it to be its purpose and policy . . . to assure so far as possible every working man and woman in the nation safe and healthful working conditions. . . .

The Congress finds that . . . an unacceptable number of consumer products which present unreasonable risks of injury are distributed in commerce . . . and . . . regulation of consumer products the distribution or use of which affects interstate or foreign commerce is necessary to carry out this chapter.

*Source:* Reprinted from The Occupational Safety and Health Act of 1970, 29 U.S.C. Sec. 651 et seq; The Consumer Product Safety Act, 15 U.S.C. Sec. 2051 et seq.

Seatbelt laws illustrate the varying conceptual approaches for injury prevention intervention strategies available to lawmakers. Various laws have required that automobiles be equipped with seatbelts or shoulder belts, funded voluntary "buckle up" programs, mandated seatbelt use and penalized nonuse, made seatbelt nonuse a form of contributory negligence in civil litigation, and otherwise used the power of government to foster seatbelt use. Mandatory seatbelt use laws may seem to be categorically distinct from more traditional public health measures. Yet any perceived difference is not because of intrinsic distinctions between the kinds of problems being addressed, but rather results from the habit of viewing injuries in terms of individual behavior and misbehavior (e.g., driver fault) and, therefore, emphasizing education and voluntary behavior change. But as noted in *Injury in America*:

Individual behavior change to prevent injuries has been more successful when the behavior was easily observable and required by law. For example, in the absence of laws requiring the use of protective helmets, only about 50% of motorcyclists voluntarily wear them, but helmet-use laws result in almost 100% use. Laws mandating individual behavior are clearly more effective than education and protect more members of society.[4(p39)]

The history of public health offers many similar examples of the superior effectiveness of legal mandates versus education by itself. For example, polio came to be recognized as a danger requiring active social intervention, including compulsory immunization laws, rather than being viewed simply as a matter of voluntary choice. Motor vehicle crashes and other injury-causing events may require similar active responses. William Haddon, Jr., Ralph Nader, and other safety leaders have consistently emphasized the effectiveness of governmental mandates in protecting the public. Most of William Haddon's 10 countermeasure strategies for reducing injury, particularly those involving the preinjury and injury phases, call for mandatory countermeasures with the force of law to support them and applying to "things" and "places." (See Chapters 2 and 6.) Law plays a significant role in implementation of such approaches, whether by banning the manufacture or sale of plastic handguns (preventing the hazard in the first place) or requiring childproof caps on medicines and household cleaners (creating a material barrier separating the hazard from that which needs to be protected).

## VALIDITY OF INJURY PREVENTION LAWS

As commonplace and extensive as injury prevention laws are, not all legislative efforts to prevent injury meet with universal approval. Although much is known about how injuries occur and about how injuries can be prevented, there are significant barriers to implementing meaningful injury prevention measures. It is not that public support for injury prevention laws is lacking; in fact, such support can be quite strong.[5] The difficulty is often that many of the most effective injury prevention efforts limit individual autonomy or threaten the profit-making practices of major corporations. This means that those who oppose injury prevention laws may be highly motivated, which in turn can lead to challenges to such measures by economically and politically powerful interests. These challenges are political, not legal; nevertheless, the injury prevention community must understand and be able to deal with them.

When new injury prevention laws are proposed, objections can be expected to arise from many quarters; some objections will be well founded, others self-serving and dubious. There are three distinct and independent objections that are often directed at existing or proposed injury prevention laws. The first is that the law would be legally invalid, that it would violate a constitutionally protected right or suffers from some other legal deficiency. The second is that, even if legally valid, the law will not work to achieve its intended purpose. The third common objection is that, even though legally valid and effective in its purpose, the law offends important philosophical, political, or economic values, such as individual autonomy or economic frugality.

The legal challenge directed at a new or proposed injury prevention law is quite likely to be one that disputes the law's legal validity. When an injury prevention law (or governmental effort to enforce the law) is challenged as being legally invalid, this means: (1) an assertion that government lacks the constitutional authority to enact a specific law or regulation or to carry out a particular action; or (2) a claim that some greater legal principle, usually involving individual rights protected by the Constititution, takes precedence over a specific law, regulation, or action; or (3) a due process argument, conceding that government did have the authority to enact a specific law or regulation or carry out a specific action, but alleging that this was not done in a proper, appropriate, and valid manner.

As has already been suggested, courts tend to uphold the validity of injury prevention laws. Local, state, and federal governments have authority to enact such laws,[6] and it is rare that legislative and regulatory bodies will exceed that authority. When an individual rights claim is made, even where constitutionally protected rights (such as First Amendment rights) are involved, the courts will balance the importance of that individual right against the needs of the society as reflected in the challenged law. This balancing is a basic feature of our legal system.

In 1905 in *Jacobson v. Massachusetts*,[7] the classic public health law decision, the U.S. Supreme Court upheld the authority of government under the police power to penalize an individual for failure to comply with a compulsory immunization statute. The Court noted that:

> Whatever may be thought of the expedience of this statute, it cannot be affirmed to be, beyond question, in palpable conflict with the Constitution. Nor, in view of the methods employed to stamp out the disease of smallpox, can anyone confidently assert that the means prescribed by the State to that end has no real or substantial relation to the protection of the public health and the public safety.[7]

The *Jacobson* Court's description of police power authority to protect public health and safety is presented in Exhibit 9–4.

Many courts have upheld compulsory seatbelt laws by using the same logic and case law. *State v. Hartog*, a decision by the Iowa State Supreme Court upholding that state's mandatory seatbelt use law as a reasonable and proper use of the state police power is typical of more recent court decisions using the logic of *Jacobson* to uphold injury prevention laws. Exhibit 9–5 presents an extended excerpt from the *Hartog* opinion.

In *Hartog* the Iowa court stated that it was following a balancing test: "does the collective benefit outweigh the specific restraint?" Similarly, the U.S. Supreme Court has balanced the individual's Fourth Amendment right to be free from unreasonable search and seizure against the reasonableness of states to conduct random sobriety checkpoint traffic stops to combat drunk driving and has concluded that the checkpoints were constitutional.

It is perhaps only in the area of due process where successful legal challenges to injury prevention laws can be found with any frequency, and then only when the authorities have not followed appropriate procedures in implementing laws. Thus, for example, administrative agencies must be able to demonstrate that they have followed all required steps in terms of notice, hearing, and full consideration before implementing new regulations. If they fail to do so, the courts may invalidate the administrative action or regulation involved.

The requirement that government afford due process by following its own rules is an important part of our constitutional system, but it is unfortunately one that can be abused by those with the resources to mount continuing due process challenges to unwanted governmental actions. The result is delay (or, worse, total obstruction) in government regulatory actions. A classic example of delaying regulation involved the attempt to require airbags in automobiles. In the words of the U.S. Supreme Court, "For nearly a decade, the automobile industry waged the regulatory equivalent of war against the airbag and lost—the inflatable restraint was proven sufficiently effective." And yet it took more than 20 years and 60 rulemaking notices and a Supreme Court decision to force manufacturers to provide airbags in a significant number of cars.[8]

This type of legalistic delay is not an example of the system working imperfectly. Quite the contrary: the legal system has traditionally served to protect the status quo. Because many public health and safety initiatives

**Exhibit 9–4**  *Jacobson v. Massachusetts*

The authority of the State to enact this statute is to be referred to what is commonly called the police power—a power which the State did not surrender when becoming a member of the Union under the Constitution. Although this court has refrained from any attempt to define the limits of that power, yet it has distinctly recognized the authority of a State to enact quarantine laws and "health laws of every description;" indeed, all laws that relate to matters completely within its territory and which do not by their necessary operation affect the people of other States. According to settled principles the police power of a State must be held to embrace, at least, such reasonable regulations established directly by legislative enactment as will protect the public health and the public safety. . . . It is equally true that the State may invest local bodies called into existence for purposes of local administration with authority in some appropriate way to safeguard the public health and the public safety. The mode or manner in which those results are to be accomplished is within the discretion of the State, subject, of course, so far as Federal power is concerned, only to the condition that no rule prescribed by a State, nor any regulation adopted by a local governmental agency acting under the sanction of state legislation, shall contravene the Constitution of the United States or infringe any right granted or secured by that instrument. . . .

We come, then, to inquire whether any right given, or secured by the Constitution, is invaded by the statute as interpreted by the state court. The defendant insists that his liberty is invaded when the State subjects him to fine or imprisonment for neglecting or refusing to submit to vaccination; that a compulsory vaccination law is unreasonable, arbitrary and oppressive, and therefore, hostile to the inherent right of every freeman to care for his own body and health in such way as to him seems best; and that the execution of such a law against one who objects to vaccination, no matter for what reason, is nothing short of an assault upon his person. But the liberty secured by the Constitution of the United States to every person within its jurisdiction does not import an absolute right in each person to be, at all times and in all circumstances, wholly freed from restraint. There are manifold restraints to which every person is necessarily subject for the common good. On any other basis organized society could not exist with safety to its members. Society based on the rule that each one is a law unto himself would soon be confronted with disorder and anarchy. Real liberty for all could not exist under the operation of a principle which recognizes the right

*continues*

**Exhibit 9–4**  continued

of each individual person to use his own, whether in respect of his person or his property, regardless of the injury that may be done to others. This court has more than once recognized it as a fundamental principle that "persons and property are subjected to all kinds of restraints and burdens, in order to secure the general comfort, health, and prosperity of the State."

*Source:* Reprinted from *Jacobson v. Massachusetts*, 197 U.S. 11, (1905)

require changes in the status quo, such efforts are at a decided legal disadvantage. Legal delays and roadblocks are a frustrating and inevitable part of the environment in which the public health and safety communities operate, calling for patience, persistence, resources, and popular support.

One frequent obstacle to enacting effective legal approaches to dealing with injury problems is the argument that industry can best regulate itself through voluntary codes or standards. This approach may be better than having no protections at all, but voluntariness means that less-responsible companies (the very ones for whom safety standards are most needed) are free to ignore industry codes. Voluntariness also means a lowest common denominator approach to developing standards. It is because of the inadequacies and inconsistencies of voluntary approaches that legal mandates are often needed to protect the public from dangerous products and conditions.

## OTHER OBJECTIONS TO INJURY PREVENTION LAWS

Even when the legal validity of an injury prevention law has been upheld, objections to the law may be raised. One quite sensible objection would be that, though valid, the law will not or does not achieve its intended purpose. Those who champion injury prevention laws, those who oppose them, and those who are affected by them all have an interest in learning whether the restrictions and costs involved are actually serving a useful function. This means that the effectiveness of every injury prevention law should be routinely evaluated. Unfortunately, this is rarely the case.

There are several reasons that we know much less than we should about the impact of injury prevention laws. It costs money to carry out such evaluation, money often not available. Moreover, those with the dollars to fund the requisite studies—the legislative bodies that enacted the laws—

**Exhibit 9–5** *State v. Hartog*

---

Hartog raises a fundamental issue: whether Iowa's mandatory seat belt law constitutes a valid exercise of the state's police power.... In support of this contention, Hartog argues that the purpose of the statute is to protect the individual from his own folly and, consequently, such purpose has no relation to the public health, safety, or welfare. Implicit in Hartog's argument is that the decision whether to wear a seat belt is a personal one affecting him only; therefore, he should be able to make that decision free of state interference. . . .

The legislature has considerable discretion in determining what constitutes the public health, safety, and welfare . . . Nevertheless, there are certain parameters to the state's police power. Those parameters were articulated in *Lawton v. Steele*. . . .

> To justify the state in thus interposing its authority on behalf of the public, it must appear, first, that the interests of the public generally, as distinguished from those of a particular class, require such interference; and second, that the means are reasonably necessary for the accomplishment of the purpose. . . .

Several courts have rejected the argument Hartog raises, that is, that his unwillingness to use seat belts places only himself at risk. These courts point out that seat belt use enhances a driver's ability to maintain control of the car and avoid injuries not only to the driver but to others. . . . Similarly, an unrestrained front seat passenger can interfere with the ability of a driver to respond to a collision. . . .

Moreover, studies have shown that such an unrestrained passenger poses danger of injuries to other occupants through direct or indirect body contact brought about by occupant kinetics. For example, instances have occurred in which a person holding a small child has been thrown forcibly against the child, crushing the child to death. . . .

It is readily apparent to us that the legislature could rationally conclude unbelted drivers and passengers endanger the safety of others. . . .

We think the seat belt law promotes the public interest in another way: reducing the public costs associated with serious injuries and deaths caused by automobile accidents. As one court has pointed out,

> the police power relates not merely to the public health and public physical safety, but also to public financial safety, and . . . laws may be passed within the police power to protect the public from financial loss. . . .

---

*continues*

**Exhibit 9–5**  continued

> Contrary to Hartog's contention, automobile occupants who do not buckle up and as a result are seriously injured may directly affect the public because
>
> > [f]rom the moment of the injury, society picks the person up off the highway; delivers him to a municipal hospital and municipal doctors; provides him with unemployment compensation if, after recovery, he cannot replace his lost job, and, if the injury causes permanent disability, may assume the responsibility for him and his family's continued subsistence. We do not understand a state of mind that permits [such a person] to think that only he himself is concerned. *Simon v. Sargent.* . . .
>
> Statistics certainly bear out the staggering direct and indirect costs attributable to injuries and deaths from automobile accidents. . . .
>
> As one commentator aptly points out:
>
> > The government provides roads as a service to its citizens, and part of that service is assuring that these roads will be safe and efficient. The motorist is not being overly imposed upon when asked to comply with minimal standards of behavior designed to reduce the dangers of his driving to other drivers. It is also difficult to object to the state's attempt to stop an individual from making the rest of society pay for the consequences of his risk-taking. Under a system of laissez-faire one could argue that a persons's risk-taking would be his own business, but our government provides services from the ambulance that delivers the injured motorist to the hospital to disability insurance. Having to buckle up may be inconvenient, but it is not an unreasonable price to pay for the use of public roads. . . .
>
> We hold that passage of [Iowa's mandatory seat belt law] was a proper exercise of the state's police power and does not violate the due process provisions of the federal and Iowa constitutions.
>
> *Source:* Reprinted from *State v. Hartog,* 440 N.W.2d 852 (Iowa, 1989) *cert. denied,* 493 U.S. 1005 (1989) *rehearing denied,* 493 U.S. 1095 (1990).

may not want to learn that legislation with which they are identified is not doing what they promised. Finally, there are considerable methodological difficulties in carrying out evaluations of the effectiveness of laws. The relevant data are limited; often the number of fatal injuries of one particular type for one particular year in one particular state is relatively small. Aggregating data from several states may be difficult because laws differ from state to state.

Laws are usually enacted in response to a particular problem. In fact, specific problems—such as drunk driving deaths—often lead to several laws being enacted at roughly the same time. Distinguishing the effect of a law passed at the height of an injury problem from the expected regression from the mean can be difficult. Even more difficult is untangling the comparative impact of several laws enacted to deal with the same injury problem. This is not to suggest that such evaluation is impossible. There is a growing literature on the subject and a growing number of relevant studies. It is important that such studies be continued, but also important that those encouraging or doing the evaluation be aware of the difficulties involved.[6,9]

A final possible objection to injury prevention laws involves the question of whether a particular law should exist at all. Even though a law may be legally supportable and even though it may be effective in reducing injuries, if it is too costly—either monetarily or in terms of individual autonomy—then maybe it ought not to exist as a law. This is a political question, not a legal or epidemiological one. But it is a question that plays a significant role in determining which laws get enacted and which do not. Chapter 14 looks at this aspect of injury prevention and injury prevention law in discussing barriers to injury prevention.

Larry Berger summarized six conditions for attempting to implement new legislation as:

> be thoroughly convinced that the bill addresses a strikingly important issue. One should have evidence that the bill's actions can be effective; support from judges and police officers that the law can be enforced expeditiously; economic estimates that excessive costs will not be involved; legal counsel confirming the constitutionality and compatibility of the proposed law with existing legislation and ordinances; and broad-based support from constituents.[10(p24)]

## PUBLIC HEALTH PRACTITIONERS AND THE LAW

What role does the public health practitioner play in dealing with legal issues in injury prevention? How is the nonlawyer to navigate in an area of possible legal challenges and arguments?

As an injury prevention practitioner, your focus should be on your injury prevention goals. Law is one *tool* to be used in achieving these goals.

Clarify your goals, then seek to determine how law might be used to better achieve them. In some cases this will mean working to see new legislation enacted (see the discussion of advocacy in Chapter 14). In other instances it may mean working to tailor the regulations that execute legislation (public health practitioners often being a source of expertise in propounding such regulations). And in some cases your contribution may be to offer help in improving enforcement efforts. Your role in determining the best use of law will involve making use of *legal knowledge, legal procedure,* and *legal advice.*

*Legal knowledge* involves understanding how the law sanctions or restricts the day-to-day functioning of your agency. You should be familiar with the injury prevention laws that exist at the local, state, and federal levels. Know what laws already exist, which are strong and which are weak, what gaps exist in the coverage of injury prevention laws, what laws exist elsewhere that might be useful models in your own jurisdiction, and how the reality of the laws as enforced compares to the theory of the laws in the statute books. Injury prevention laws form an unplanned hodge-podge or patchwork and a goal for the injury prevention professional is to steadily push this flawed system toward a more rational, comprehensive future.

Being knowledgeable about existing law also means knowing what gaps there are in existing laws. It is the public health practitioner who is best able to recognize that present laws are not working and that changes are needed. For example, are there significant gaps in the coverage of your state's mandatory child restraint use law?

You should be able to do much of your background research. Law libraries are a useful reservoir of secondary source material: law review, encyclopedia, and treatise articles that summarize the current state of the law and that often suggest new legal approaches to dealing with problems. Especially with the help of law librarians, this material is quite accessible to the layperson. When what you need is legal information, you can rely on the law library, professional and other national associations, and the like.[11]

*Legal procedure* refers to the general principle that in all of your work you must follow established procedures and document, document, document, i.e., keeping written records of everything that you do that may have law-related repercussions. This might include confidentiality procedures followed during data collection or expert advice provided to advocacy groups involved in lobbying for new injury prevention legislation.

*Legal advice* is what legal counsel provides to you. Aspects of legal challenges to public health measures require reliance on legal counsel, such as defending the constitutionality of a local handgun ordinance before a state supreme court. Dealing with such difficult challenges requires the skills of trained attorneys. Obviously an attorney must be consulted when an adverse legal proceeding, such as a lawsuit, has been initiated. It is wise to do so as well when a lawsuit is threatened. And legal help is also called for when meeting with parties with potentially adverse interests. But perhaps the most useful input from legal counsel can be in offering legal predictions or interpretations. If a law intended to achieve a certain result is enacted and is challenged, will the courts uphold it? How could the law best be tailored to ensure that the courts will uphold it? Will enforcement of the law create unwanted legal complications? It is in providing such predictions of how the legal system is likely to react to new inputs for which legal expertise can be most useful.

Whether you are enforcing existing laws or considering the need for changes in existing laws, you will be interacting with legal counsel. You should be able to do this in plain, understandable, nonlegalistic language. Working with legal counsel should not be a quiescent process. Most important of all, do not passively accept the argument that "the law" prevents you from doing what seems the most sensible way to deal with an injury problem. Insist on finding out exactly why this may be the case and how the law could be used to achieve your injury prevention goal.

Make your injury prevention goals clear and then work with lawyers to tailor optimal legal approaches to achieving those goals. Your role as the public health practitioner is to define the problem to be solved and the end to be achieved by any proposed legislation, regulation, enforcement action, lawsuit, or other legal action. It should be noted here that new legislation is not always the best approach to dealing with an injury problem. Better or more creative approaches to enforcement of existing laws may be more useful (or at least more feasible) than legislation. For example, in some states police have used enforcement of laws requiring seatbelts for each seating location in a motor vehicle as a way to deal with the dangerous practice of people riding unrestrained in the cargo area of pickup trucks. This may be a more direct approach to the problem than trying to enact new legislation on the subject.

The injury prevention practitioner's responsibility is not done after injury prevention laws are enacted. Passage of a law is a first step; implementing the law is more difficult. A law in the statute books is meaningless unless it is enforced. It is important to work with those responsible for enforcement—state police, inspectors, prosecutors—to help them understand why a particular law was enacted in the first place and why its enforcement is worth the time and energy required. Provide enforcement personnel with feedback on the impact of various laws on injury rates. (Of course, police agencies often are involved in supporting enactment of injury prevention laws in the first place, since they are on the front lines in dealing with many injuries, including motor vehicle and firearm injuries.)

## TORT LAW

A different type of legal approach to injury prevention is private litigation, or tort law. The law of torts determines when one person (including groups of persons, corporations, or government) must pay compensation for civil, noncontractual wrongs caused to others. Tort lawsuits serve not only to compensate victims of negligence but also to deter individuals and companies from acting negligently in ways that could harm the public. A company tempted to market a tractor with a tendency to roll over will know that it risks serious monetary consequences unless it redesigns its product or adequately warns users of the hazard. Several public health law experts suggest that the tort lawsuit can play a valuable, positive role in forwarding injury prevention goals by making manufacturers and sellers aware of the severe monetary consequences that might flow from careless marketing of products with the potential to injure the public.[12-14] As one court explained it:

> public policy demands that responsibility be fixed wherever it will most effectively reduce the hazards to life and health inherent in defective products that reach the market. . . . It is to the public interest to discourage the marketing of products having defects that are a menace to the public. If such products nevertheless find their way into the market, it is to the public interest to place the responsibility for whatever injury they may cause upon the manufacturer, who even if he is not negligent in the manufacture of the product is responsible for its reaching the market.[15]

Product liability lawsuits can be brought for defects in manufacture, defects in design (such as the failure to make cars crashworthy by failing to incorporate known safety features), or failure to adequately warn of hazards. Although injury prevention laws and regulations are the most direct way to bring about a safer environment, it may not always be possible politically to get such laws enacted. In such cases, tort lawsuits may serve to fill the void. Of course, this is not the favored approach, because the impact of such lawsuits is limited in time and clarity. Still, tort lawsuits have played a notable role in some areas of injury. Products that have been the focus of successful tort lawsuits include unstable hot water vaporizers, particularly dangerous farm machinery, cars without airbags, and BB guns without mechanisms to indicate whether the gun is loaded.

## CONCLUSION

Law is part of the political process—not an abstract set of principles. But intimidating legal mystique (most legal sentences, a law professor once observed, "have a way of reading as though they had been translated from the German by someone with a rather meager knowledge of English"[16(p121)]) often prevents nonlawyers from dealing with legal principles and concepts in the same way they would deal with other political issues. Instead, law is seen as a mystery understandable only to those who have dedicated their professional careers to the task. This is an inappropriate approach to any area of endeavor. Surely law can be understandable to the nonlawyer. This is not to say that there is no role for the legal expert or that there are not subtle and complex areas of law. But it does mean that the nonlawyer can research, understand, discuss, and debate legal issues.

Working with the legal profession should not mean abdicating responsibility to them. Public health practitioners can and should discuss legal issues with legal counsel, colleagues, legislators, and others. Public health practitioners can help develop and implement injury prevention laws in the same way that they deal with other aspects of the never-ending battle for a safer and healthier environment.[17]

---

## NOTES

1. Lescohier D. *A Review of Legislation and Literature Pertaining to the Prevention of Unintentional Childhood Injury in Massachusetts.* Boston: Massachusetts Committee on Children and Youth; 1981.

2. *Queenside Hills Realty Co., Inc. v. Saxl, Commissioner of Housing and Buildings of the City of New York.* 328 U.S. 80, 1946.

3. Robertson LS. *Injuries: Causes, Control Strategies, and Public Policy.* Lexington, MA: Lexington Books; 1983.

4. Committee on Trauma Research, Commission on Life Sciences, National Research Council and Institute of Medicine. *Injury in America: A Continuing Public Health Problem.* Washington, DC: National Academy Press; 1985:39.

5. Fergusson DM, Horwood BA, Shannon FT. Attitudes of mothers of five-year-old children to compulsory child health provisions. *N Z Med J.* 1983;96:338–340.

6. Christoffel T, Teret SP. *Protecting the Public: Legal Issues in Injury Prevention.* New York: Oxford University Press; 1993.

7. *Jacobson v. Massachusetts.* 197 U.S. 11, 1905.

8. *Motor Vehicle Manufacturers Association v. State Farm Mutual Automobile Insurance Company.* 463 U.S. 29, 1983.

9. Robertson LS. *Injury Epidemiology: Research and Control Strategies.* 2nd ed. New York: Oxford University Press; 1998.

10. Berger LR. Childhood injuries: Recognition and prevention. *Curr Problems Pediatr.* 1981;12:24.

11. Christoffel T. Using the Law Library. In: *Health and the Law: A Handbook for Health Professionals.* New York: The Free Press; 1982:433–436.

12. Teret SP. Injury control and product liability. *J Public Health Policy.* 1981;2:49–57.

13. Teret SP. Litigating for the public's health. *Am J Public Health.* 1986;76:1027–1029.

14. Teret SP, Jacobs M. Prevention and torts: The role of litigation in injury control. *Law Med Health Care.* 1989;17:17–22.

15. *Escola v. Coca Cola Bottling Co. of Fresno.* 24 Cal.2d 453, 150 P.2d 436, 1944.

16. Rodell F. *Woe Unto You, Lawyers!* New York: Berkeley; 1980.

17. Christoffel T. The misuse of law as a barrier to injury prevention. *J Public Health Policy.* 1989;10:444.

# PART III

# Practical Knowledge, Skills, and Strategies

CHAPTER **10**

# Injury Prevention:
# The Role of Public Agencies

"[G]overnments at all levels have an irreplaceable role to play in assuring conditions in which people can be healthy."

Committee for the Study of the Future of Public Health,
*The Future of Public Health*, 1988

## WHAT THIS CHAPTER IS ABOUT

In *Injury in America* it was noted that "injury is the principal public health problem in America today."[1(pv)] A distant observer might conclude, therefore, that injury should be a principal concern of public health agencies, but this is not the case. Why not? Perhaps injury is not preventable, or at least is not very amenable to traditional public health assessment and intervention. Perhaps other public health concerns are easier to deal with effectively. Perhaps injury can more effectively be handled by nonpublic health agencies and institutions —or perhaps governmental priorities are simply not established in a purely logical manner.

We do not really have to debate these matters in this chapter. It is enough to note that there are things that public agencies, particularly public health agencies, can and are doing to reduce the toll of injury in America. In this chapter we will outline what this has meant in terms of state and federal injury prevention activities, while in the next chapter our focus will shift to developing injury prevention programs at the local level. Our concern is to better understand *existing* governmental injury prevention activities and programs, expanding the reader's knowledge of who the major injury prevention players are at the state and federal levels of government and what they do.

Unfortunately, governmental injury prevention efforts do not form a coordinated system. Instead, they are more like a patchwork quilt. Still, it is important to know what resources are available from existing governmental programs. This will become especially relevant in the next chapter, when we look at the steps that need to be followed in establishing and developing your own injury prevention program.

## INTRODUCTION

Although perhaps best remembered for his role in campaigning against tobacco use by the young, former Surgeon General C. Everett Koop also advanced the cause of injury prevention. In particular, Dr. Koop produced a landmark report that established violence as a public health issue.[2] He also provided much-needed visibility for the area of child injury prevention, noting that if "a disease were killing our children in the proportions that accidents are, people would be outraged and demand that this killer be stopped."[3]

Perhaps ironically for a Reagan-appointed Surgeon General, Dr. Koop called attention to the fact that government—federal, state, or local—and public health agencies can play a positive role in improving the health of the public. There are negatives limiting that role—insufficient funding, the patchwork quilt of agencies, lack of a master plan, gaps in focus and authority, and a media-fueled negative image for government agencies, but there is a critical role for government in protecting the public's health, and those in the field of public health need to make the most of that role.

*The Future of Public Health* organized the role of public health agencies around three core functions: assessment, policy development, and assurance.[4] When it comes to injury prevention, attention and resources have been directed primarily at the assessment level: getting federal and state agencies to systematically collect, assemble, analyze, and make available information on injury occurrences, behavioral risk factors, and the like. The development of comprehensive injury prevention policies has had less emphasis. And the assurance function—which encompasses direct services and programs as well as health promotion, disease prevention, environmental health, and health education functions, has remained on the back burner. All and all, however, injury prevention has been made legitimate as part of the governmental public health role.

## THE STATE PLAYERS

State-level injury prevention activities have come a long way since the 1950s, when such efforts were largely restricted to inspecting people's homes for safety hazards. In particular, recent national planning efforts have increased the emphasis placed on injury prevention by state health agencies. Even so—and despite the extent of the injury problem—injury prevention is not yet an integral part of state or local public health practice. Most states have not yet addressed injury systematically as a major public health problem. With a few exceptions, the same is even more true of local health departments. At best health agencies are in the initial planning phases for comprehensive injury prevention programming, with activities that tend to be fragmented and with competing health priorities inhibiting resource and staff allocation.

And yet, state agencies are an essential component of injury prevention. They coordinate, train, and provide data and technical assistance at the local level, which is where injury control efforts must ultimately be based. It is at the local level that needs are identified, data collected, community support garnered, and interventions implemented.

### State Health Departments

In the last decade, much of the emphasis of state health agencies concerned with unintentional and intentional injuries has been on infrastructure support rather than intervention programs: creating injury surveillance programs, studying the epidemiology of injury, improving the availability of injury data, funding research studies, and developing state planning documents.

Inventories of state injury prevention activities has been limited to a 1987 survey of all state health agencies and a 1991 survey of the maternal and child health (MCH) agencies in each state health department. Since 1981, the number of states maintaining injury programs has tripled, from 12 to 32 states, with a variety of state health department divisions being involved. These include epidemiology, environmental health, maternal and child health, health promotion and chronic disease prevention, and emergency medical services. Still, the 1987 survey found that only 10 states had a separate injury program or unit with a comprehensive focus, all states spent less than 1% of their total health department budget on injury prevention, and the national average for staffing was 4.7 full-time equivalent personnel devoted to injury prevention per state.[5]

The 1991 survey found that 42 MCH agencies reported having injury prevention interventions in place, although in 35 of these, interventions could best be described as having general, nonspecific targets. Nearly half of the MCH agencies had a designated injury prevention coordinator and nearly two thirds dedicated some funds to injury prevention efforts (with amounts ranging from $4,000 to $619,000 with a median of $90,000). Twenty-two states reported using these funds for staff and materials in the state MCH office, 7 to support activities in other agencies within the health department (including epidemiology and health promotion), and 10 to support the injury prevention work of an agency or program outside the health department (such as a poison control center or the department of education).[6]

While the leadership in most state health departments are convinced that injury prevention is an important topic, they have not been able to develop a strategic plan for moving forward. Continued reliance on federal funds awarded for specific activities, such as research and surveillance, has made it harder for state health departments to develop other crucially needed injury prevention services and programs.

Individual state health agencies may or may not have an established injury prevention program or a full-time staff person devoted to injury prevention, but every state health agency does have a designated representative for the State and Territorial Injury Prevention Directors Association (STIPDA). This association, which was created in 1994, is made up of health department representatives from each state. For those states without a formal injury prevention program, STIPDA helps their representatives address infrastructure issues in anticipation of establishing an injury prevention program, redirect injury issues in the absence of such program or staff, prepare grant applications to secure program funding, and develop basic injury data for the state at minimal staff-time costs. STIPDA sees its mission as one of sustaining, enhancing, and promoting the ability of state, territorial, and local health departments in reducing death and disability from injury. This means focusing on (1) expanding the ability of public health agencies to develop injury-related policy, conduct research, and design, implement, and evaluate interventions; (2) providing training and education for injury prevention practitioners; and (3) coordinating and collaborating with other agencies and organizations to expand injury prevention activities.[7]

This fledgling organization recently received funds from the Centers for Disease Control and Prevention (CDC) and the Maternal and Child Health Bureau to establish a permanent office, hire an executive director, and expand its activities. STIPDA has been involved in the development of a Safe States Initiative, an action plan to integrate and expand core public health functions in injury prevention so as to create comprehensive, community-based, fully integrated prevention programs. The core components of this initiative include data collection and analysis, program design and implementation, program evaluation, intrastate and interstate coordination and collaboration, technical support and training, and public policy analysis to support legislation and regulations. STIPDA has identified eight core functions of a state injury control program. These core functions are state and local injury data collection; statewide coordination, leadership, and administration; program development and implementation; policy development; evaluation; professional training and education; public information and educational programs; and ensuring the protection and health of the population by investigating injury clusters or events. See Exhibit 10.1 for fuller descriptions of each.

## State Highway Safety Offices

Because of federal funding inducements, every state has a state highway safety office (SHSO) that is the administrative unit in the state charged with highway safety as its primary function. The SHSO develops a state highway safety plan describing how federal highway safety funding will be implemented in the state and providing a summary of highway safety goals and objectives for the coming year. The SHSO allocates funds to other state agencies, local governments, law enforcement agencies, public service groups, and other organizations to allow them to implement programs and projects according to these plans.

The SHSO may be located in any one of several different state agencies, including the departments of transportation, public safety, motor vehicles, or public works. The SHSO is run by the state governor's highway safety representative (GHSR), a gubernatorial appointee who serves as—and has the authority to be—the focal point for state highway safety activities. The GHSR plays a key role in coordinating highway safety program activities

**Exhibit 10–1** State Injury Control Program: Core Functions

The following eight functions should be considered core functions of a state injury control program. Assessment and quality assurance of each of these functions should be a priority.

*Statewide and local injury data collection.* Public health surveillance and monitoring of health behavior and conditions form the basic foundation of public health; regular collection and analysis of information related to emerging patterns of injury morbidity, mortality, and disability, associated costs, and prevalence of injury-related risk factors and behavioral patterns is essential. Outcomes of program interventions are often evaluated by surveillance data.

*Statewide coordination, leadership, and administration.* The injury problem is too large and too diverse for any one group to address alone and there are many other disciplines, agencies, and organizations currently involved and important in injury prevention, education, and policy development. State and local health departments have been charged with responsibility for the frontline defense of the public's health. Because public health addresses the diverse causes of injury (e.g., traffic, falls, sports, violence, drowning) and because of an existing and established leadership role, state health departments are the appropriate group to coordinate or facilitate state and local injury prevention efforts. A byproduct of this statewide coordination is the prevention of fragmentation and duplication of prevention activities.

*Program development and implementation.* Today, with widespread implementation, there are many proven effective and cost-effective injury prevention strategies that could greatly reduce injury incidence and associated societal costs. Injury prevention program development and implementation is based on local and state data and, in general, is delivered at the community level. Successful programs are multifaceted and use a combination of approaches. The involvement of communities in program planning, implementation, and evaluation is critical. Surveillance data are integral, not only in the development of prevention programs, but also in the evaluation of such programs.

*Policy development.* Public health policies may be reflected in legislation, or the establishment of regulations or standards; this may occur on many levels. Injury surveillance data is critical to drive the development and

*continues*

**Exhibit 10–1** continued

evaluation of policy initiatives. There have been many successful injury prevention policy efforts (i.e., mandatory child restraint legislation, flame-retardant clothing), however, there is great potential for new policy initiatives that can be initiated at the state and local level.

*Evaluation.* Accountability and quality assurance activities are necessary and integral components of any state and local injury prevention efforts. The evaluation is designed as a part of the program design or policy initiative. While statistical reduction in injury morbidity and mortality may not be feasible at the community level, other outcome measures (impact–bicycle helmet use, smoke detector prevalence) should always be evaluated. When feasible, states should determine cost-benefit and cost-effectiveness of injury prevention programs.

*Professional training and education.* Because of the diversity of potential professionals addressing injury prevention (i.e., emergency medical services, law enforcement, schools), a special emphasis is needed on training public health and other professionals from all relevant disciplines regarding the comprehensive public health approach to injury prevention. Links between education and practice settings are crucial in order to serve competency-based, cost-beneficial injury prevention programs.

*Public information and educational programs.* An important population-based function of public health programs is to serve as the health educator of the public. To reduce injury risk factors, the public must be alerted regarding the potential adverse outcomes of high-risk behaviors and benefits of safety behaviors; these efforts can perhaps be best targeted to children, but also must target legislators and the public at large.

*Ensuring the protection and health of the population by investigating injury clusters or events.* An important function of statewide injury surveillance data is to alert injury control officials regarding injury clusters or real and/or potential injury hazards; these events must be thoroughly investigated to identify risk factors and appropriate action taken to ensure the protection of the public's health. To be effective, these processes need to occur on a timely basis.

*Source:* State and Territorial Injury Prevention Directors' Association at http://www.stipda.org/stipda/core.htm. Used with permission. For more detailed information, see *Safe States: Five Components of a Model State Injury Prevention Program and Three Phases of Program Development* or contact STIPDA at stipda@mindspring.com.

across a variety of other state agencies, such as the state police, emergency medical services, transportation and health departments, and the courts.

SHSOs receive funding from the National Highway Traffic Safety Administration (NHTSA), according to a formula that combines road mileage and population. Federal Alcohol Incentive Grant funds are also allocated to states according to set criteria, such as the state's legal blood alcohol concentration (BAC) definition of intoxication. At least 40% of federal funds allocated by SHSOs must be used to address *local* traffic safety problems.

It is important that health agencies be aware of the state highway safety plan so that they can determine how they may supplement their motor vehicle injury prevention efforts with assistance from the SHSO. State and local health departments often compete for SHSO-controlled funding to undertake programs such as infant car seat loaner programs for low-income populations, bicycle safety programs, or incentive programs to reduce drinking and driving. Safe Communities, a new NHTSA-funded priority area, offers many opportunities for health department and SHSO collaboration.[8,9]

Similar structures for other unintentional injuries and violence prevention do not exist within state health departments (e.g., federal funds do not come to the states for allocation specifically for product-related injury prevention). Federal funds would only be available for such purposes at the local level if a state chose to use some of its federal block grant funds, state appropriations, or research grant funding for such purposes. Knowing what will work to reduce injury is most meaningful when there is a mandate to implement such measures and resources earmarked to do so.

## Other State Agencies

Injury prevention does receive attention from a variety of other state agencies, notably the offices of the state fire marshal, the attorney general's office, the governor's office, and—somewhat less frequently—a state child death review team or state medical examiner.

### State Fire Marshal's Office

The duties of the state fire marshal vary, but most collect data from local fire departments, usually on a voluntary basis. This information may be compiled and made available as an annual report. In at least one state, the fire marshal's office also oversees the state-mandated burn registry. Although epidemiologists need to be wary of the incompleteness and other limitations of such data sets, if they are examined carefully they can be quite useful. (See Exhibit 10–2.)

### State Attorney General

There are a number of attorneys general who have been interested in injury prevention and who have sought to incorporate the expertise of public health in working toward this goal. Because of the powers invested in the office, the state attorney general can be a particularly good ally in pursuing injury prevention goals. The attorney general is the chief lawyer and law enforcement officer of the state, and may also be charged with the responsibility for

- state consumer protection
- consumer complaints and product safety issues
- enforcement of fair labor and business practices, including investigating violations of child labor laws and work-related injuries to minors
- criminal investigations, including some violence prevention initiatives related to the family and community (e.g., youth, gangs, child abuse, domestic violence, and victim compensation)
- insurance issues, including requirements for community benefits programs, injury prevention being a possible strategy

Many attorney general offices are particularly active in the area of domestic violence, where they may organize training programs for law enforcement officers, prosecutors, health care providers, community groups, and others to review domestic violence developments and enforcement issues. Some examples of specific injury prevention activities initiated by state attorneys general offices are presented in Exhibit 10–3.

### Governor's Office

State governors may create task forces related to injury prevention, based on personal interest, public pressure, and/or a series of well-publicized events. Even if state and local public health agencies are not formally represented on such task forces, it is critical that the public health community educate task force members on the public health perspective on injury prevention. Often public health will become most involved when task force attention is focused on implementation.

**Exhibit 10–2** Working with the State Fire Marshal's Office

---

The research analyst who compiled data into an annual report in one state's fire marshal's office was very concerned that locally submitted data never got used and that registry reporting was incomplete. This concern led to cooperative activities with the state health department's injury staff, who assisted the fire marshal's office in developing a brochure and fact sheets presenting their data and incorporating it into prevention recommendations. A dissemination plan was developed that included involving local fire departments and providing them with feedback on the data they submitted. This in turn improved reporting and increased involvement in prevention at the local level. This partnership also resulted in the state fire marshal and commissioner of public health jointly sending a letter to hospitals thanking them for their participation with the burn registry, reminding them of the reporting requirement and highlighting how what was learned had been useful for prevention purposes. This all came about because injury program staff in the health department made the calls to ask the fire marshal's staff some questions about data in their annual report and inquiring about data collection cooperation with local fire departments.

---

An example of one such task force is provided by the experience in Maine, where the governor established a Children's Cabinet composed of the following department commissioners: human services, education, corrections, mental health, mental retardation and substance abuse services, and public safety. The purpose of the Children's Cabinet was to create and promote coordinated state policies and service delivery systems in those areas that served and supported children and families. A number of task force subcommittees were created, including one on youth suicide, which issued a report containing 10 global recommendations for action, along with a summary of research supporting the recommendations. The recommendations included developing community-based awareness programs, developing a uniform training program for all service providers, encouraging schools to establish student assistance teams, providing a single core team for individual adolescents in need, and improving law enforcement collaboration with other agencies serving youth. These recommendations were reviewed by the Children's Cabinet, which delegated the job of implementing and working out the many details and specifics to two working groups, one on data and evaluation and the other on information dissemination and training development. At this stage the injury prevention

**Exhibit 10–3**  State Attorney General Injury Prevention Initiatives: Selected Examples

- Implemented a smoke detector public information campaign with a smoke detector giveaway through the attorney general's office as part of an effort to address home insurance issues.
- Conducted a public information campaign to eliminate the sale of dangerous infant furniture.
- Requested state injury prevention program staff to obtain rates of suicides and suicide attempts, detailed by mechanism employed, with the information presented at an attorney general's press conference related to firearms issues.
- Held educational forums and a domestic violence conferences in conjunction with President Clinton's domestic violence hotline (1-800-799-SAFE).
- Held a domestic violence symposium for teachers, health care workers, and clergy focusing on the legal process, community resources available for victims and perpetrators, the effects of domestic violence on children, and cross-cultural perspectives.
- Sponsored legislation to ban assault weapons.
- Developed police training for children and guns, hate crimes and children, and children witnessing domestic violence, with the goal of enhancing the skills of police officers who handle cases involving juvenile offenders and victims.
- Sponsored an elder abuse hotline.
- Sponsored legislation to revise child labor laws, using teen work injury data and poor school grades as the rationale.
- Promulgated regulation requiring all handguns offered for sale in the state to meet specific quality standards and carry childproofing features, use-limitation devices, and a load indicator to make guns more inaccessible to children and safer for their lawful owners.
- Proposed mandatory violence prevention education in schools to give children the skills they need to handle conflicts appropriately and to resolve disputes without violence.
- Published a safe schools newsletter to provide educators with up-to-date information on new laws, new cases, and new initiatives in the area of school safety.
- Established a crime and violence prevention center out of the attorney general's office to provide information, technical assistance, and high-quality resources in the areas of family violence prevention, safe schools, general violence prevention, drug and alcohol abuse prevention, community policing, and youth gang prevention.

program staff within the state department of public health became very active in providing information and leadership in support of several of the recommendations, specifically

- planning, evaluation, and surveillance activities
- identifying state-of-the-art approaches (by consulting with other states and national resource centers)
- identifying realistic process and outcome benchmarks for policy implementation
- developing a specific youth suicide prevention plan

Emphasis was placed on strategies that were research based, integrating such strategies into existing prevention programs and coordinating efforts between different state departments.

There are three practical points to be noted in this task force example.

1. Public health usually does get invited to the table to discuss injury issues, especially when implementation steps are being considered.
2. It is up to injury staff within health agencies to examine recommendations from state task forces, identify how they fit into a broader injury prevention agenda, and then proactively communicate this insight to the relevant policy makers.
3. Process may be prolonged—in this case three years—and bureaucracy cumbersome, but patience has its rewards. (Maine now has a comprehensive youth suicide prevention implementation plan with designated lead agency roles for the bureau of health as well as for the departments of mental health and public safety.)[10]

### *Child Death Review Teams*

Recent years have seen the development of state-level, multiagency, multidisciplinary child death review teams, which can routinely, systematically, and professionally gather data on the circumstances surrounding injury-related deaths of children, with the goal of determining how each death occurred and how it might have been prevented. Creation of these review teams often resulted from instances of child abuse deaths that had been initially misdiagnosed.

Almost every state now has some kind of multidisciplinary child fatality review team, although some are not housed in a specific state agency. Traditionally child death review teams were part of the state child protective agency, but more recently teams have been located administratively in the governor's office, public health or law enforcement agencies, or in the state office for children. Teams frequently have representation from the state medical examiner, attorney general, state law enforcement, the courts, district attorneys, probation officers, social services, pediatricians and other health care providers, mental health and child protective services, public health, emergency medical services, and others.

State child death review teams identify and investigate risk factors that lead to child deaths, and they recommend policies and programs to prevent future fatalities. The field of public health brings to this coordinated approach expertise in the areas of sudden infant death syndrome, injury prevention in general, and violence prevention in particular. It is important for injury prevention programs to be active on these teams. The public health role would include provision of vital records and development of epidemiological risk profiles of families for early detection and prevention of child death and serious injury. Child fatality review team data could be presented in conjunction with state injury prevention plans, *Healthy People 2000* goals, maternal and child health block grant needs assessments, and other measures of preventive services. Injury prevention program staff can then coordinate multiagency prevention programs, including such things as child safety seats for automobiles, drowning prevention, and limiting firearms access for suicide prevention. Program staff can also identify outreach opportunities for injury prevention in families that are beyond the coverage of mainstream community medical providers.

State child death review teams may be coordinated by a state agency such as the medical examiner's office or department of social services, by an outside agency, or by a special commission established by state or local statute. Child death review began as a method to address suspected child abuse and neglect cases. The teams have focused primarily on suspicious deaths, particularly where homicide is suspected, but they are increasingly investigating unintentional injury deaths. As such, they are an untapped general resource for the injury prevention staff in state health agencies. Teams may investigate all deaths of children under a certain age, all injury-related child deaths, deaths as well as near-deaths due to serious injury, or only deaths occurring to children who were previously known to child protective services. See Exhibit 10–4 for an example.

Because of their newness, the benefits of death review teams are only beginning to be realized and their long-term effectiveness has yet to be

**Exhibit 10–4** Child Death Review Teams

The Pennsylvania Child Death review team, along with the state chapter of the American Academy of Pediatrics, has examined adolescent motor vehicle fatalities and found that speed is a significant risk factor. The team provided information on circumstances of these deaths to drivers education teachers to improve the development of those specific skills most needed by young drivers. With support from the Pennsylvania Department of Health, user-friendly software is being developed to assist both state and local teams in gathering data on child deaths. Some states also have county- or local-level child death review teams. For example, California has such a team in each county. A few of these localized teams are now expanding to examine domestic violence–related adult deaths in addition to deaths of children.

determined through evaluation studies. Potential outcomes of such inter-agency teams include

- reduced misclassification of cause of death
- reduced duplication of effort
- increased attention to and specific targeting of prevention
- improved interagency communication for management of future cases
- increased accuracy for criminal, civil, and social intervention
- development of profiles of families at risk
- better targeting of interagency services
- evaluation of the impact of specific risk factors, including substance abuse and domestic violence
- improved data collection for surveillance of deaths or special studies on certain categories such as burns or bathtub drownings
- improved training of agency staff
- increased use of the media to provide public education on injury prevention[11]

### *Coordination and Outreach Role of Public Health*

Whichever state agency is involved in dealing with injury prevention, it can make a difference as to whether the agency's efforts are integrated into existing programs or operate as a separate program. It also makes a difference as to which of several cooperating agencies is the lead agency and which are supporting agencies, a point discussed at length in Chapter 11. An important role for public health is outreach to other agencies (i.e., learning what others are doing so as to avoid duplication and turf battles). This is also the way to identify collaborative opportunities that will strengthen existing injury prevention efforts and avoid development of new injury prevention initiatives in isolation from that already going on. In some states this coordination has been formalized by establishing a working coalition of relevant state agencies to better coordinate their various efforts, improve and share existing sources of injury data, develop a state injury prevention plan, and build coalitions on particular injury topics. In other states coordination has simply meant having two people on the same administrative level—not necessarily the uppermost levels—communicate regularly and informally about their agency's injury prevention activities. This type of coordination is important, yet it is often neglected because attention is focused on the immediate crises of the day.

Exhibit 10–5 lists the state agencies most likely to be involved with injury prevention programs.

## THE FEDERAL PLAYERS

Federal agencies concerned with injury prevention focus primarily on specific causes of injury or on certain groups at high risk for injury. Agencies that relate to specific causes of injury include the National Highway Traffic Safety Administration, the Occupational Safety and Health Administration, and the Consumer Product Safety Commission. Agencies that target certain high-risk groups include the Maternal and Child Health Bureau and the Indian Health Service. The mandates of agencies that focus on specific injury causes usually include an orientation toward regulation and the development of safety standards. The federal injury prevention agenda was broadened to include increased research and program development as a result of the release of *Injury in America* in 1985[1] and the subsequent establishment of an injury control program at the CDC. This expansion—and specifically the high-profile involvement of the CDC—helped establish injury prevention as a legitimate topic with a scientific basis to be addressed within the public health arena. This section describes some of the major federal injury prevention players with statutory authority to address injury prevention. As with other areas of public health, federal health agencies often have overlapping mandates to address the same issues, each

**Exhibit 10–5**  State Agencies Involved in Injury Prevention

---

**EXECUTIVE BRANCH**

- Department of Public Health
  - Adult Health
  - Alcohol and Substance Abuse
  - Emergency Medical Services
  - Environmental Health/Community Sanitation and Code Enforcement
  - Epidemiology
  - Food and Drug
  - Health/Vital Statistics
  - Health Promotion and Disease Prevention
  - Maternal and Child Health
  - Occupational Health
- Department of Transportation
  - Motor Vehicles Licensing and Registration
  - Highway Department
- Office of the Attorney General
- Secretary of State
  - Motor Vehicle Licensing and Registration
- Department of Labor
  - State Occupational Safety and Health Administration
  - Workers' Compensation
  - Wage and Hour Division
- Department of Agriculture
- Department of Public Safety/Crime Control
  - Corrections
  - State Fire Marshal
  - State Offices of Emergency Management
  - State Police
- Department of Mental Health
- Department of Consumer Protection
- Department of Natural Resources
- Department of Education
  - Comprehensive School Health Education
  - School Bus Transportation
- Department of Elder Affairs
- Department of Social Services
- Department of Youth Services

---

*continues*

**Exhibit 10–5** continued

- Governor's Office of Highway Safety/Governor's Highway Safety Representative
- State Offices for Victim Assistance
- Office of the State Medical Examiner

**LEGISLATIVE BRANCH**

- Committee on Health (and Environment)
- Committee on Public Safety
- Committee on Criminal Justice
- Committee on Ways and Means
- Special Commissions

**JUDICIAL BRANCH**

- Courts
- Jails
- Probation

with its own orientation, target population, purpose, and program activities. A 1994 report to Congress concluded that duplication is not rampant.[12]

Federal agencies play a variety of important roles in injury prevention. In addition to administering their own programs and enforcing their own standards and regulations, they direct federal resources to the states, including resources for training and program development and for injury research. Federal agencies also provide policy direction and leadership in applying the results of research to policy, and they stimulate the state and local public health community.[13]

Recommendations to federal agencies from a 1987 state health agency needs assessment are still quite relevant today. They include

- increasing seed money for injury prevention programs at state and local levels
- assisting state injury staff in obtaining higher-level administrative support for injury prevention within state agencies
- disseminating information on successful and unsuccessful aspects of federally funded injury prevention projects

- developing or fostering training programs for injury prevention practitioners on both program content, development, implementation, and evaluation
- taking the lead in increasing public and professional awareness of injury prevention and the cost-effectiveness of various injury prevention approaches
- fostering linkages among public health and other disciplines working in the areas of public safety, criminal justice, and social services
- providing technical assistance in developing feasible reporting systems for state and local injury morbidity
- conducting surveys of state health department activity to be able to address their injury program needs[5]

Several federal agencies will be described in the following pages. The first to be discussed are those within the Department of Health and Human Services (DHHS). Then descriptions of the injury activities of agencies in other Cabinet departments and of independent federal agencies will be presented.

## Department of Health and Human Services

### National Center for Injury Prevention and Control (NCIPC)

The CDC is known for its epidemiologic expertise, its established working relationships with state and local public health departments, and its financial and technical support of interventions to prevent and control disease. In recent years the CDC has broadened its focus to encompass injury as well as disease. In 1985 the CDC was identified as the lead agency for injury control within the federal government. In 1992 its injury prevention program was elevated to the stature of a center and became the NCIPC. This designation was meant to concentrate and strengthen a federal role in injury prevention that had been limited and scattered across several agencies.

There are three branches of the NCIPC that carry out its mission of providing leadership in preventing and controlling injuries.

1. Division of Unintentional Injury Prevention
2. Division of Violence Prevention
3. Division of Acute Care, Rehabilitation Research, and Disability Prevention

NCIPC activities center on research, surveillance, program implementation, program evaluation, and public education. NCIPC programs cover all injuries and phases of injury control: prevention, acute care, prevention of disabilities, and rehabilitation.

The CDC and NCIPC are in a unique position to coordinate injury prevention activities across a wide spectrum of government and private agencies and organizations, each of which works on one type of injury or one phase of injury prevention. NCIPC activities have included the development of a national injury prevention planning document, sponsorship of an extramural research program, sponsorship of national injury prevention conferences on a periodic basis, and provision of core funding for 10 injury prevention research centers at leading universities (see Exhibit 10–6).

Recently the NCIPC launched a special initiative, a five-year project designed to put into place the systems and the infrastructure needed to lower injury rates. The four goals of the initiative are: (1) to reframe the message of injury prevention in order to generate greater public awareness of the problem of injury, focusing on the themes of safe at home, safe at work, safe on the move, safe in the community, and safe in school; (2) to create public/private partnerships to stimulate new funding for more community-based injury prevention programs and public education; (3) to increase communication and identify priorities and problems in the field of injury prevention; and (4) to lower injury morbidity and mortality.

Despite being the lead agency for injury prevention and control, limited funding from Congress has hampered the NCIPC's role. Because of limited staff and limited surveillance capacity, as well as a need to develop real world programs that can be implemented at the local level, much NCIPC intramural research is done through partnerships with state and local governmental agencies. The NCIPC concentrates its efforts on nonoccupational injuries, since occupational injuries are within the purview of the CDC's National Institute of Occupational Safety and Health.

### *National Institute of Occupational Safety and Health (NIOSH)*

NIOSH was created by the Occupational Health and Safety Act of 1970 to serve employers and employees in the areas of injury, safety, and ergonomics by focusing on research and training related to occupational safety and health. NIOSH, which is an institute within the CDC, is charged with making research-based recommendations to the federal Occupational Safety and Health Administration (OSHA), a regulatory agency. NIOSH

**Exhibit 10–6**  Injury Control Research Centers

According to the National Center for Injury Prevention and Control, "Injury Control Research Centers conduct research in all three core phases of injury control (prevention, acute care, and rehabilitation) and serve as training centers as well as information centers for the public. Research design in these centers is interdisciplinary and incorporates the fields of medicine, engineering, epidemiology, law, and criminal justice, behavioral and social sciences, biostatistics, public health, and biomechanics."

Injury control research centers are located in the following institutions:

- Colorado State University
- Harborview Medical Center
- Harvard University
- Johns Hopkins University
- University of Alabama at Birmingham
- University of California, Los Angeles
- University of California, San Francisco
- University of Iowa
- University of North Carolina, Chapel Hill
- University of Pittsburgh

*Source:* Reprinted from http://www.cdc.gov/ncipc/res-opps/icrcs.htm, National Center for Injury Prevention and Control.

works to better understand the multiple causes of worker deaths and injuries. It conducts intramural research and surveillance and also funds extramural research. Several surveillance systems for fatal and nonfatal occupational injuries are maintained by NIOSH (see Chapter 12). The NIOSH Division of Safety serves as the focal point for injury prevention and worker protection research. It is the only federal agency that awards training grants specifically for injury prevention and control. Unfortunately its scope is currently restricted to occupational injury for the health professions.

NIOSH's activities include

- investigating specific hazardous working conditions on request
- evaluating and identifying general hazards in the workplace
- carrying out research, including support for Agricultural Safety Research Centers
- supporting training of health professionals and funding of university-based Educational Resource Centers

- developing educational materials and recommendations for worker protection
- publishing results of investigations through *NIOSH Alerts* (including prevention recommendations for the public)

Recent NIOSH initiatives include efforts to promote adolescent worker safety (involving community-based health education demonstration grants) and developing a national occupational research agenda.[14]

### *Division of Adolescent and School Health (DASH), National Center for Chronic Disease Prevention and Health Promotion, CDC*

DASH is charged with identifying risk behaviors of young Americans, monitoring the prevalence of these risk behaviors, assessing intervention priorities, implementing national programs to reduce these risk behaviors, and evaluating and improving these and related programs. Behaviors related to unintentional injuries and violence are one of DASH's six priority areas. Risk behavior prevalence is monitored through a national data collection effort—the Youth Risk Behavioral Surveillance System—which is also used to examine trends in risk behaviors over time. Another national data collection effort—the School Health Policy and Programs Study monitors what schools and education agencies are doing to promote healthy behavior and to prevent unhealthy behavior through school policies, teacher training, and risk reduction curricula. Both of these monitoring systems include injury-related questions.

The Division of Adolescent and School Health provides direction and leadership for school health programs, which includes developing and implementing an agenda in the area of injury prevention. Current activities include the development of a registry of injury prevention evaluation research to make information accessible to practitioners. In addition, DASH is working closely with adolescent risk behavior experts, other federal agencies, state agencies, and national organizations to develop guidelines for school and community programs to promote lifelong safety practices and prevent injury and violence.

### *National Center for Health Statistics (NCHS)*

The NCHS focuses exclusively on monitoring U.S. health data trends by compiling mortality statistics and data on illnesses and injury. The data is collected through several national surveys that are conducted annually (see

Chapter 12). The NCHS, which is a center within the CDC, produces a wealth of data relevant to injury prevention. Within the NCHS, its National Committee on Vital and Health Statistics has been in the forefront in efforts to improve the reporting of external causes of injury in hospital discharge data. Recent NCHS activities have included an injury chartbook as a feature of *Health, United States, 1996–97*,[15] special reports on specific injury topics (such as firearms), a redesign of ongoing surveys to incorporate a focus on injury, and leadership for an international collaborative effort on injury statistics, the mission of which is to promote international comparability of injury statistics.

### *Maternal and Child Health Bureau (MCHB), Health Resources and Services Administration (HRSA)*

The Health Resources and Services Administration provides services to low-income and high-risk populations, develops health resources and manpower for these same populations (including funding for education and training of health personnel), and provides financial assistance to support health services through grants and contracts to state and local government and private health care institutions. The HRSA supports a variety of programs aimed at improving the health of the nation by harnessing and coordinating available resources to promote access to quality health care and to improve service delivery, primary care education and practice, and services to underserved and vulnerable populations.

The MCHB was created to advance the health of mothers and children. It serves women of childbearing age, mothers, children, youth, and families. Its primary focus is on supporting states and communities in their efforts to plan, organize, and deliver primary and preventive health care. A large part of its charge involves promoting comprehensive services to meet the health care needs of its target population, especially those most vulnerable to problems in accessing quality health care because of income level, geographic location, age, gender, disabling condition, and race. Because of its charge, the MCHB reaches especially high-risk populations for injury and violence prevention and directly works with state health agencies on injury prevention issues. Because unintentional injuries and violence are the leading killer of children and adolescents, it makes sense that a significant proportion of MCHB resources be devoted to this problem area. The MCHB's injury prevention program supports the acquisition and dissemination of knowledge about the incidence of injury and violence, the contributing factors, and effective interventions.

To assist states in developing programs that improve maternal and child health, the MCHB provides funds to improve state programs and activities that address health issues affecting the target population. States receive support via two mechanisms: MCHB block grants and 15% set asides to fund Special Projects of Regional and National Significance (SPRANS) and Community Integrated Service Systems (CISS). Many state MCHB programs have incorporated injury and violence prevention efforts into their activities funded under the MCHB services block grant and have used these funds to support a staff position dedicated to injury and violence prevention and/or to fund mini-grants to localities. Beginning in the 1980s, SPRANS funds were used to support state-specific injury and violence demonstration projects. Exhibit 10–7 presents information on one SPRANS-funded injury prevention effort.

In 1995 Congress mandated the Office of Adolescent Health within the MCHB to coordinate and provide mechanisms for collaborative adolescent health activities. The Office of Adolescent Health was directed to assist public health agencies and practitioners in fulfilling the core public health functions of assessment, policy development, and assurance as they related to adolescent health. They were to make research findings available, encourage establishment of partnerships, sponsor consensus meetings, and develop evaluation efforts. This program funded adolescent health coordinators in 41 states to guide the implementation of innovative adolescent health programs and to help build state and local coalitions to address such problems as teen pregnancy, human immunodeficiency virus and acquired immune deficiency syndrome, and violence and injury prevention. The keystone of this approach was integration of effort (e.g., improve access to health care for adolescents by promoting school-linked and school-based health centers).

The MCHB also supports a separate emergency medical services for children program to improve the way in which children are served in emergency situations. The program addresses the whole range of children's emergency services, from trauma to illness and from prevention to acute care to rehabilitation. When Congress authorized this program in 1984, it recognized that the lack of prompt emergency transportation, medical services, special pediatric equipment, and adequate training for health professionals compromised the unique emergency medical service needs of children. Under the program, grants are provided to universities and state and local agencies for research, continuing education, and the development, planning, implementation, and enhancement of state emergency medical

**Exhibit 10–7** The Children's Safety Network

---

Since 1991, Special Projects of Regional and National Significance funds have been used to support the Children's Safety Network National Injury and Violence Prevention Resource Center. The Children's Safety Network is a group of organizations working to assist maternal and child health and related agencies to prevent child and adolescent injuries by

- serving as a source of information for professionals on all causes of injury, both intentional and unintentional
- providing technical assistance, training, and resources to help integrate injury and violence prevention into existing maternal and child health programs
- facilitating the development of new injury prevention programs
- conducting research and policy activities that improve the state-of-the-art of injury and violence prevention
- serving as advocates with national and federal agencies on behalf of state and local injury prevention practitioners

As part of these efforts, special attention is given to rural injury prevention, adolescent violence prevention, injury data for state-level needs assessments, and assistance to practitioners, insurers, and others in using injury data, estimating costs, and being strong advocates for program and policy initiatives.

---

services for children (EMS-C) systems. These grants have supported many injury prevention projects at the state and local level. The MCHB also funds an EMS-C technical assistance and resource center that assists grantees in developing new programs and works with professional organizations to develop training efforts and help the public understand the problems of emergency medical services for children and to build coalitions to support EMS-C efforts. Most recently, the MCHB began to administer a traumatic brain injury (TBI) program that will include state demonstration grants to improve the delivery of services to individuals sustaining TBI.

### *National Institutes of Health (NIH)*

NIH conducts and sponsors biomedical, social, and behavioral research and training at its component institutes. Several of these institutes concern themselves with aspects of injury.

- The National Institute for Child Health and Human Development conducts research related to child development and injuries, including the mechanisms of childhood injury and interventions aimed at prevention.

- The National Institute on Aging carries out research on injuries related to the aging process, specifically from falls and motor vehicle crashes.
- The National Institute of Arthritis, Musculoskeletal and Skin Diseases concerns itself with research on those injuries that result in arthritis, particularly injuries resulting from participation in sports.
- The National Institute of Neurological Diseases and Stroke is concerned with the study of brain and spinal cord injury.
- The National Institute of Mental Health is interested in child abuse and, until recently, had a violence and traumatic stress branch. Research interests include suicidal youths, perpetrators and victims of violence, and children and adolescents who are at risk for serious mental disorders and learning disabilities (e.g., survivors of unintentional injuries and violence).
- The National Heart, Lung, and Blood Institute examines sleep disorders (e.g., sleep deprivation) that could affect driving safety and work safety.
- The National Institute on Disability and Rehabilitation Research, the National Institute on Alcohol Abuse and Alcoholism, and the National Institute on Drug Abuse also carry on work that relates to the prevention of injury.

Despite the fact that injury, as the leading cause of productive years of life lost, is a major health problem in the United States, there is no national institute on injury. This is the result of political judgments and has clear repercussions for injury prevention.[16]

### *Substance Abuse and Mental Health Services Administration (SAMHSA)*

SAMHSA develops programs to prevent and treat alcohol, substance abuse, and mental health problems. Part of its mission is to provide financial assistance through grants and contracts that support health services to state and local government and private health care institutions. These efforts have clear implications for injury prevention.

### *Indian Health Service (IHS)*

The IHS is concerned with the health care needs of Native Americans (American Indians and Alaska Natives). Since midcentury, traumatic injury has been recognized as the leading cause of death in the majority of the communities served by the IHS. Since the 1960s, the IHS has focused attention on the prevention of injuries, concentrating originally on health education approaches that admonished unsafe behaviors. In the 1980s, with Native American motor vehicle crash fatalities many times the nation average, the IHS intensified its efforts to stem these deaths and disabilities from traumatic injury, beginning with an injury surveillance system to identify the most severe injuries and target intervention efforts based on epidemiological data. In 1987 an injury prevention specialist fellowship and an injury prevention practitioners course were started. These were "capacity building" efforts to address the needs of health professionals and field practitioners. In 1990 an injury prevention program five-year plan was created.

Based on early successes, Congress appropriated funds in 1990 that enabled the establishment of full-time injury prevention specialists in all 12 IHS areas. Additional congressional resources have provided funding for tribes to target specific injury problems through community-specific solutions. In 1997, the IHS issued its first request for proposals to address tribal infrastructure in injury prevention. Recent years have seen improvements in injury mortality and morbidity for Native Americans, but the rates are still unacceptably high.

## Other Federal Agencies

The federal government's injury prevention activities discussed so far are centered in the Department of Health and Human Services, but there are many important agencies in other parts of the federal structure that play key roles in the field of injury prevention.

### *Consumer Product Safety Commission (CPSC)*

The CPSC was established by Congress in 1972 as an independent regulatory agency, which means that rather than being part of a Cabinet department, it is overseen by commissioners appointed directly by the president. The CPSC is charged with protecting the public from unsafe consumer products. "Consumer product" is broadly defined to include any article produced or distributed for sale for a consumer's personal use, consumption, or enjoyment, in or around a household or school, in recreation, or otherwise. This small regulatory, research, and educational agency has jurisdiction over some 15,000 consumer products, from coffeemakers to fireworks, from lawnmowers to toys. Excepted from its jurisdiction are products covered by other federal agencies: motor vehicles (regulated by the Department of Transportation), food and drugs (regulated by the Food and Drug Administration), and alcohol, tobacco, and firearms (regulated for tax purposes by the Treasury Department). The CPSC is responsible for enforcing six federal statutes: the Consumer Product Safety Act, the Federal Hazardous Substances Act, the Fire Safe Cigarette Act, the Flammable Fabrics Act, the Poison Prevention Packaging Act, and the Refrigerator Safety Act.

Although categorized as a regulatory agency, the CPSC takes a comprehensive approach that includes education, product testing, dissemination of information, hazard identification and analysis, hazard assessment and reduction, compliance and enforcement, development of guidelines, standard setting, and cooperation with community groups. Using the classic techniques of public health, the CPSC uses an interdisciplinary approach, drawing on the perspectives of epidemiologists, engineers, economists, physicians, and policy analysts—all working toward the end of developing effective prevention strategies.

CPSC activities include conducting research on potential product hazards; developing educational materials for and educating consumers about potential hazards; banning, recalling, or requiring repair of hazardous products; developing voluntary standards with industry; operating the National Electronic Injury Surveillance System (a surveillance system for product-related injuries and deaths [see Chapter 12]); and operating a toll-free hotline for consumers to report unsafe products or product-related injuries (1-800-638-2772). Issuing and enforcing mandatory standards is a last resort that is seldom employed by the agency.

The CPSC maintains regional offices, but the bulk of its work is carried out in Washington, D.C. It does not provide grant funding to outside agencies, states, or universities. Its in-house research includes collecting and analyzing economic and hazard exposure information on products, investigating specific injury cases to determine their causes, and maintaining chemistry and engineering laboratories to test consumer products. Much of its work is directed at efforts to mobilize industry into developing voluntary standards (as was done, for example, with disposable cigarette lighters that are now child resistant). Notable CPSC successes include reduced injuries and deaths through design changes in cribs, hair dryers, playpens, bean bag chairs, drawstrings on children's outer garments, electric heaters, toys, garage door openers, and product packaging (child-resistant closures). The CPSC has propounded only a few product bans, including bans of infant cushions, lawn darts, and refuse bins.

### Occupational Safety and Health Administration (OSHA)

Created by the Occupational Safety and Health Act of 1970, OSHA is part of the Department of Labor. OSHA establishes occupational safety and health standards, ensures compliance with these standards by means of a workplace inspection program, and assesses penalties for violations. The agency has limited resources and relies heavily on self-reporting and sporadic inspections. Moreover, not all employee groups are covered by OSHA; as many as one third of U.S. workers may not fall within its protective jurisdiction. OSHA relies on the scientific findings of the NIOSH to develop the occupational safety and health standards it seeks to enforce.

### National Highway Traffic Safety Administration (NHTSA)

NHTSA was established in 1970 to carry out safety programs under the National Traffic and Motor Vehicle Safety Act of 1966. It is responsible for reducing deaths, injuries, and economic losses resulting from motor vehicle crashes, including those involving bicyclists and pedestrians. The agency's major work is carried out by setting and enforcing safety performance standards for motor vehicles.

NHTSA provides technical assistance, training, data, and informational materials specific to its mandate. It oversees databases such as the Fatality Analysis Reporting System (FARS) and the National Automotive Sampling System, both of which are described in Chapter 12. NHTSA has been working to link medical with traffic safety databases. Safety information made available to the public by NHTSA, including crash test data, is broken down according to make and model of vehicle (unlike the CPSC, which is not permitted to routinely identify products by manufacturer, thus greatly limiting the value of its data for public protection).

NHTSA helps state and local governments and national organizations to conduct effective local highway safety programs by providing them with grant funding. It has 10 regional offices that coordinate work with the states. NHTSA funds research and provides money at the state and regional level for programs that address its national traffic safety priorities. Current priority areas include occupant protection, alcohol and other drugs, police traffic services, traffic records, emergency medical services, motorcycle safety, pedestrian/bicycle safety, and roadway safety. Funds are given out in several ways. The Section 402 State and Community

Highway Safety Grant program is equivalent to public health service block grants, in that (1) 402 funds are awarded on the basis of state population and (2) the states decide how to allocate these funds based on state-level problem identification consistent with the national priorities. NHTSA also supports a Section 403 Highway Safety Research and Development program, which provides grant moneys to public and private organizations for demonstration projects, outreach to national organizations, materials development, and training and education. An Alcohol Incentive Grants program enables states to address problems associated with alcohol-impaired driving (states are eligible if they have met specific criteria, e.g., sanctions for repeat offenders, administrative driver license sanctions, graduated licensing systems for youth). NHTSA also sponsors a competitive and comprehensive research program on vehicle safety that encompasses human factors (e.g., driver fatigue and inattention), crashworthiness (e.g., airbags), crash avoidance (e.g., braking, intelligent transportation systems), and crash testing. NHTSA provides core funding for transportation safety research institutes at the University of Michigan and the University of North Carolina.

A new NHTSA focus called the Safe Communities initiative began in 1995. It seeks to get health care professionals to work side by side with law enforcement, business, local government, school, and other community and agency personnel. The Safe Communities initiative is based on the idea that communities are in the best position to design innovative solutions to deal with their entire injury problem. Four things are required to qualify as a safe community:

1. data linkage among traffic safety and health sources to define the community's injury problem
2. expanded partnerships, especially with the health care sector
3. citizen involvement and input in program design and implementation
4. integrated and comprehensive injury control system incorporating prevention, acute care, and rehabilitation

NHTSA provides designated Safe Communities with leadership guidance, 402 funds, and technical assistance to enhance community action and engage new stakeholders.

Exhibit 10–8 lists the various federal agencies having some involvement with injury prevention (some substantial, others quite limited).

**Exhibit 10–8** Federal Agencies Involved in Injury Prevention

---

## DEPARTMENT OF HEALTH AND HUMAN SERVICES, PUBLIC HEALTH SERVICE

- Centers for Disease Control and Prevention
  1. National Center for Injury Prevention and Control
     –Division of Unintentional Injury Prevention
     –Division of Violence Prevention
     –Division of Acute Care, Rehabilitation Research, and Disability Prevention
  2. National Institute of Occupational Safety and Health
  3. National Center for Chronic Disease Prevention and Health Promotion
     –Division of Adolescent and School Health
  4. National Center for Health Statistics
- Health Resources and Services Administration
  1. Maternal and Child Health Bureau
- National Institutes of Health (some funding of injury-related research)
  1. National Institute on Aging
  2. National Institute on Alcohol Abuse and Alcoholism
  3. National Institute of Arthritis, Musculoskeletal and Skin Diseases
  4. National Institute of Child Health and Human Development
  5. National Institute on Disability and Rehabilitation Research
  6. National Institute of Neurological Diseases and Stroke
  7. National Heart, Lung, and Blood Institute
  8. National Institute of Drug Abuse
  9. National Institute of Mental Health
- Substance Abuse and Mental Health Service Administration
  1. Center for Substance Abuse Prevention
- Indian Health Service
- Administration on Children, Youth and Families
  1. Children's Bureau
     –Office on Child Abuse and Neglect

## DEPARTMENT OF TRANSPORTATION

- National Highway Traffic Safety Administration
- Federal Highway Administration

## DEPARTMENT OF LABOR

- Bureau of Labor Statistics
- Mine Safety and Health Administration

---

*continues*

**Exhibit 10–8** continued

- Occupational Safety and Health Administration
- Office of Safety and Health
- Wage and Hour Division

**DEPARTMENT OF JUSTICE**

- Drug Enforcement Agency
- Office of Justice Programs
  1. Bureau of Justice Assistance
  2. Bureau of Justice Statistics
  3. National Institute of Justice
     –National Criminal Justice Reference Service
  4. Office of Juvenile Justice and Delinquency Prevention
  5. Office for Victims of Crime

**DEPARTMENT OF THE INTERIOR**

- Bureau of Indian Affairs
  1. Indian Highway Traffic Safety Programs

**DEPARTMENT OF EDUCATION**

- Drug Free Schools and Communities Division

**OTHER**

- Consumer Product Safety Commission
- National Transportation Safety Board
- Federal Emergency Management Administration

## CONCLUSION

There are many governmental agencies working to reduce the number and severity of injuries in America. These agencies exist at the local, state, and federal levels and, together, they form an interconnected system. We have looked at some state and federal agencies that make up this system; these agencies carry out a broad range of programs and provide funding and assistance to local health departments. How these local departments use this support is the subject of the next chapter.

When this patchwork injury prevention system works well, public agencies can cooperate synergistically to achieve their common goal. When the system does not work well, problems can fall into the cracks of bureaucracy. It is important that the injury prevention practitioner understand this patchwork of agencies and programs so as to make best use of all potential assistance and resources. Used to fullest advantage, the network of injury prevention agencies can provide a coordinated approach to protecting the public from injury.

---

## NOTES

1. Committee on Trauma Research, Commission on Life Sciences, National Research Council and Institute of Medicine. *Injury in America: A Continuing Public Health Problem.* Washington, DC: National Academy Press; 1985.

2. Surgeon General's Workshop on Violence and Public Health, Leesburg, VA, October 1985. Papers appear in Rosenberg ML, Fenley MA. *Violence in America, A Public Health Approach.* New York: Oxford University Press; 1991.

3. Statement by C. Everett Koop, MD, ScD, Surgeon General, U.S. Public Health Service, Department of Health and Human Services before the Subcommittee on Children, Family, Drugs, and Alcoholism, U.S. Senate, February 9, 1989, Washington, DC.

4. Committee for the Study of the Future of Public Health. *The Future of Public Health.* Washington, DC: National Academy Press; 1988.

5. Harrington C, Gallagher SS, Burgess LL, Guyer B. *Injury Prevention Programs in State Health Departments: A National Survey.* Boston, MA: Harvard School of Public Health; 1988.

6. Children's Safety Network. *Injury Prevention Outlook: An Assessment of Injury Prevention in State Maternal and Child Health Agencies—Background Report.* Newton, MA: Education Development Center; 1992.

7. See http://www.stipda.org.

8. "Program Resources for a Safe Community" at the NHTSA Safe Communities web site. http://nhtsa.dot.gov:80/safecommunities/ServiceCenter/default.asp.

9. Education Development Center, University of Illinois at Chicago. *Who's Who in Traffic Safety.* Newton, MA: Education Development Center; July 1996.

10. Children's Cabinet Information Dissemination and Training Development Work Team and Data and Evaluation Work Team. *Maine Youth Suicide Prevention Implementation Plan.* Augusta, ME: Maine Department of Human Services; May 1998.

11. Durfee MJ, Gellert GA, Tilton-Durfee D. Origins and clinical relevance of child death review teams. *JAMA.* 1992;267:3172–3175.

12. Public Health Services Agencies Use Different Approaches To Protect Public against Disease and Injury. U.S. GAO: April 1994, GAO/HEHS-94-85BR.

13. Gallagher SS, Messenger KP, Guyer B. State and local responses to children's injuries: The Massachusetts Statewide Injury Prevention Program. *J Soc Issues.* 1987;43:149–162.

14. National Institute for Occupational Safety and Health. *National Occupational Research Agenda.* Cincinnati, OH: NIOSH; 1996.

15. Fingerhut LA, Warner M. Injury chartbook. In: National Center for Health Statistics. *Health, United States, 1996–97 and Injury Chartbook.* Hyattsville, MD: U.S. Public Health Service; 1997.

16. Terris M. The paradox of the missing Institute. *J Public Health Policy.* 1983;4:394–397.

# CHAPTER 11

# Developing a Public Health Agency Injury Program: A Systems Approach

"Health departments should be seen as crucial but not sufficient. . . . They must develop the stabilizing interest to sustain a search for answers into the future."

William H. Foege, Preface to *Violence in America*, 1991

## WHAT THIS CHAPTER IS ABOUT

Injury is a major public health problem. Fortunately it is one that is, to a large extent, preventable using the classic public health approaches of surveillance, epidemiological analysis, and educational, environmental, and legal interventions. How can these public health approaches best be developed, organized, and implemented to reduce injuries?

The previous chapter reviewed existing governmental injury prevention programs at the state and federal levels, but most public health activity in the United States is carried out on the state and local levels. How have health departments dealt with the relatively new area of injury prevention? How have state and local agencies worked together on this issue? What are the best ways for public health agencies to create and develop injury prevention programs? How can the lead agency responsible for injury prevention activities most effectively collaborate with other governmental agencies? What resources are required to undertake meaningful injury prevention activity? How can support from colleagues and the public be established for agency injury prevention efforts? These and related issues are the subject of this chapter. Our goal is to suggest effective strategies for developing and implementing public health agency responses to the problem of injury at the state and local levels.

## INTRODUCTION

Public health agencies are well positioned to develop and implement injury prevention strategies and programs. They are well equipped to do so because they are already in the prevention business and have the tools of the trade (i.e., public health agencies have long been developing and implementing strategies for disease prevention). Public health agencies have experience in

- gathering and using data
- reaching high-risk populations through targeted service delivery (e.g., women, infants, and children nutrition programs [WIC], new immigrants)
- working at the grassroots level in the communities being served
- building coalitions

State health departments are mandated to carry out surveillance on public health hazards. Traditionally, their programs have been adapted as new health hazards have been recognized. The classic public health approach as applied—first to infectious diseases and later to chronic diseases—is the same approach that provides the most logical framework for dealing with injury, one that uses data collection, biostatistics, epidemiology, health education, and the other tools of public health. The skills and resources needed to effectively deal with injury do not have to be created de novo; they already exist, busily working away within local and state health departments.

The goal of agency-centered injury prevention efforts is to develop and implement a prevention strategy that can bring about meaningful reductions in morbidity and mortality and an enhancement in life quality. This is usually done by measuring the extent of a health problem, identifying risk factors, developing and implementing preventive interventions to change human behaviors or the environment, and evaluating the resulting effects, all with the goal of reducing the incidence of the problem. Health departments combine regulatory authority, program funding, provision of services at the local level, and public education.

Although injury prevention programs can be most effective when directed at the local level, state health departments can provide the leadership and expertise needed to inspire, support, and guide local efforts. State health departments must have trained staff to provide in-house expertise in injury prevention; assess and analyze injury risks to specific populations at the local level; publish and disseminate such data on a timely basis; know and support effective intervention strategies; supply tools and materials to make it as easy as possible for local practitioners to integrate injury and violence prevention within their setting; provide leadership to multiple federal, state, and local agencies involved in eliminating injuries and fostering safety in their state; and develop a legislative, regulatory, and budgetary strategy to institutionalize injury prevention within the state.[1] (Exhibit 11–1 reviews the core functions of a state injury control program.)

Despite the fact that injury is a major public health problem, state health departments spend only about 1% of their combined budgets on injury prevention. Most state and local health departments lack a division or unit dedicated to injury prevention. Despite the proven cost-effectiveness of most injury prevention programs, injury prevention has had a low priority within public health. Why is this the case? More to the point, how can it be changed?

To succeed in reducing injuries and their consequent costs, a major initiative is needed to institutionalize injury prevention activities, encompassing surveillance, service delivery, and policy formation. Recommendations from a 1987 assessment of state health agency programs are still very relevant.[2] These recommendations included

- establishing a separate and comprehensive injury control program as a focal point
- establishing a coordinating body to lead injury prevention activities
- organizing a statewide injury prevention task force to collaborate with other state and local agencies
- developing a state plan for injury control
- expanding programs to target intentional injuries, including suicide and other forms of violence
- attending to those types of unintentional injuries that have received little program attention in the past, such as pedestrian, fall, and sports-related injuries
- implementing multiple strategies, with increasing emphasis on legislation and enforcement, environmental alteration, and product modification
- creating educational efforts for policy makers to develop knowledgeable advocates for injury prevention

**Exhibit 11–1**  State Injury Control Program Core Functions

It would be useful to recall the core functions of a state injury control program developed by the State and Territorial Injury Prevention Directors Association. These functions were described in detail in Exhibit 10–1.

1. statewide and local injury data collection
2. statewide coordination, leadership, and administration
3. program development and implementation
4. policy development
5. evaluation
6. professional training and education
7. public information and educational programs
8. ensuring the protection and health of the population by investigating injury clusters or events

*Source:* State and Territorial Injury Prevention Directors' Association at http://www.stipda.org/stipda/core.htm. Used with permission.

- improving use of existing resources, such as established guidelines, available data, technical assistance, and private and block grant funding
- incorporating realistic evaluation components into programs as they are designed
- increasing networking with those with more expertise in injury prevention programs in order to avoid having to constantly "reinvent the wheel"
- developing strategies to expand state supported and state funded injury prevention efforts

This may seem complicated and overwhelming, but as with so many challenges, the trick is to approach the effort one step at a time. This chapter will look at three important aspects of developing an injury prevention initiative: (1) getting on the agenda, (2) starting up with a lead agency, and (3) focusing on those factors most critical to a successful injury prevention program.

## GETTING ON THE AGENDA

How can health departments move ahead with injury prevention? If no injury prevention program exists, who is to bring it into being? Is it necessary to have a management-level person as the initiating and driving force? Just how does one begin? To get to the starting point with any health problem, that problem must be on the public health agency agenda. Unfortunately this is an area in which inertia plays a big role; traditional programs continue of their own volition because they have the staff, the support network, the public image, and established funding sources. These factors obviously do not favor public health initiatives in new areas such as injury prevention.

There are, however, some external forces that can help get new initiatives onto the public health agenda. An important source of such external pressure is found in the Year 2000 Health Objectives, which constitute a cornerstone for prevention programs in federal, state, and local health agencies. A series of injury-related year 2000 objectives outline specific target reductions in the areas of motor vehicle injury prevention, prevention of violence and injuries due to violence, home and leisure injury prevention, occupational injury prevention, and acute care and rehabilitation. (The text of these objectives can be found at the ends of Chapter 4—objectives related to unintentional injuries—and Chapter 5—objectives related to intentional injuries). In addition to the injury-related Year 2000 objectives, the Centers for Disease Control and Prevention (CDC) injury prevention plan—*Injury Control in the 1990s: A National Plan for Action*—complements the injury-related Year 2000 objectives.[3] Health objectives developed for the year 2010 will continue this approach.[4]

A logical first step in getting injury prevention onto the public health agency agenda is to describe the expected "payoff" of injury prevention interventions. A comprehensive listing of injury prevention benefits is one that would include—but not be limited to—reductions in injury rates, longer life, less disability, and so on. Other benefits would include cost savings for both government and the private sector, reduced demands on the health care system, improved trauma response, and an enhanced sense of community; however, it is a common mistake to simply provide data demonstrating need and assume this will drive the agenda-setting process. *Data alone will not secure a place on administrative and policy agendas.*

It is possible to imagine word coming down from on high—a governor or mayor, state legislature or city council, or a board of health—mandating the development of injury prevention initiatives, but in the real world, programmatic initiatives emerge in this way only in the aftermath of a well-publicized tragedy, and few such directives come with resource support and long-term commitment. Instead, agency staff usually must lay the groundwork for new initiatives. And new initiatives don't come from already overburdened staffs asking for additional burdens, so there must be some sense that new resources will be forthcoming or that injury prevention efforts will help further existing objectives (including professional ones). Or there must be some expectation that outside funding will assist the initiation of new programmatic efforts. Most important of all, there must be a strategy.

The way injury prevention is presented is key to getting on agendas. Oftentimes getting on the agenda can be facilitated by *not* seeking a separate new program but, rather, through *integration* (i.e., integrating injury prevention into existing programs). For example, most states have early intervention (EI) programs supported by maternal and child health funds. These programs target young children with developmental delays or children living in families with serious social problems. These are children who are at high risk for both unintentional and intentional injury. EI staff who do home visits or who offer support to parents are in a position to provide counseling or to point out hazards. These staff members should receive training about injury prevention and understand the opportunity they have to deal with this issue. Exhibit 11–2 provides an outline of the injury prevention component of an actual citywide EI program. One way to have injury prevention addressed within EI or other existing programs might be to work with the state-level manager of the program. You can have injury prevention identified as an unmet need that should be included in the grant writing process when the existing EI programs apply for state funding support.

Integration of injury prevention into existing public health programs can be both a fiscally and politically advantageous way of getting on the agenda. But there are some significant barriers to such an approach. Many government and private funders are primarily interested in distinct, controlled projects that link outcomes to a given intervention. Although this is useful for research purposes, it greatly complicates attempts to integrate injury prevention into other funded programs.

Funding restrictions can present other problems. Funders of new injury prevention initiatives often want to see efforts made to increase the visibility of the topic, such as local or statewide injury prevention conferences. This could be helpful in getting injury prevention on the agenda. But such conferences can also turn out to be a poor use of staff time, with speakers

**Exhibit 11–2** Step 1: Early Intervention—Integrating Injury Prevention

These are the goals that were developed by the Step 1 Early Intervention Program after it was decided that injury prevention should become an integral part of Step 1 activities.

**TARGET POPULATION**

1. 7,500 families with children ages 0–19
2. parents who are teens, cognitively limited, emotionally disturbed, or stressed
3. families with developmentally delayed children
4. senior citizens

**PROGRAM ACTIVITIES**

1. Train staff in injury prevention.
2. Address injury prevention in parent support groups.
3. Conduct home safety inspections of 75% of enrolled families.
4. Distribute safety supplies on sliding fee scale.
5. Eliminate environmental risks of injury in all three Step 1 center sites.
6. Collaborate with 16 other area early intervention agencies.
7. Provide training to reduce environmental risks in clients' homes.
8. Mail injury prevention materials to area health care providers.
9. Develop public awareness programs targeted to specific seasons.
10. Use parent trainers as peer educators.
11. Link injury prevention interventions with local regulatory and licensing agencies.

preaching to the choir of the already convinced. It makes the most sense if such educational efforts are focused on getting injury prevention on the agenda of other professional conferences and meetings—school health nurses, day care providers, licensing inspectors, case workers who transport children in cars, adolescent health and family planning staff, domestic violence workers, childbirth educators, early intervention staff, English as a Second Language teachers, and lead-reduction paint staff.

All in all, a much better job needs to be done of getting injury prevention integrated into other health department programs. Table 11–1 provides a useful framework for integrating childhood injury prevention activities and topics into other programs and settings. The chart suggests age-appropriate injury prevention topics for a variety of settings, such as prenatal care clinics, hospitals, primary health care settings, WIC clinics, parenting classes, and schools. Tapping into these valuable services and environments can provide ideal opportunities to educate families about child safety as part of a broader child health approach.

Actual examples of this integration approach include

- a home visiting program that conducts child safety screenings in the homes of pregnant and parenting adolescents
- a county WIC clinic that screens pregnant and parenting women and girls for signs of abuse
- a child death review team that investigates motor vehicle–related deaths of adolescents
- a school-based health center that regularly counsels students about safety belt use, impaired driving, on-the-job hazards, and child labor laws
- a school health unit that includes a chapter on injury and violence prevention in its Statewide School Health Manual
- a school-based health clinic that counsels boys at risk for perpetrating dating violence
- a home lead screening program that trains its home visitors to identify and respond to signs of family violence

As these examples illustrate, health departments can find innovative ways to incorporate injury prevention messages into diverse agency programs. State and local health agencies must continue to identify those places where injury control fits into existing programs (and how such integration can be institutionalized at low cost in their routine activities). In particular, state and local agencies should ask themselves

1. Which existing health department programs could have an injury control component?
2. How can injury prevention be incorporated into the state health plan or into block grant service plans?
3. What kind of program-specific protocols can be developed to (1) provide a framework for content, (2) maintain high quality, (3) serve as a teaching tool for service providers, and (4) assist in information sharing across program areas?

**Table 11–1** Examples of MCH Settings for Addressing Injury Prevention Topics

| | Prenatal Care | Hospitals | WIC Parenting Classes | Primary Health Care Settings | Home Visiting Programs | Schools | Day Care Centers |
|---|---|---|---|---|---|---|---|
| Bike safety, helmets | | X | | X | X | X | X |
| Child abuse | X | X | X | X | X | X | x |
| Child safety seats | X | X | X | X | X | | X |
| Drownings | X | | X | X | X | | X |
| Farm machinery | | | | X | X | X | |
| Firearms | X | | X | X | X | X | X |
| Home safety | X | X | X | X | X | | X |
| Injuries from farm animals | | X | X | X | X | X | |
| Motorcycle helmets | | X | | X | | X | |
| Parenting skills | X | X | X | X | X | X | X |
| Pedestrian | | | | X | | X | |
| Playground safety | | | | | X | X | X |
| Safety belts | X | X | X | X | X | X | X |
| Sports | | | | X | | X | |
| Suicide | | X | | X | X | X | |
| Violence prevention | X | X | X | X | X | X | |
| Work-related injuries | | | | X | | X | |

*Note:* MCH, maternal and child health.

*Source:* Adapted from Children's Safety Network, *A Data Book of Child and Adolescent Injury,* 1991, National Center for Education in Maternal and Child Health.

4. How can the injury prevention training of other agency staff be improved?
5. What other groups can be collaborated with to provide additional settings for incorporating injury prevention messages?

The second question above—how can injury prevention be incorporated into the state health plan or into block grant service plans—is critical to ensuring that injury prevention does not slip through the cracks of public health programs. It is very important that states have a specific section of the state health plan that addresses injuries and lays out clear goals and measurable objectives. For example, Washington state developed a public health improvement plan that devotes an entire section to violence and injury control, including a subsection on suicide among youth and young adults. The plan uses *The Future of Public Health* document as its framework and outlines the specific responsibilities of both state and local public health agencies.[5]

The Emergency Preparedness and Injury Control (EPIC) Program of the California Department of Health Services, a five-year strategic plan dedicated to injury prevention, gives a fuller idea of how injury prevention can be incorporated into a state health plan. The strategic plan for 1993–1997 contained 52 objectives for reducing injury morbidity and mortality and suggested ways that the activities could be incorporated into other health department programs. California's planning model is particularly noteworthy in its attention to process. EPIC begins its strategic planning during the annual California Conference on Childhood Injury Control, seeking input from practitioners and researchers across the state. The State Injury Control Task Force then works with the EPIC program to formulate a plan, which is reviewed by participants at the next annual conference. Such a consensus building process is a critical phase of injury prevention planning, as it encompasses the input, needs, and realities of the local program staff who will be implementing the plan, thus ensuring "buy-in" from them and investing them in its successful outcome.[6]

Under the California approach, a specific injury prevention plan is formulated for a number of service programs: adolescent family life program, Black infant health project, comprehensive prenatal services, high-risk infant follow-up program, family planning program, rural health care system, primary health care system, and the women, infants, and children program. Each program has an objective with an implementation activity, a responsible staff person, a timeline, and an evaluation measure. Guidebooks have been developed to use in each setting. The plan exemplifies the use of Maternal and Child Health Block Grant funding to address childhood injuries.[7]

Injury prevention can be integrated into a variety of other state agencies, for example, the state office of elder affairs or the state office of social services. Interagency cooperation at the state level is most common between the state highway safety agency and the state public health agency.[8] Injury prevention should be integrated within agencies that are credible to target populations, where injury prevention will be perceived as compatible with the agency's primary role, can easily incorporate injury prevention into existing activities, and have organizational structures that can facilitate such integration into their daily operations.

Getting on the agenda also means building a broad base of support outside of the health agency, such as with professional associations, the media, citizen groups, and state legislators. It may take several years to create such a constituency. One does not need to be at a management level to get the ball rolling. The experience in several states has underscored that the persistence of program staff is a critical factor in success.

Throughout the process of seeking to introduce a new area of responsibility within public health you will need to keep in mind that conflict is essential and that it should not be shied away from. Conflict creates controversy. Controversy attracts attention. And attention often leads to constructive change.

## STARTING UP: THE IMPORTANCE OF THE LEAD AGENCY

A 1987 national survey found that only 10 states had a separate injury program or unit with a comprehensive focus, and the situation does not seem to have improved greatly since then.[2] In many of the state health departments with established injury prevention programs, the programs are limited to particular subpopulations, such as children. Another survey found that nearly half of state maternal and child health (MCH) agencies did have a designated injury prevention coordinator and nearly two thirds dedicated funds to injury prevention efforts. Of this latter group, 22 used their injury prevention funds for programs, staff, and materials in the state MCH office, 7 to support activities in other agencies within the health department (including epidemiology and health promotion), and 10 to support the injury prevention work of an agency or program outside the health department (such as a poison control center or department of education).[9]

According to the most recent survey data, the state health department divisions most likely to be involved in injury prevention include epidemiology, environmental health, maternal and child health, health promotion and chronic disease prevention, and emergency medical services. Injury prevention should certainly be integrated into all these settings. But one division must be designated as the lead agency to coordinate—not control—the various players. The determination of which division should take the leadership role should focus not only on resources available but also on enthusiasm for the issue.

The National Committee for Injury Prevention and Control noted that "a lead agency or organization can serve as a community or statewide focal point for injury prevention expertise, offering assistance and resources."[10(p22)] *Preventing Childhood Injuries: A Guide for Public Health Agencies*, a start-up guide developed from the experiences of injury prevention practitioners in three states (California, Massachusetts, and Virginia), suggests that a local lead agency serve "as the regional focal point for injury prevention activities [guiding] its community's governmental, professional and private agencies towards a shared goal, utilizing common strategies for injury control." Without such a lead agency, "Time, energy and money will be expended on isolated efforts, but the critical mass of resources needed to be effective will not be brought together."[11(p28)]

State lead agencies can assist local injury prevention efforts in several important ways, including the provision of resources and guidance. Of course, to serve in this role a state agency must have a minimal level of injury prevention expertise and resources. It needs to have the expertise necessary to maintain an injury surveillance system. It must also be able to assist local agencies in accessing state resources, both within and outside of the state health department. The injury prevention specialists who developed *Preventing Childhood Injuries* recommend that a state lead agency begin by targeting childhood injuries before expanding to dealing with injuries in other age groups.[11(pp35–36)]

The lead agency for injury prevention should serve as a coordinating body, rather than being a controlling force within a health department. It should provide focus, reduce duplication, and improve the use of existing resources. The lead agency must provide direction, structuring the big picture, the strategic thinking needed to get injury prevention on the map within the health department, as well as within other state agencies and with external public and private agencies. In so doing, it will be responsible for: (1) identifying injury problems and the specific needs for injury prevention programs, policies, and services within the state; (2) keeping abreast of developments within the field of injury prevention and sharing this information with others; (3) understanding where injury prevention fits into what other agencies are doing, serving as a coordinating force that brings different players to the table; and (4) building a solid constituency for injury prevention activities within the state.

*Preventing Childhood Injuries* describes the responsibilities of the local injury prevention lead agency as

- determining the extent and nature of the injury problem within the region
- establishing the key target injuries on which control efforts will be focused
- establishing goals for the injury control effort
- identifying alternative strategies and courses of action that will meet the goals established
- determining existing and additional resources needed to implement the identified injury control plan
- monitoring implementation of the plan and providing technical assistance
- evaluating the plan's impact and revising strategies[11(pp28-29)]

We would add to the above: Identifying the right mix of agencies to be involved and coordinating their efforts. It takes a certain level of skill to coordinate without control and without becoming bogged down in turf issues.

If these lead agency responsibilities are carried out well, increased visibility and increased funding can result. Unfortunately, in many states the lead agency role has been reduced to pursuing and writing grants to be able to do whatever categorical program for which funding is available, rather than developing the infrastructure needed to establish a firm and effective base for injury prevention, one that is capable of enduring.

It is extremely important that lead agency staff understand that they cannot do the job alone. For effective leadership, lead agency staff must have small egos, think for the common good, put turf issues aside, be persistent for the long term, and be politically savvy. A recently published study indicates that the greatest influence on the success of program implementation is the extent and efficacy of constituent support and advocacy.[12]

Other divisions within the state health department with an interest in injury issues can identify how to integrate injury prevention within their routine activities—at both the state and local levels—to complement the work of the lead division. Given the magnitude and diversity of the injury problem, it is not appropriate for those working in state health agencies to neglect the injury problem within their own setting simply because there is a "designated lead agency" located in a different division. Each division within the state health agency needs to ask itself: "What should I be doing to address this significant public health issue?" See Exhibit 11–3 for an example.

So, how do you get things going? What is the start-up process for establishing an injury prevention program coordinated by a lead agency? Starting an injury prevention program in a state or local health department requires effective problem identification (and, of course, creative and steady leadership). Problem identification is a necessary component of setting goals and objectives and of focusing implementation. It goes well beyond looking at injury rates in a community. The National Committee for Injury Prevention and Control described problem identification as "the process of deciding which injury you want to prevent in what population and with what resources," a process consisting of several key tasks, namely "to determine the nature of the injury problem, the characteristics of the population, the resources available to address it, the community's perception of the problem, and the political environment."[10(p23)]

The injury prevention specialists who developed *Preventing Childhood Injuries* recommend a series of 11 start-up steps.[11] They are:

1. Gather and analyze data on injuries in your region.
2. Select and prioritize your target injuries and population, looking at such factors as severity of injury, medical and social costs, and availability of interventions.
3. Determine your intervention strategies and implementation methods. Consider available and proven strategies, support already existing in the community, potential implementation barriers, and the political feasibility of the strategies and methods.
4. Develop an implementation plan with specific and measurable goals and objectives.

**Exhibit 11–3**  Injury Prevention within a State Maternal and Child Health Agency

---

The Children's Safety Network National Injury and Violence Prevention Resource Center has characterized nine key activities that form the framework for injury prevention within a state maternal and child health (MCH) agency. These components include:

1. designation of an injury prevention coordinator within the MCH division with broad-based training in the concepts of injury prevention and program development
2. dedication of MCH funds to support a basic level for injury prevention activities within existing services
3. advocacy within state government and among the public for injury prevention efforts aimed at children and adolescents
4. assessment of MCH program needs based on analysis of state and local injury mortality and morbidity rates, high-risk behaviors in youth (e. g.seatbelt use, weapons carrying, use of protective equipment such as helmets or shin guards), and available services
5. participation in efforts to improve data sources and the availability and quality of injury data
6. development of an injury prevention service plan for the MCH population that targets key injuries, uses proven strategies, and integrates injury prevention into existing MCH services
7. support and guidance for local MCH programs by providing locally specific data, information, and materials on the injury problem and prevention strategies, training, and technical assistance
8. evaluation of injury prevention program processes and outcomes to determine effectiveness of programs and as a management tool
9. collaboration with other relevant government and private agencies and academic institutions to address childhood injuries from multiple perspectives

Many of these components are universal and should be considered for adoption regardless of the health agency's particular sphere of responsibility

Courtesy of Education Development Center, 1992, Newton, Massachusetts.

---

5. Identify, select, and commit community agencies and individuals to carry out the prevention program and obtain a broad base of support (a step best realized by developing and maintaining a coalition[13]).
6. Develop protocols and materials (educational, legislative, technologic) needed for program implementation.

7. Orient and train agencies and individuals to carry out the intervention plan.
8. Implement the plan.
9. Monitor and support the program, providing feedback and technical assistance in an ongoing fashion.
10. Evaluate and revise the program.
11. Share lessons learned with other programs.

## CRITICAL FACTORS

In a recent study, Cassady et al surveyed all U.S. state health departments to identify the characteristics of a successfully implemented state injury prevention program. They identified "five activities that were felt to be critical indicators of successful implementation: legislative activities, surveillance, monitoring and evaluation, community involvement with the injury program, and the ability to create a permanent place for the program within the state agency (institutionalization)."[12] They concluded that:

> In general, successful implementation of injury prevention programs in state agencies is related to constituent participation, administrative control, organizational capacity, and the attributes of relevant policies. Constituent participation, that is, the extent and efficacy of constituent support and advocacy, had the greatest influence on the success of program implementation. Hence, the activities of advocacy coalitions are instrumental in securing and sustaining program funding, evaluating program performance, and encouraging greater involvement of other community groups.
>
> Another critical factor is the extent to which program managers have administrative control over resources and the setting of program priorities.[12]

The remainder of this chapter will review factors critical to a successful injury prevention program. The discussion will focus on: (1) a systems approach, (2) funding, and (3) collaboration.

### Systems Approach

Perhaps the most important determinant in establishing an injury prevention program is developing a systems approach to program implementation. More states may be doing more things to reduce injury, but most states have not addressed injury systematically as a major public health problem and are only in the initial planning phases for comprehensive injury prevention programming. Achieving injury reduction requires a system, rather than a fragmented approach.

Because of limited resources and other factors, injury prevention has been piecemeal and fragmented. There are unnecessary divisions between research and programs, disciplines (e.g., behavioral psychologists and epidemiologists), agencies with similar goals (e.g., public health and traffic safety), prevention programs and infrastructure development, lead and supporting agencies, various levels of government, and educational, environmental, and regulatory approaches. These divisions produce narrowly focused perspectives, which, in turn, hamper the ability to advance the field of injury prevention.

Systems thinking is a conceptual framework that helps in understanding how events are interrelated, connected into patterns, and organized into a totality, rather than being fragmented, unrelated happenings. As applied to injury prevention, systems thinking requires a coordinated effort of public health, medical, law enforcement, political, community, and other players, organized and united into a planned approach. "The efforts of each agency and individual in the system should be directed toward achieving the overall goals of the program. The systems approach includes five phases: analysis, design, development, implementation, and evaluation."[14] Exhibit 11–4 presents a checklist of "Measurements of Key Activities in a Systems Approach to Developing a Comprehensive Injury Prevention Program."

Although quite common in business, systems thinking has only recently been applied to public health and injury prevention. For the systems approach to operate effectively, there must be an established organizational structure responsible for directing the system and for establishing and nurturing linkages with other entities. This is where the multidisciplinary tradition of public health should come in. At the operational level, creating, maintaining, and improving a comprehensive systems approach is the job of an injury control program manager. This requires both the time and the ability to step back, look at the big picture, create linkages, and coordinate resources into a unified effort. It requires a logical planning and implementation effort, one in which epidemiological factors are analyzed, target injuries identified, effective intervention strategies selected, and impeding factors and organizational roadblocks identified.

**Exhibit 11–4** Measurements of Key Activities in a Systems Approach to Developing a Comprehensive Injury Prevention Program

## I. MEASUREMENTS INDICATING KEY ANALYSIS/ ASSESSMENT ACTIVITIES ARE TAKING PLACE

A. Data collection and analysis
  • Morbidity data used to define problems and evaluate strategies.
  • Mortality data used to define problems and evaluate strategies.
  • Efforts underway to improve the quantity and quality of morbidity data.
  • Agencies that collect data are coordinating activities.

B. External and internal environmental analysis
  • State demographics available and current.
  • Analyses of ethnic composition, occupational status, and economic levels of various local communities are completed.
  • Key legislative committees and supporters identified.
  • Complementary activities in health department and community identified.
  • Groups likely to oppose or be in competition with prevention efforts identified.
  • Task force to advise injury activities operational.

## II. MEASUREMENTS INDICATING KEY DESIGN/ DEVELOPMENT ACTIVITIES ARE TAKING PLACE

A. Development of comprehensive plan
  • Plan with goals and measurable objectives.
  • Plan time bound and specific.
  • Plan developed through group consensus.

B. Targeting of high-risk groups and injuries
  • Proposed interventions based on mortality and morbidity behavioral risk factor data for the defined geographic area/target group.
  • Proposed interventions based on analysis of injuries by age, race, and economic status.

C. Identification and involvement of key individuals
  • Advisory committee or task force in place.
  • Members drawn from both inside and outside the health department.
  • Members clear on roles.

*continues*

**Exhibit 11–4**  continued

D. Selection of effective interventions
- Interventions based on current research and literature.
- Interventions appropriate to the community or population being targeted.
- Interventions combine education, environmental modification, and legislation/regulation.

## III. MEASUREMENTS INDICATING KEY IMPLEMENTATION ACTIVITIES ARE TAKING PLACE

A. Collaboration
- Community, grassroots coalition in place.
- Activities planned or ongoing.
- Working relationships among various agencies and groups established.

B. Staff training
- Workshops, professional education, materials available to staff.
- Staff with previous experience in injury control, public health education
- Technical assistance provided to local programs.

C. Integration
- Existing health department programs with an injury control component.
- Injury prevention identified in the State Plan.
- Protocols exist for information sharing across program areas.
- Injury prevention included in the training of other health professionals in health agency.

D. Use of appropriate strategies
- Materials checked for reading level and cultural appropriateness.
- Interventions multifaceted.
- Safety devices affordable.
- Legislative/regulatory initiatives feasible.

## IV. MEASUREMENTS INDICATING KEY EVALUATION ACTIVITIES ARE TAKING PLACE

A. Evaluation planned from the beginning
- Evaluation plan in place prior to implementation.
- Data to be collected consistent with program objectives.

*continues*

**Exhibit 11–4** continued

- Data collection instruments and protocols in place.
- A person responsible for evaluation designated.

B. Project monitored and tracked
- Data collection instruments and protocols correctly used by practitioners.
- Adjustments to program being made based on findings as necessary.
- Percent of target being reached can be determined.
- Amount of resources being used can be determined.

C. Outcome evaluation completed
- Sound evaluation methodology used.
- Changes in knowledge, attitudes and/or behaviors can be determined.
- Changes in injury rates can be determined or inferred from changes in knowledge, attitudes, behavior.
- Changes in public policy can be determined.

Courtesy of Education Development Center, 1990, Newton, Massachusetts

## Funding

No matter how perfect a systems approach to injury prevention may be, it will be merely an abstraction unless adequate funding exists. When state health departments are asked what they need to improve their injury prevention efforts, they consistently say they need more money for the kind of comprehensive programs they want and need to do. States are often criticized for not allocating more state funds for injury prevention programming. Why, then, don't states contribute more resources?

To begin with, state practitioners face the standard funding obstacles: lack of public and legislative awareness of the injury problem, lack of media coverage compared to other public health issues, and lack of advocacy around the issue. Despite what most of those immersed in the field may believe, the public is generally not aware that there is such a field as injury control. State legislators, too, are often not aware that injuries are a public health problem, especially unintentional injuries, which are still viewed as "accidents" by the majority of the population.

Injury prevention does not have its own line item in most state budgets. Rather, it is usually hidden within large, multimillion dollar "family and community health" or "preventive health services" line items, which, to the average state legislator, connotes such things as immunizations and prenatal care. This precludes policy makers from viewing injury prevention as a discrete public health issue and does not provide a ready, easy mechanism with which to earmark dollars for injury control. Without such a mechanism, budget expansion is generally reserved for more visible issues such as human immunodeficiency virus prevention and substance abuse, and money available for injury prevention programs is often diverted to other areas for political reasons.

To secure state and local funding and support for injury prevention activities, health departments need a recognizable constituency to keep the pressure on policy makers; however, they face a number of barriers to cultivating these much-needed champions. State health commissioners are essential allies but are not the complete solution; they generally have firm agendas to promote, sometimes at the expense of other, less popular or easily understood programs such as injury control. They must champion all public health issues, and the relatively new field of injury control can slip through the cracks.

Ideally, health departments need a dedicated injury prevention coordinator to be the advocate within the department and community to build a grassroots constituency and to influence change. Through the State and Territorial Injury Prevention Directors Association (STIPDA), the CDC provides some financial support to link injury prevention representatives from each state. A lead injury prevention representative has been designated in each state to be a member of STIPDA. The association fosters the sharing of successes in overcoming barriers and provides money for conference attendance and other training opportunities. Most states also have a local or state SAFE KIDS coalition, which could be a valuable asset as a constituency to support funding for injury prevention.

Funding to support core staff must come from the health department itself, but there are numerous supplemental funding sources in addition to those from the health department budget to carry out research or demonstration projects or specific intervention activities. However, without an influx of federal dollars, the critical mass to create the changes needed in injury prevention will be slow in developing. Exhibit 11–5 lists the federal

**Exhibit 11–5**  Federal, State, and Private Funding Sources: Some Examples

---

**FEDERAL AGENCIES**

- National Center for Injury Prevention and Control
- Office of Disease Prevention and Health Promotion
- Health Resources and Services Administration
- Maternal and Child Health Bureau
- National Institute on Occupational Safety and Health
- Office of the Assistant Secretary of Health
- Office of Minority Health
- National Highway Traffic Safety Administration
- Department of Justice
- Department of Education
- National Institutes of Health
- Alcohol, Drug Abuse, and Mental Health Administration

**STATE AGENCIES**

- Governor's Highway Safety Bureau
- Department of Education
- Department of Labor and Industries
- Department of Mental Health

**PRIVATE AGENCIES**

- California Wellness Foundation
- Allstate Insurance
- Community Foundations
- Commonwealth Fund

---

agencies that provide funding for state and local injury prevention activities. Attention should be paid in particular to the CDC National Center for Injury Prevention and Control and the Maternal and Child Health Bureau (MCHB). Currently most CDC injury control funding comes in the form of categorical grants. For example, the CDC recently released requests for proposals for two injury areas: (1) bicycle helmet promotion and (2) residential fire-related injuries. The agency will award a total of 10 state grants to cover either topic area. For the fire-related injury grants, the states will replicate a smoke detector education and monitoring program initially developed and implemented by the Oklahoma health department. Demonstration projects such as these, with clear outcome measures and demonstrated success, are certainly a sound public health approach, especially in terms of their research value. To address the immediate needs of states and their *community-specific* injury mortality and morbidity rates, however, states also need to be equipped to address the specific injuries that are most harming their populations.

The CDC has taken an important step in this regard by offering grants for basic injury program development and planning, which enables states with little to no injury prevention programming to build basic capacity and begin to examine and address injuries. This funding structure has left an important gap, however. States with more advanced injury control programs, but whose data do not show high rates of bicycle- or fire-related injuries, fall between these two alternatives. Information on CDC funding opportunities can be found at http://www.cdc.gov/ncipc/res-opps/grants1.htm.

The MCHB has been especially successful in providing seed money to enable state and local projects to build momentum around an issue, create a core constituency, demonstrate success, and thereby convince state policy makers to fill funding gaps. For example, the MCHB's Healthy Tomorrows program, a partnership with the American Academy of Pediatrics, provides seed money to innovative programs that prevent disease and disability among children. After the first year of federal funding, each Healthy Tomorrows project is required to obtain two thirds of its total operating budget from nonfederal sources. The increased use of MCHB and preventive health block grant dollars for injury-related activities indicates that states are increasingly savvy about using federal funds for injury prevention.

Information on MCHB funding opportunities can be found at http://www.hhs.gov:80/hrsa/mchb/guidance.htm. Federal funding of various technical assistance and resource centers, such as the Emergency Medical Services for Children (EMSC) National Resource Center funded by MCHB, National Highway Traffic Safety Administration's Safe Communities service center, Center for Substance Abuse Prevention's National Clearinghouse for Alcohol and Drug Information, and the MCHB's Children's Safety Network, have also given states resources to help them make the most of the funding and structures they do have.

The goal in developing funding is to move from research, demonstration, and pilot projects to routine practice across all programs. Education and constituency building is critical here. Injury prevention requires strong state-level support, which can only be won by developing state and local advocates and creating a presence that can't be ignored by state legislators who control the purse strings. Outside groups can be invaluable in promoting injury prevention goals, effectively presenting their thoughts at public hearings. The common practice of soliciting input on the use of a state's MCHB or preventive health block grant funds is a concrete example of what needs to be done more often in injury prevention. It is necessary to identify decision makers, educate them, and cultivate relationships that go beyond a one-time meeting or contact. For example, parent groups and other advocacy groups concerned with rare medical conditions use such mechanisms quite successfully to keep the funds for services flowing in their direction. Unbelievably, this doesn't seem to happen for a very common disabler: injury.

## Collaboration

Another critical factor in forwarding injury prevention programs is to develop successful alliances and collaborative initiatives. Collaboration can make possible data sharing, access to other networks and areas of expertise, more effective interventions based on the complementary approaches and expertise of different agencies, reduced duplication and fragmentation (allowing for cost-effectiveness), and a united front that impresses the legislature and other public officials and adds muscle to advocacy.

A unique aspect of injury control is the array of disciplines that are necessary for a successful approach to the problem. Partnerships are essential. Biomechanics, epidemiology, medicine, education, and social and behavioral sciences are essential for defining the injury problem, but their efforts need to be supplemented by also involving manufacturers, advocates, law enforcement, parents, teachers, fire fighters, bartenders, and youth groups. No one group can do it alone. The list of possible collaborators is almost endless. Exhibit 11–6 lists some obvious examples.

Coordinating such disparate groups to find a rallying point and get people moving in the same direction obviously takes skill and experience. In addition, collaboration needs to occur across geographical levels—lo-

**Exhibit 11–6**  Potential Collaborators in Building Support for Injury Prevention Programs

- Elected/appointed officials (and their staffs)
- Physician organizations
- Dental organizations
- Nursing organizations
- Other health professional organizations
- Business organizations
- Labor organizations
- Religious organizations
- Law enforcement departments
- Fire departments
- Hospitals/hospital associations
- Foundations
- Managed care groups and organizations
- Insurance companies
- Health professional schools
- Departments of transportation/motor vehicles
- Departments/boards of health
- Mental health departments and agencies
- Social service departments and agencies
- Substance abuse departments and agencies
- Schools/school boards/education departments
- Teacher organizations
- Youth groups
- Parent groups
- Other governmental agencies
- Volunteer agencies
- Advocacy groups
- SAFE KIDS coalitions
- Planners
- Architects
- Poison control centers
- Newspaper reporters and editorial boards
- Broadcast journalists
- Universities, colleges, think tanks, etc.
- Alcohol servers

cal, state, and national—and needs to happen not only governmentally, but also in private groups—such as professional associations (e.g., the American Academy of Pediatrics)—that have state and, sometimes, local chapters. It has been difficult to build this type of collaboration, especially with government agencies that tend to be viewed simply as sources of funding and sources of regulatory requirements, but it is important to understand the substantial contributions these agencies can offer in technical assistance, training, and knowledge of recent developments in the field.

Several factors can limit collaboration. These include:

- Lack of time: There often seems to be no time to attend meetings. The ironic result is that frequently people from the same state have their initial meeting at conferences convened by others outside the state.
- A narrow focus: Focusing on a specific injury issue to the exclusion of all other injury interests can hinder collaboration.
- Turf issues: Competition for resources and credit can lead to lack of coordination and interaction between agencies, an unwillingness to try new approaches, and a lack of a lead agency to serve as a neutral party and initiate collaborative activities. Sharing credit and learning from others can surmount ego and turf problems.
- Limited resources: Here the problem can be an attitude of "we will collaborate after we get our funding." There can also be a problem with funding criteria that lack the flexibility to support collaborative projects.
- Differing perspectives and orientation: Jargon and bureaucratic and professional ideologies often inhibit collaboration, stereotype other agencies, and lead to lack of understanding about what each potential collaborator brings to the table.
- Data linkage problems: Inconsistencies in hardware and types of data collected by different agencies often make it difficult to compare data.
- Attitudes: It is possible to believe "we know best" even when one has only recently discovered the injury prevention field.

It takes a great deal of work to overcome barriers that detract from the real task of reducing injuries. To make collaboration work, agencies must commit to attending regular meetings called by others, to learning one another's perspectives, language, and terminology, to sharing data, to serving on each other's boards and task forces, and—most important—to establishing an identified liaison for purposes of regular communication.

Collaboration implies an equal partnership. It means trusting in the motives and intelligence of people from different backgrounds with different roles and experiences, be they public health, law enforcement, engineering, or some other field. A successful leader can bring others together for cooperative planning, serve as a facilitator for change, listen and be a cheerleader for innovative ideas and approaches, be inclusive rather than exclusive, and work as a partner, not as the expert that knows exactly what to do and how to do it.

According to *Preventing Childhood Injuries: A Guide for Public Health Agencies*, a key element in successful community-based injury prevention is a "properly chosen and structured advisory board . . . to provide you with both technical and program implementation assistance."[11] This can best be done through subcommittees to an overall advisory board, namely a technical committee and a program committee.

> The Technical Committee's role is to provide credibility to your program. . . . Representatives of the following disciplines or professions are good choices for membership in the Technical Committee: an epidemiologist, a biostatistician, a physician specialist in the target injuries (e.g., burns, poisonings), an administrator from other Maternal and Child Health programs, . . . a health educator, an engineer, and a member representing the local chapter of the Academy of Pediatrics. . . .

> Good choices for membership on the Program Committee are representatives of the groups through which you plan to implement your program. These may be a local pediatrician, individuals representing community clinics, day-care centers, local government, voluntary agencies, a parent, a respected business leader and a representative of broadcast or print media. This committee should be task-oriented and expect to assist your program staff on a day-to-day basis during implementation.[11(pp37–38)]

An alternative to advisory boards is to work with community-based coalitions, either ongoing groups or groups established with assistance from the health department. Such a coalition might be generally focused on injury prevention or it might concern itself with particular injury problems, such as fires, drunk driving, or childhood injuries. The National Committee for Injury Prevention and Control noted that "it is important to discover what concerns engage and motivate the community. . . . It is important to find out what kinds of injury prevention projects have been tried before in the community, whether they have worked, and whether they are still in place."[10(pp24–25)]

Finally, it should be noted that a part of collaboration is the effective use of volunteers. Assistance by unpaid volunteers can be invaluable; it can also be a severe drain on the agency. Critical factors in determining what impact volunteers will have are the selection and training processes used. The goal should be volunteers that can function effectively with minimal supervision but within well-understood parameters.

## CONCLUSION

*Injury Prevention: Meeting the Challenge* was developed by the National Committee for Injury Prevention and Control to aid local and state health departments to appropriately organize their injury prevention efforts.[10] It is a useful source of inspiration and guidance: inspiration in that it is filled with stories of successful efforts to implement injury prevention interventions and guidance in that it explains how to work to achieve similar successes.

Injury prevention on the part of state and local health departments may be relatively new, but much has happened in just the last decade. The most sensible course for everyone in the injury prevention field is to learn from the successes, as well as the missteps, of those who have gone before. This is possible through such publications as *Injury Prevention: Meeting the Challenge*[10] and *Preventing Childhood Injuries: A Guide for Public Health Agencies*[11] and through such groups as the State and Territorial Injury Prevention Directors Association, the Children's Safety Network, and the Injury Control and Emergency Health Services Section of the American Public Health Association. The suggestions offered in this chapter provide a starting point to be pursued in conjunction with the collective experience of all who have labored to reduce the toll of injury in America.

Much of what is helpful in initiating a new injury prevention program is having a sense of what does and does not work. Fortunately, this information is being shared. Some of the effort of the National Center for Injury Prevention and Control is aimed at disseminating examples of successful intervention programs. Another particularly useful source of real world examples is the World Wide Web site maintained by the Harborview Injury Prevention and Research Center (at http://weber.u.washington.edu/~hiprc/childinjury), as well as other sites to which this site is linked.

---

## NOTES

1. Gallagher SS, Messenger KP, Guyer B. State and local responses to children's injuries: The Massachusetts Statewide Childhood Injury Prevention Program. *J Soc Issues.* 1987;43:149–162.

2. Harrington C, Gallagher SS, Burgess LL, Guyer B. *Injury Prevention Programs in State Health Departments: A National Survey.* Boston, MA: Harvard School of Public Health; 1988.

3. *Injury Control in the 1990s: A National Plan for Action.* The Report to the Second World Conference on Injury Control was coordinated by the Centers of Disease Control and Prevention but represent the views of the various individual contributors. Printed by the Association for the Advancement of Automotive Medicine for the Second World Conference on Injury Control, May 1993.

4. See http://odphp.osophs.dhhs.gov/pubs/hp2000/210.htm.

5. Washington State Department of Health. *Public Health Improvement Plan.* Olympia, WA: Washington State Department of Health; 1994.

6. California Department of Health Services. Injury Control Task Force. *Strategic Plan for Injury Prevention and Control in California, 1993–1997.* Sacramento, CA: California Department of Health Services; 1992.

7. California Department of Health Services. *Injury Prevention Plan of the Primary Care and Family Health Division, 1993–1995.* Sacramento, CA: California Department of Health Services; 1992.

8. National Highway Traffic Safety Administration. *Motor Vehicle Injury Protection: An Assessment of Highway Safety and Public Health Activities in Selected States.* DOT HS 808 150, August 1994, NTS–22.

9. Children's Safety Network. *Injury Prevention Outlook: An Assessment of Injury Prevention in State Maternal and Child Health Agencies—Background Report.* Newton, MAzional Committee for Injury Prevention and Control. New York: Oxford University Press. *Injury Prevention: Meeting the Challenge.* Published as a supplement to the *Am J Prev Med.* 1989;5:22–25.

11. Adapted with permission from S. Micik, J. Yuwiler, and C. Walker, *Preventing Childhood Injuries: A Guide for Public Health Services,* 2nd edition, p. 42, © 1987, North County Health Services. For information on obtaining this publication, please contact the California Center for Childhood Injury Prevention, 619-594-3691.

12. Cassady CE, Orth DA, Guyer B, Goggin ML. Measuring the implementation of injury prevention programs in state health agencies. *Inj Prev.* 1997;3:94–99.

13. Cohen L, Baer N, Satterwhite P. *Developing Effective Coalitions: An Eight Step Guide.* Pleasant Hill, CA: Contra Costa County Health Services Prevention Program; 1994.

14. Micik S, Miclette M. Injury prevention in the community: A systems approach. *Pediatr Clin North Am.* 1985;32:251–265.

# CHAPTER 12

# Injury Surveillance: A 10-Step Plan

"Development of effective intervention strategies requires an adequate national surveillance system for monitoring injuries, their causes, and their short-term and long-term consequences."

Committee on Trauma Research Commission on Life Sciences, and the National Research Council and the Institute of Medicine, *Injury in America*, 1985

## WHAT THIS CHAPTER IS ABOUT

The first step in addressing any public health problem is collecting the data that helps you describe and understand the extent and nature of the problem. This requires systematic surveillance. Experience with monitoring infectious diseases provides useful guidelines for developing injury surveillance systems.[1] Such surveillance systems must then be tailored to the special needs of injury prevention. Unfortunately, much of the work in the injury field has focused on developing injury surveillance systems that end up being too expensive. More sustainable systems must be developed. This chapter will introduce you to some of the important issues in developing and maintaining practical injury surveillance systems. We will review what you will need to master to conduct injury surveillance systems without having to become an epidemiologist or a researcher. We will outline the key steps in developing an injury surveillance system. We will also discuss sources of data for such systems and the use of E codes.

## INTRODUCTION

Surveillance means different things to different people. According to Webster's, "surveillance" means "a watch kept over someone or something." In the criminal justice field, surveillance refers to monitoring the behavior of suspicious individuals. To others, it implies the global positioning of satellite systems for spying.[2] But to members of a community coalition concerned about injuries, "surveillance" can often produce blank stares.

Surveillance means collecting and assessing data. In the public health arena, surveillance has been defined as the "ongoing and systematic collection, analysis and interpretation of health data needed to plan, implement, and evaluate public health programs."[3] A strong surveillance system is an essential part and foundation of any public health activity, assessment being one of the three core functions for public health agencies at all levels of government.[4] *Healthy People 2000*, *Injury in America*, *Injury Prevention: Meeting the Challenge*, and the CDC National Injury Plan—all of these national resource documents recognize the need for improved surveillance of injuries at the national, state, and local levels.

## WHAT DATA DO YOU NEED?

There are five main purposes for an injury surveillance system: (1) to understand the injury problem well enough to design programs that are correctly targeted to injury causation, specific risk factors, population at greatest risk, geographical location, and temporal issues; (2) to track progress and monitor trends in the magnitude and distribution of injury morbidity and mortality and identify new and emerging hazards in a timely fashion; (3) to make an assessment of the global impact of a program; (4) to generate hypotheses and develop a database for future prevention efforts with a sample size large enough to be useful for research; and (5) to describe injury patterns that justify the need for a prevention program.

At the national, state, and local levels, government agencies need injury data to identify injury problems, assist in decision making, and monitor progress, but it has been difficult to conduct population-based studies on the causes of injury because of the lack of appropriate databases. Many state and local agencies lack a full capacity for surveillance.[4] Developing the capacity to perform injury surveillance and obtain injury data at the local or state level is indeed a challenge. Finding the appropriate level of injury surveillance is not an easy task. For example, what causes will be included in the definition of injury—intentional only or intentional and unintentional? What level of severity should be captured: Deaths? Hospitalizations? Emergency room patients who are treated and released? Ambulance calls? Minor injuries treated at home? What sources of centralized data already exist at the state level? At the local level? What resources are available to conduct injury surveillance, including staff, funds, and computers? How can the administrative and maintenance costs of surveillance be kept low and realistic?

So where does one start? While the injury surveillance task may seem overwhelming, experience shows that it can be done. In the pages that follow we suggest a 10-step plan to help structure your injury surveillance system. The steps are

1. Define the objectives for the injury surveillance system.
2. Form a data committee.
3. Identify existing data sources.
4. Determine the strengths and limitations of each potential data source.
5. Conduct preliminary data analysis.
6. Reevaluate objectives for the surveillance system based on steps 3 through 5.
7. Consider linking information from existing data sources.
8. Perform validation studies to evaluate the injury surveillance system.
9. Develop a dissemination plan for sharing data.
10. Tie surveillance to action and funding.

The amount of time it will take to complete each step will vary widely depending on resources and the number of potential data sets you wish to examine, but it will take some time to get the process moving. For this reason, the early steps in the process—particularly step 3, identify existing data sources—will be described in considerably more detail than the latter steps. In approaching any of these steps, it would be wise to check with others with experience for technical assistance and advice.

## STEP 1: DEFINE THE OBJECTIVES FOR THE INJURY SURVEILLANCE SYSTEM

An injury surveillance system can serve a number of purposes, including problem definition, prioritizing injury problems, identifying data sources, linking data sources, supporting intervention efforts, and disseminating data from the surveillance system. But system objectives must be kept simple if the injury surveillance system is to be practical and sustained over time. The first priority is having a clear idea of what will be done with the data. The more specific you can be, the more manageable the system. Do you want to get an overview of the leading causes of injury in the community? Do you want to clarify the magnitude and nature of an injury problem that continually surfaces in the news media or at community meetings? Do you want to better understand injuries that occur in a particular location—highway, home, work, school, or recreation areas? Do you want to know which injuries make the greatest contribution to health care costs? Do you want to plan and guide your prevention efforts? By attending to these questions early, you can make certain that you collect the right information from the start.

How will you define injury? It is paramount that a clear definition, one comparable to definitions of the same condition used in other localities and at other times, be adopted and applied consistently. A case definition would consider specific types or causes of injury, injury severity, intention, age groupings, and whether all cases or only a sample will be included in a surveillance system. Selecting the causes of injury or the age span that will be included is usually not a problem. The biggest decision usually is the level of severity to be captured. Start with deaths and the most severe injuries, but make a plan to phase in other levels later. **Do not** try to do everything at once. A guiding principle in all data collection should be to "start small." You can work on prevention projects without knowing everything about every injury in your community. Capturing information on even the most minor injuries (or even near-misses that may not require medical attention) can be an overwhelming task. In addition, it may not give you the information you need. For example, many childhood injuries are minor and may be an important and normal part of children's experimentation with the environment rather than a focus of public health intervention.

The most commonly used model of injury severity is an iceberg or pyramid. Increasing severity, as measured by increasing levels of medical intervention, represent greater forces of energy at work: deaths at the top tip, followed by hospitalizations, then emergency department treatment, and, finally, all episodes reported. (See Figure 12–1.) Whatever type of injury surveillance system you design needs to be flexible to accommodate the various levels of the severity pyramid.

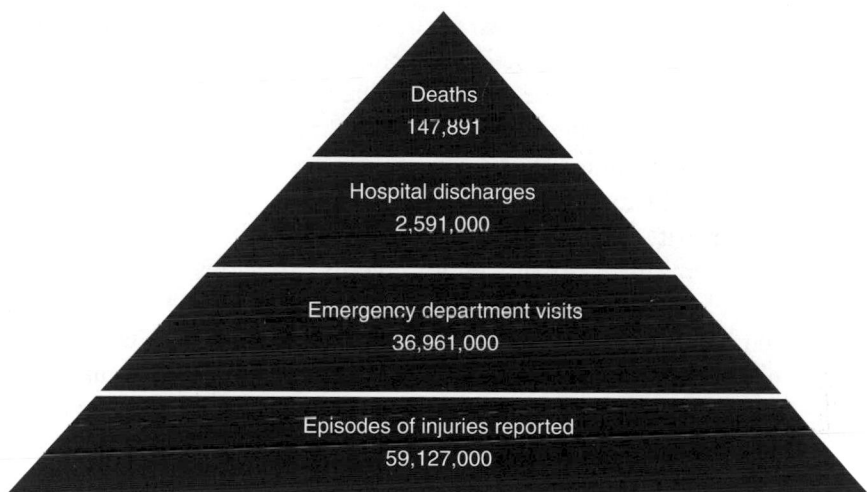

**Figure 12–1** Burden of Injury: United States, 1995. *Source:* Reprinted from L.A. Fingerhut and M. Warner, Injury Chartbook, in *Health, United States, 1996–1997,* p. 18, 1997, National Center for Health Statistics, U.S. Public Health Service.

Keep in mind that injury deaths are rare events and they therefore provide a skewed picture of the injury problem. Most people who are injured do not die. Mortality data reflect less than 1% of all injuries and are not a good guide for ascertaining either the overall incidence of injury, the medical consequences of injury—such as long-term disability—or the cost of injury. Yet, surveillance of fatal injuries using death certificate data has been the norm in the injury field because death certificates can be obtained readily and inexpensively for the entire population. Moreover, death certificate data will always include the cause of death from injury. But despite such advantages, mortality data are not sufficient to properly define the injury problem. At the community level there are simply too few cases of injury deaths to adequately profile the injury problem and target local prevention efforts. In a population-based study of child and adolescent injuries in Massachusetts, 96.5% of all injury cases were treated and released from an emergency room, 3.4% were admitted to a hospital, and less than one tenth of 1% resulted in death.[5] Nonfatal injury data are essential for gaining support for injury prevention at the local level. Thus the absence of population-based data on nonfatal injuries at both the national and the local level is of considerable concern.

Data on both fatal and nonfatal injuries provide a picture of the injury problem and set priorities for action. A comparison of the leading causes of fatal and nonfatal injuries shows they are often different from one another. For example, in the Northeast Ohio Trauma Study, falls were the number one cause of injury, but ranked fourth as a cause of injury death (behind motor vehicle collisions, suicides, and assaults).[6,7]

Relative severity may be a less critical data issue. There are several classification systems used to assess injury severity. Surgeons and trauma specialists use physiologic systems (Glasgow Coma Scale, Revised Trauma Score, Pediatric Trauma Score) and anatomic systems (Abbreviated Injury Score and Injury Severity Score) to (1) estimate the severity of injuries, (2) make clinical treatment decisions at the scene of an emergency or at the hospital, (3) examine quality of response retrospectively, and (4) assess impairment and disability. Some systems are based on the injured person's initial diagnostic evaluation and early neurological findings. Originally these systems were developed to facilitate triage of motor vehicle collisions in the field, but they are now applied to all injuries. This type of trauma severity scoring is less useful for general injury surveillance, but may help in examining what happens to patients when they are discharged from a hospital and what the costs are to society. The purpose of surveillance is to better understand the distribution and etiology of injuries, and categorizing injury by severity may make an important contribution in this regard.[8–16]

Identifying such difficult variables as alcohol involvement, relationship of perpetrators to victims, or preexisting conditions would not seem to be a sensible initial objective of an injury surveillance system. These variables should wait until there is a better understanding of the big picture. In developing initial data objectives, get the basics, identify gaps in the data collected, and then work on reducing gaps.

## STEP 2: FORM A DATA COMMITTEE

Accurate and comprehensive injury data will be difficult to collect without broad support and participation from relevant organizations. Fortunately, public health agencies can provide an umbrella for gathering groups together, making it possible to achieve goals otherwise out of reach of a single agency or organization. For example, law enforcement agencies and public health agencies have an overlapping objective: to reduce motor vehicle injuries. Police reports provide one source of information on motor vehicle–related incidents. But police reports tend to underreport injuries and, when they do report, do not include information on the type of injuries sustained or on the medical treatment and costs involved. Hospital records, on the other hand, contain detailed information on both the medical aspects of the injury (nature and severity) as well as the costs of the medical treatment. But unlike police reports, hospital records do not include information on such things as seatbelt use or road conditions. The logical way to overcome these drawbacks is for data collectors to benefit from each others' data. This requires a forum in which data collectors and users can define their common data collection needs, develop linkages, and disseminate linked data reports. A data committee can provide the appropriate device for such collaboration.

A data committee is a mechanism or forum for the coalition building necessary for developing an effective injury surveillance system. A data committee should include any and all organizations that record injury data, as well as all community members who may use the data. A data committee or coalition can help mitigate turf issues, improve data sharing cooperation and collaboration, enhance the capacity for injury surveillance, and—ultimately—reduce injuries. Coalitions are essential to institutionalizing injury surveillance as an ongoing part of injury prevention efforts. Advocacy by a coalition of groups may be the only way that access can be gained to data from local emergency departments or school systems or that a data form may be changed. Exhibit 12–1 suggests potential members for a local data committee.

Community members and agencies that collect data may not be familiar with the public health approach to data and the notion of studying data to determine injury patterns and prevent future occurrences. For example, schools may record student injury incidents and file written reports, but without attention to future prevention. They may only examine such data in cases where litigation is feared. As the initiator of a data committee, be prepared to describe some short- and long-term objectives of data collection to the committee, emphasizing both benefits to the community and benefits to participants. It helps to have a chart or grid handout developed that describes known data sources and invites additional sources of information.

**Exhibit 12–1**  Potential Members of a Local Data Committee

- Epidemiologist (health department or university)
- Fire department
- Emergency medical service provider
- Health maintenance organization
- Hospital (particularly departments such as emergency room, medical records, community health education, community health planning, pediatrics)
- Injury survivors/family members
- Local expertise such as harbormaster or 4-H representative
- Mental health
- News media
- Physician
- Poison center staff
- Police (traffic reports, criminal arrests)
- Public health agency
- Schools (nurse, coach, athletic trainer, risk manager)
- Social service organizations (child abuse/domestic violence)
- State health department injury prevention program*
- Suicide hotline
- Youth sports organizations

  *Ideally with capability to provide information on centralized injury data resources connected to the health department and other state agencies such as the poison center, vital statistics, health and risk behavior surveillance, workers' compensation, medical examiner files, child fatality review team, fish and game (hunting and firearms).

## STEP 3: IDENTIFY EXISTING DATA SOURCES

Injury data are collected by several entities, including public health, health care delivery, and public safety agencies. In many instances, data collection is instigated for purposes far removed from injury prevention. An injury surveillance system should be able to take advantage of such currently available data sets even though they undoubtedly will have limitations. Existing data sources must be identified and then examined to determine availability and access, format (e.g., can the data be accessed electronically?), collection and reporting methods, demographic data elements, injury data elements, coding schemes, principal contacts for data requests, policies on release of data, and confidentiality requirements. Data collected for purposes other than injury prevention will not be a perfect fit, but much can be achieved using such "inadvertent" data. These other data sources include law enforcement, criminal justice, fire safety, traffic safety, product safety, occupational health and safety, workers' compensation, medical examiner/coroner, vital statistics, trauma registry, hospital discharge, emergency department, ambulatory clinic, emergency medical services, ongoing periodic health and risk factor surveys, and news media files. Of course, any individual data source may or may not contain information useful for prevention.

## National Data Sources

There are a number of national data sources that can provide the "big picture" of injury trends in the United States. A few of these national data sources can also provide data at the state-specific level. But while useful for highlighting the importance of the injury problem and serving as a benchmark measure against which to compare your state, national data sources generally are not sufficient for developing state and local injury prevention programs that target the major causes and risks for your area. In fact, many national data sources were designed or established for purposes other than monitoring injuries and associated health outcomes. Consequently, they do not provide standardized or comprehensive injury data on the circumstances of the injury event, information crucial for injury prevention. There are other weaknesses from a local injury prevention perspective. Because of national sampling strategies, often data cannot be reported for state and local areas without significantly compromising accuracy. Some national data systems rely on voluntary reporting, rather than a statistical sample of localities. Federal agencies with injury data sources include the Bureau of Justice, National Center for Injury Prevention and Control, Consumer Product Safety Commission, Department of Labor, Federal Bureau of Investigation, Federal Emergency Management Agency, Indian Health Service, National Center for Health Statistics, National Highway Traffic Safety Administration, National Institute of Drug Abuse, and National Institute of Occupational Safety and Health. There are also several private organizations that compile national injury data, often in annual publications such as the National Safety Council's *Accident Facts*[17] or as part of voluntary registries on specific cause of injury, such as the National Burn Registry or the National High School Athletic Injury Registry.

Information on some of the key national sources follows.

### National Electronic Injury Surveillance System

Data on injuries related to consumer products or recreational activities are compiled by the Consumer Product Safety Commission (CPSC) by means of statistical samples from approximately 100 emergency departments throughout the country. The data set customarily excludes alcohol, tobacco, firearms, automobiles, motorcycles, trains, boats, aircraft, pesticides, and occupationally related and violence-related injuries (suicide attempts and assaults). Unlike comparably collected federal motor vehicle data, identification of specific name brands is not permitted. You can contact the CPSC for summaries of specific categories of products that appear in this data set. CPSC also has data derived from special studies, newspaper reports, and consumer reports. State-specific information is not available.

### Vital Statistics

This source of information on all deaths in the United States is compiled by the National Center for Health Statistics (NCHS). It includes external cause of injury codes (E codes). Data are abstracted from death certificates submitted by state vital statistics offices. Annual reports summarizing vital statistics data are available with about a two-and-one-half-year delay. More specific analyses are available on request and are also produced on a periodic basis (e.g., *Health, United States, 1996–97*).[18] Requests for data for only your state should be made to your state office of vital statistics.

### National Hospital Discharge Survey

This NCHS sample of inpatient records from short-stay hospitals provides estimates of inpatient care and hospital utilization. Annual summaries are published. They have not included external cause of injury codes. Because of the sample size, reliable data are not available on specific injuries or for specific states; however, multiple years can be combined to improve reliability. Requests for data on your state should be made to your state hospital association or state health agency.

### National Health Interview Survey

This continuous survey is conducted by the NCHS on about 48,000 U.S. households annually, asking for information on injuries occurring within the last two weeks and on hospital episodes within the last year. Until recently, the type of injury rather than the cause was recorded—now all injuries receive an E code. Supplemental health interview questionnaires periodically monitor some of the *Healthy People 2000* health objectives, including seatbelt and helmet use, firearm safety, home safety issues, use of protective sports equipment, and the like. In 1996, the core questions were redesigned to include a significant injury component, focusing on injuries requiring medical attention in the previous three months and including details on the circumstances surrounding the injury events. Acute condition data are published annually (e.g., *Current Estimates 1997*). Other results may be published periodically in special supplements. State-specific information is not available.

### National Ambulatory Medical Care Survey

This annual NCHS survey samples office-based physician visits for a randomly assigned seven-day period and includes information on injury and injury type. Participation is voluntary. Information on the cause of injury, place of injury, and work relatedness has also been collected since 1995. Findings are published annually. State-specific information is not available.

### National Hospital Ambulatory Medical Care Survey

This annual NCHS survey of health care provided by hospital emergency and outpatient departments is drawn from a sample of approximately 500 hospitals and includes cause of injury codes. Participation is voluntary. Information on work-, firearm-, and violence-related injuries has been collected since 1995. Published reports appear annually. State-specific information is not available.

### Fatality Analysis and Reporting System (FARS)

This is a compilation by the National Highway Traffic Safety Administration (NHTSA) of motor vehicle–related crashes in the United States that occur on a trafficway and result in at least one fatality within 30 days of the crash. FARS includes information on all persons involved in the fatal crash, the motor vehicle, and the circumstances of the crash. Excluded are intentional crashes related to homicide, suicide, or police intervention; crashes resulting from natural disasters; and crashes that do not occur on a trafficway. Limitations of FARS include the fact that it is not E coded to make it comparable to death certificate data and it contains a minimal amount of medical information. Published reports are available annually and include information at the state, county, and local level.

### National Automotive Sampling System (NASS)

This is a sample of motor vehicle–related crashes compiled by NHTSA in 17 states from (1) local police traffic crash reports submitted to a central state agency, (2) medical records, and (3) physical evidence obtained at the scene or by interview. Reports are included where either an injury or property damage occurred and at least one vehicle was towed. Published reports are available with national estimates. State-specific information is not available.

### Census of Fatal Occupational Injuries

This is a compilation of work-related fatalities prepared by the Bureau of Labor Statistics (BLS) and drawn from multiple data sources at the state and federal levels, including death certificates and workers' compensation reports and claims. This is perhaps the most comprehensive source of occupationally related deaths. The BLS produces an annual national report. State-specific and metropolitan statistical area–specific data are available. Many states also produce their own state-specific fatal occupational injury reports.

### Survey of Occupational Injuries and Illnesses

This BLS survey is based on a sample of job-related injuries and illnesses obtained by surveying U.S. employers in private industry. The sample is drawn from cases required to be reported to the Occupational Safety and Health Administration and includes injuries resulting in death, loss of consciousness, restricted work activity, transfer to another job, or medical treatment beyond first aid. This may well be a low count of the actual number of occupational injuries. The data system provides national and state data, and an annual summary is prepared. Many states also produce state-specific reports.

### National Traumatic Occupational Fatality Surveillance System

This is a compilation of all work-related injury deaths for workers 16 years of age or older with an external cause of injury code. It is prepared by the National Institute for Occupational Safety and Health (NIOSH) and is drawn from death certificates from all 50 states, New York City, and the District of Columbia, using those death certificates that contain a positive response to the "injury at work" item. It includes standard codes for the cause of injury (E code), the occupation (Bureau of the Census), and the industry (Standard Industrial Classification). However, worker deaths are underrepresented and the compilation is not as comprehensive as other sources. Summaries of the data can be found periodically in journal articles.

### Census of Agriculture

This is a Department of Commerce compilation of injuries and deaths connected with farm or ranch work, as reported by responses to a mail survey of all farm operators in the United States. Injuries that result in paid medical care or lost work time are included. However, information is not obtained on the nature, cause, and severity of the injuries or the persons injured.

### Uniform Crime Reporting System

This is a Federal Bureau of Investigation (FBI) compilation of national crime statistics voluntarily reported by state and local law enforcement agencies. Reports must meet a set of minimum standards to ensure accuracy and consistency. A physical injury need not have occurred. Agencies report aggregate data (e.g., total number of arrests made in a specific month), which makes it difficult to obtain more useful subcategory information. Reports are published annually.

### National Incident-Based Reporting System

This FBI compilation contains crime statistics for 46 specific crimes voluntarily reported by state and local law enforcement agencies from jurisdictions with populations of 100,000 or more people. Data on injuries are limited and based on law enforcement officers' observations. The system is an improvement over the traditional uniform crime reports because (1) information is submitted on individual crimes rather than in aggregate, (2) it includes more detailed information on assaults, sex offenses, and homicides, and (3) information is submitted in an electronic format. Only about 20% of states participate, but the ultimate goal is to replace the current uniform crime reporting system.

### National Crime Victimization Survey

The Bureau of Justice Statistics interviews a sample of households to provide this national estimate of crime and crime victimization. The survey includes crime victims over 12 years of age for certain criminal offenses, including rape, robbery, assault, and domestic violence, and includes both completions and attempts, whether or not they are reported to the police. Murder and kidnapping are not included. A survey is conducted annually, with special supplements focusing on particular issues. Published reports are available on the annual overall results and on specific topics. State and local data may be available as special reports, but the sample design does not make this a good source.

### National Child Abuse and Neglect Data System

This is a compilation of reports and referrals for investigation of *alleged* child maltreatment (sexual abuse, child abuse, family violence) voluntarily submitted by child protective service agencies in all 50 states. Prepared by the Office of Child Abuse and Neglect, it includes a summary data component of key aggregate indicators and outcomes of investigations and a separate detailed case data component of more detailed case-level data. The latter is provided by a smaller subset of states. Not all states have the same definition of child maltreatment case dispositions. Duplicate reporting may occur on the same child. An annual report is published for the summary data component and occasional reports are published from the more detailed component. Some states publish annual compilations of child abuse and neglect reports.

### National Incidence Study of Child Abuse and Neglect

This is a periodic survey by the Office of Child Abuse and Neglect drawn from child maltreatment reports by community professionals. The survey is based on a probability sample of counties. Data are collected on cases of child maltreatment from local child protective services staff and a broad spectrum of community agencies (e.g., schools, juvenile probation officers) for children under age 18 years. National estimates are generated.

### Behavioral Risk Factor Surveillance System

This is a random-digit telephone survey of adults age 18 and older living in households in all states. It is conducted by the National Center for Chronic Disease Prevention and Health Promotion. Behaviors related to the leading causes of death are included. Many of the items are useful for monitoring the *Healthy People 2000* prevention objectives.[19] An injury module was developed for the survey in 1988, but only a few states have used it. In 1993, a few questions on child safety were added to the core questionnaire. Reports are issued periodically in *Morbidity and Mortality Weekly Report*.[20] Make requests for data from your state through your state health agency.

### Youth Risk Behavior Surveillance System

This National Center for Chronic Disease Prevention and Health Promotion compilation is based on school surveys self-administered to approximately 12,000 students, primarily in grades 9 to 12, to examine the prevalence of risky behaviors associated with the leading causes of morbidity and mortality. Forty-three states and 13 cities participated in 1993. Injury risk surveys include seatbelt use, motorcycle and bicycle helmet use, drinking and driving, weapon carrying, fighting, and suicide attempts. Many of the items were developed to monitor the Year 2000 Health Objectives. States and schools have the option of omitting questions, and many do not ask about suicide, sexual behavior, and weapon carrying. Reports are issued periodically and state-level data are available. Because some school districts use this questionnaire to conduct their own surveys, information may be available at the school district level.

Exhibit 12–2 gives further information on federal data sources.

## State and Local Data Sources

There are not many state or local nonfatal injury surveillance systems that collect to a centralized location. But where they do exist, state and local sources are much more likely than national sources to reflect local injury problems and are therefore more useful in setting program priorities and evaluating the impact of injury prevention programs. Nothing generates support better than local data. Local injury reports, even from newspapers, are useful to spark interest in program implementation.

In most states, data may be available directly from local agencies that perform data collection, such as police departments or hospitals. State agencies often collect data at the community level, using local sources, then compile it for the entire state. State aggregations are usually large enough to provide enhanced statistical representativeness of injury problems.

Standardization of reports from community to community or from state to state may be an issue. Also, despite the advent of the computer age,

**Exhibit 12–2** Federal Data Sources

---

A minimum of 31 federally funded systems have been identified, 8 of which provide data on work-related injuries and deaths, 13 of which provide information on intent, and 3 of which provide information on the cost of injury. More detailed information on federal injury data systems can be found at:

- National Center for Injury Prevention and Control, *Inventory of Federal Data Systems in the United States*, available at http://www.cdc.gov/ncipc/pub-res/federal.pdf

  Also see:

- Annest JL, Conn JM, James SP. *Inventory of Federal Data Systems in the United States for Injury Surveillance, Research and Prevention Activities*. Atlanta, GA: Centers for Disease Control and Prevention, National Center for Injury Prevention and Control; May 1996.
- Posner M. *Youth Violence: Locating and Using the Data*. Newton, MA: Children's Safety Network, Education Development Center, Inc.; March 1996.

---

many local and some state sources still are not computerized; you may have to retrieve data by sorting through paper copies filed in boxes. You will be able to obtain reports at the state level for death certificates, hospital discharges, and police and fire reports. Several states have implemented centralized reporting of data from prehospital emergency medical services providers and from trauma registries; others are in the process of doing so. Unlike infectious diseases, for which there are 49 diseases with a mandate for state and local reporting, mandates requiring physicians to report injuries are very limited. A few states have injury registries or require the reporting of specific injuries or injury causes (e.g., burns, head and spinal cord injuries, gunshot wounds, teenage work-related injuries). Even in those instances, reporting compliance levels may be uncertain and resource limitations may mean that annual reports may not be available.

State and local sources for injury surveillance will have problems with quality, completeness, and timeliness (as do national sources). There have been some attempts to develop nationally standardized definitions for the collection of data in trauma registries and prehospital provider data sets, but because of the many variables involved, this proves to be costly and it seems unrealistic to expect widespread implementation in the near term.

Information on some key state and local sources follows.

### Vital Statistics and Death Certificate Data

This information, which is available on 100% of injury-related deaths, is generally of high quality and is verified and coded to provide information on both the etiology and the nature of the injury and on victim age and gender. It is also inexpensive to obtain. An analysis of 5 to 10 years of this mortality data is useful in determining trends and planning injury prevention programs. Injury deaths are coded using the external cause of injury codes from the International Classification of Disease Codes (ICD-9), which are discussed below. Annual reports are published for state vital statistics. You may often obtain community-specific data most expeditiously at the local or county offices, which compile and submit that data to the state vital statistics office.

### Medical Examiner and Coroner Reports

These reports may be available for people whose deaths resulted from an unintentional injury, violence, or suicide. The reports, which are usually in narrative form, can be a rich and detailed source of information on injury deaths. But access to these reports may be hampered because not all states maintain a centralized file, let alone one that is computerized. And medical examiner and coroner report data may not be as complete as vital records, because these officials are not called in to investigate all deaths. There is quite a bit of variability from state to state on the quality of medical examiner and coroner reports, the policies on which types of injury deaths get included for death investigations, the percentage of reports based on full autopsies, and the release of these reports. These data are usually not aggregated or published.[21] The offices of your state medical examiner should provide guidance on how to access this type of data.

### Hospital Discharge Data

Collected for purposes of reimbursement, planning, and cost containment on 100% of injured patients who are discharged from a hospital, this is a valuable source of injury data if collected in a central location in a standardized format. Hospital discharge data allow you to compare the consequences and costs of different causes of injuries with those of other diseases and medical problems. Currently, about 35 states require that hospitals submit summary data on their discharges, which are then aggregated at the state level as a uniform hospital discharge data set. State hospital associations may also collect and analyze such data. The major limitation of hospital data remains the fact that few hospitals code the cause of injury.

In an ideal world, every medical record would include a nature of injury code (N code) accompanied by an external cause of injury code (E code). The role and value of E codes were discussed in Chapter 3, but a few words should be added here regarding the role of external cause of injury coding in injury surveillance.

Since the late 1980s, the need for E codes has been highlighted in national documents, including *Healthy People 2000, Injury Prevention: Meeting the Challenge*, and the *National Agenda for Injury Control*, and is now supported by policy statements from the National Health Information Management Association (the professionals who perform the actual coding in hospitals) and related organizations. Getting both the cause and place of injury routinely included in medical records has been a lengthy and uphill struggle, one that is finally achieving success. The major impediments to E code adoption have included the fact that E codes (unlike N codes) are not required for reimbursement, the long-term lack of a separate space to record this variable on most billing forms, the lack of any incentive to record (and, in fact, a disincentive in that E coding adds to costs without direct provider benefit), the perceived lack of interest in their use, and inadequate documentation by medical staff—making it difficult for hospital information management specialists to provide a specific code, for example, fall in sports due to pushing, shoving, colliding, or tackling (E886.0) instead of a vague code such as fall and hit head (E888).

The year 1992 was a landmark for E codes. After years of public health practitioners advocating for the use and inclusion of E codes on hospital billing forms, the U.S. Department of Health and Human Services' Health Care Financing Administration (HCFA) included a labeled space (albeit one for voluntary use) for one E code on the uniform billing form for hospitals. This change had taken a coordinated national effort to fundamentally redesign the standard patient record form. As of 1998, 23 states have mandated hospital reporting of E codes. The new era in data reporting was confirmed when E codes appeared as the focus of a column by humorist Dave Barry, who elaborated on official government classifications of bad things that could happen on one's vacation—everything from shark bite (E906.3) to being butted by an animal (E906.8) to getting a marble in the nose (E912).[22]

E code information in the hospital discharge data set is powerful when combined with information from vital statistics. Even if hospitals do not code the cause of the injury, the total number of injury admissions can be determined using the nature of injury codes and identifying ZIP code areas with high-frequency injury rates. Some states produce annual summaries and some will do customized data runs for a fee. In some areas, it may be possible to obtain some community-specific aggregated injury data directly on request to an individual local hospital.

### Trauma Registries

Trauma registries are generally maintained by hospitals that specialize in the care of acute injuries. They use registry data to ensure quality of care and to assess effectiveness of various treatments. The data collected and the format used may not be consistent among registries. Trauma registries will usually include a broad array of data on a limited number of injury types. Drownings, poisonings, and burns are often excluded. Most registries are now computerized and include an external cause of injury code (E code) and an injury severity score. Although there is no national aggregation of trauma registry data, there are 24 state trauma registries that may produce annual reports. You may be able to obtain some community-specific data directly on request from an individual trauma registry, but because many trauma center patients are referred from a broad geographic area, data may not be representative of the local community. Unfortunately, it seems to be easier to get funds for an institutional trauma registry that is not population based; statewide systems are not as likely to receive funding.

### Other Special Registries

Some specialized registries are maintained to collect information regionally about a particular injury, cause of injury, injury risk group, or to aid in the evaluation of patient care. Data on head and spinal cord injuries, burns, and gunshot wounds are available in a few states. Most were established because of concern over the severity of the particular injury type involved and the medical care costs involved.

### Emergency Medical Services Data

These data are generally collected on a form known as a "run sheet" or "trip report" by emergency medical technicians who respond to calls in the field. This data set is therefore limited to injured patients transported to medical facilities by ambulance, not those transported by family and friends in private vehicles. Most emergency medical services (EMS) data are not standardized, computerized, or centralized at the state level. Because of this variability, a National Highway Traffic Safety Administration consensus conference has developed 81 recommended data elements to encourage the creation of a uniform EMS data set. "Run sheets" often have information on circumstances at the injury scene, information that will not be recorded in the emergency room. In most areas, EMS data will need to be requested from individual EMS services. In some states, statistics will be available through the office of emergency medical services, which can be a good source for local data (but one that is often underutilized). In some larger cities, EMS may use a tracking system known as geographic information systems mapping and you may therefore be able to obtain a map of where injury calls occurred.

### Emergency Department Data

The vast majority of medically treated injuries are seen in an emergency department (ED) and a record is created there. Patient visits registered in ED logs routinely include narratives of a patient's chief complaint, but often without any indication of whether the visit is injury related and, if it is, what the cause of injury was. In the past, ED data were not computerized and data collection was very labor intensive. Even computerized ED systems may not be searchable by cause of injury, type of injury, or location of injury. Such variations make it difficult to obtain local injury data reports or to develop a statewide ED database modeled after the existing hospital discharge database. Currently about 12 states have data sets with emergency department visits aggregated at the state level. The level of inclusion of E-coded data on injury is unknown.

Statewide and citywide ED surveillance systems encompassing all injuries are confined to a few special studies, such as those from Massachusetts,[5,23] Northeast Ohio,[6,7] Harlem,[24] Philadelphia,[25-27] Washington, D.C.,[28] and Orange County.[29] Although it is an attractive data source for nonfatal injuries, the sheer volume of traffic in EDs, the number of injury cases seen in the ED, and variations in structural features of ED information management systems present a considerable challenge to creating a computerized ED database for injuries. Still, it would not hurt to make your interest in injury data known to your local hospital ED. If a hospital ED information system is being computerized or an existing computer system upgraded, you may want to encourage incorporation of software that can work with injury data identified by cause.

### Physician Office Visit Data

Some medical and surgical specialists do have unique injury data sets that will not be seen at an ED. For example, if injuries to the eyes, teeth, or from sports are of special interest, you may need to collect data from ophthalmologists, dental offices, and sports medicine clinics. But in most cases physician offices are not the place to start your search for useful existing data and should only be phased in after other sources are up and running in a surveillance system. Most of the injuries seen in physician offices are minor. Collecting this data will be extremely difficult, as physicians are seldom willing to permit direct access to their records, voluntary reporting tends to be unreliable, and confidentiality issues are a concern. The increase in health maintenance organizations and managed care organizations may make this type of data collection more efficient by merging the records of many physicians, but the other problems mentioned above will still remain. (A few research projects, such as the Pediatric Practice Research Group in Chicago, have sought to aggregate patient data from multiple private practice offices voluntarily participating in selected research projects.)

### Police Reports

Police incident and arrest reports can be a useful supplement to medical information on injuries from violence, motor vehicle collisions, and pedestrian and bicycle injuries. Individual law enforcement officers file these reports with their departments (or their precinct in large cities). They may be maintained by city and county police, sheriff's departments, state police, or highway patrol agencies. Records involving juveniles will be difficult to obtain because of state confidentiality laws regarding minors. Reporting by police agencies to state systems is often voluntary. The data may be aggregated at the state level with a yearly summary from the state police, department of public safety, or registry of motor vehicles. In some states, law enforcement agencies compile lists of intersections or street addresses where collisions take place. These are useful to locate "hot spots" where attention on prevention should be focused. At the same time, there are limitations in police data. The police are known to underreport traffic injuries resulting in medical treatment.[30] And there are many informational items of interest to injury prevention experts, such as where firearms used in injury events were obtained, that police do not (and often cannot) routinely collect.

### Fire Reports

Local fire departments keep records on fires and injuries. Local fire departments often work in conjunction with EMS. Reporting of fire-related injuries to a state system is often voluntary. Such reports may be aggregated at the state level and compiled into an annual report by the state fire marshal.

### School Reports

Public schools usually maintain records of injuries received on school premises. They also maintain records of disciplinary or suspension records for assaults. This information is often in narrative form, is rarely computerized, and is extremely difficult to access because of confidentiality and litigation concerns. But some schools or school districts may be willing to aggregate data and share it. Exhibit 12–3 provides an example.

### Child Protective Services

The biggest problem with this source of data for child abuse and neglect is the difficulty of gaining access. Under most circumstances, confidentiality concerns and regulations are extreme and make the data unavailable to those outside the system.

### Poison Control Center Data

Many states have regional or statewide poison control centers located in hospitals. Records of calls for help to these centers can provide information on numbers of incidents, including those that occur and are treated at home and substances involved (e.g., over-the-counter medicine, vitamins, cleaners).

**Exhibit 12–3** School District Injury Surveillance

Like many school districts, the town of Needham, Massachusetts, finds itself with a growing school population and aging school facilities. As a result, many of the schools are undergoing large-scale renovations, including new carpeting, fresh paint, and new heating and ventilation systems. These renovations have brought with them some unanticipated health and safety outcomes. Many students attending classes in the renovated school buildings presented to the school nurse with headaches, allergy symptoms, and other health complaints. Investigation revealed that fumes from paint and new carpeting were the culprits. As a result of these incidents, the town's health officer, in cooperation with the school nurses, instituted a surveillance system to track health and safety complaints and incidents at the schools. Injuries are 1 of 10 categories included in this surveillance system. Although not originally designed as an injury prevention tool, this surveillance system has become a valuable source of information about injuries and has resulted in several preventive measures.

Every school is required to complete a school accident report form for all serious injuries that occur within the school building or on school grounds. The school nurse is responsible for ensuring that the information on the forms is accurate and complete. Each month, the school nurse conducts a simple analysis of frequency and circumstances of injuries (and other health and safety incidents or complaints) occurring in the school environment. The results of each school's analysis are presented at the monthly meeting of the school's Health and Safety Committee, whose members include the school principal, representatives from the faculty, parents, students, and a school nurse. The committee discusses the cause of the injuries and potential strategies for prevention. When possible, the committee recommends amendments to the physical environment or school policy to lessen the chances of these injuries recurring. Examples of changes that have been implemented as a result of data collected through this surveillance system include, at the elementary school level, repair and replacement of playground equipment, the addition of teacher aides on playgrounds to enhance supervision, and a bike helmet program. At the high school level, athletic trainers have used these data to improve conditioning regimens and to make modifications to the gym environment to enhance safety.

The American Association of Poison Control Centers has a standardized data collection form, but not all centers use it.

### Child Death Review Teams

Some states require the formal review of all child deaths or at least suspicious child deaths. Child death review teams, which may operate at the county or state level, examine multiple data sources using representatives of law, social services, medicine, criminal justice, mental health, and public health. Such teams may detect causal information on injury deaths that are very useful for prevention purposes; they may also uncover deaths that have been misclassified as to cause. Individual case data are not available. Some states and counties publish annual reports.

### Other Sources

There are a number of other possible local and state data sources, but these greatly underreport injuries, may not have information on the cause of injury, and may be difficult to access. These sources have not been well studied and their advantages and limitations are unclear. These sources include

- workers' compensation data through the state department of labor
- insurance companies
- unions
- local parks and recreation departments
- behavioral risk factor surveillance
- youth risk behavior surveys
- news media files

## STEP 4: DETERMINE THE STRENGTHS AND LIMITATIONS OF EACH DATA SOURCE

Working with existing data sets makes great sense. While creating a new injury surveillance system can provide you with more control over data content, format, variables to be collected, population base, and the quality of the data, this approach suffers from extreme expense, length of time required to get a new system up and running, possible duplications of effort, and technical and political complications. The logistical difficulties of developing, operating, and maintaining a new data system cannot be overestimated. Usually it will require the cooperation of other agencies. Real world experience suggests that consolidating, evaluating, and improving *existing*, easily available sources of injury data should be the priority in any injury surveillance program. Using data already collected by another organization will be less complicated, less expensive, and less time consuming than undertaking your own data collection. Of course existing sources have their own disadvantages. They may lack variables of major interest, be incomplete, not cover the appropriate geographic area, not be computerized, not be in the desired format, be of uneven quality, and be difficult and costly to manipulate. They may also create problems regarding confidentiality of records and linkage of data.

In short, no approach to data collection is perfect: Each will have its own advantages, limitations, and costs, and its own levels of quality and reliability. The advantages and limitations of each source of data must be considered and weighed against the practicalities and realities of resource limitations, keeping uppermost in mind your data collection needs and objectives (as discussed in step 1). Important considerations in selecting a data approach include usefulness for injury surveillance, research, and practice; estimates of accuracy, completeness, and representativeness; timeliness, resource requirements; simplicity; and potential biases if the data are incomplete or not population based. Familiarity with such factors is essential before analyzing and reporting injury data. Technical guidelines for evaluating surveillance systems in general are available from the Centers for Disease Control and Prevention (CDC).[31]

Yet despite the disadvantages of using existing data sets, this is usually the most sensible approach to employ. It is, however, not an approach to be taken blindly. There are several critical questions to ask in evaluating possible data sources. Ask data providers to describe their data collection objectives, data sources, the data collection process, the elements collected and their definitions, the way the data are managed, and their methods for quality assessments. A matrix table, such as that presented in Table 12–1, may be helpful in making a comparative analysis of potential data sources.

Other questions to ask about existing data sources include

- Are the data computerized or must they be manipulated manually?
- What period of time do the records span?
- How often are data collected: annually, monthly, continuously, periodically?

**Table 12–1** Potential Data Sources: A Matrix

| Agency | Each Record in File Equals an Individual | Each Record in File Equals an Event | U.S. Standard Classification Code Used | Records Computerized | Machine Readable Copies of Records | Hard Copy Custom Tabulation Available | Access to Original Documents | Records Span What Years? (C = Computerized) | Restriction on Access to Your Records? Yes/No | Fee for Data | Comments |
|---|---|---|---|---|---|---|---|---|---|---|---|
| Bureau of Vital Records and Health Statistics* | Yes | No | ICD9 NESCA U.S. Census Bureau | Yes | See comments | Yes (city/ county/state) | No | 1800–present C: 1969–present | Yes† | No unless unusually extensive | Tape/disk available depending on nature of research project |
| Chief Medical Examiner* | Yes | No | No | In progress | In progress | | Yes | 9/86–present | Yes† | No | |
| Health Services* Planning and Review | Yes | No | ICD9 (E Codes) | Yes | Yes | Yes (city/ county/state) | No | 7/84–86 Updates 2X/year | Yes† | No fee for state agencies | Outside agencies contact N.H. Hospital Association |
| National Head Injury Foundation–N.H. | Yes | No | ICD9 | Yes | No | No | No | 1/85–12/85 | | No | |
| N.H. Alliance for Safety Belts | No | Yes | No | No | No | No | No | 1985–1988 | No | No | |
| Division Enforcement/ Department of Safety* | No | Yes | No | No | No | Yes (city/ county/state) | Yes | 1/74–present | No | No fee for public agencies | |
| Marine Patrol/ Department of Safety* | No | Yes | | No | No | No | No | 7 years–present | Yes† | | Statistics available on individual basis |
| Department of Resources and Economic Development* | Yes | No | No | No | No | No | No | 1985–present | Yes† | $.10/page | |
| Bureau of Emergency Medical Services* | Yes | Yes | No | No | No | No | Yes | Variable | Yes† | No | |
| Fire Marshal's Office* | No | Yes | Fire Rep. Sys. FEMA/USFA | Yes | Contact office | Yes (city/ county/state) | Contact office | 1981–present C: 1984–present | Yes† | No | Sample report forms are available. Not all towns currently reporting |
| OHRV Section/Fish & Game Department* | Yes | No | No | Yes | No | Yes (city/ county/state) | Yes | 1970 (Part)–1988 C: 1987–1988 | Yes† | $1.00 | Sample OHRV accident report form available |
| Poison Information Center | Yes | Yes | AAPCCGC | Yes | No | No | No | C: 1986–1988 | Yes† | | Annual Stat. Report AVA beginning with 1987 stats |

*Note:* AAPCCGC, American Association of Poison Control Centers/Genetic Codes; ICD9, International Classification of Diseases, Ninth Edition; FEMA, Federal Emergency Management Agency; USFA, United States Fire Administration; OHRV, Off-highway recreational vehicle.

*State agency.

†For specific details concerning access and/or confidentiality of records, contact agency.

Courtesy of Education Development Center, 1988, Newton, Massachusetts.

- Are the data disseminated regularly?
- How are data disseminated?
- Are the data available on tape or CD-ROM?
- What is the most recent year of data available?
- Is reporting of data voluntary?
- How much time is there between the date of the injury and its availability for surveillance purposes?
- Is there a code book that defines variables and coding of variables?
- Are analyses available on request?
- Can custom tabulation be done?
- Is access to original documents possible?
- Are there any restrictions on access to records?
- Is there a fee for the data?
- Is there a report with the latest results?
- To what level of geographic specificity is the data available: national, regional, state, county, city, census tract, ZIP code?
- What type of data is obtained: mortality, morbidity, incidence, prevalence, nature of injury, severity of injury, anatomic location, treatment, length of hospitalization, level of impairment or disability, expected source of payment, cost/charge information, surgical and medical procedures performed?
- What demographic information is available: age (actual years or grouped category), date of birth, sex, race, ethnicity, marital status, occupation, industry, education, income, place of residence?
- What data are available on the circumstances surrounding the injury event: date of injury, time of injury, place of occurrence (home, school, work), intent, product involved, type of weapon involved, and external cause of injury code (E code)?
- Which activities were associated with the injury: sports, work, day care, boating, home, recreation, farm, domestic violence, child neglect or abuse?
- Is a narrative description available?
- Are data included on contributing behaviors: seatbelt use, airbag installation, smoke detector installation, drug and alcohol involvement, riding with a drinking driver, bicycle helmet use, motorcycle helmet use, protective equipment for sports, unsupervised swimming, swim-

ming pool fencing, firearm storage, swimming ability, weapons carrying, physical fighting, previous suicide attempt?

- What other barriers are there to use of this data?

Regardless of how effective you are in identifying potential data sources, the fact is they were created for purposes other than your own and will not be perfectly aligned to your needs. Examine data variables, considering which variables the different potential sources of data have in common, which they differ on, and how these compare to the ideal data source. Looking more carefully at specific variables allows you to reduce duplication in incidence, obtain more detailed information on cases that are included in different sources (e.g., police report of motor vehicle crash with resulting injuries), get estimates of injury at different levels (e.g., emergency room treated and released), and assess the potential for data linkage. There is software available to assist in matching data from different sources in order to eliminate duplication. Definitions for injury may vary from one data source to another, making it difficult to compare or group information from different sources. For example, age may be available, but only in aggregate groupings that vary from one source to the next.

It is best to start your exploration of data sources on a small scale. You could begin with the three data sources that almost universally exist in all states in centralized locations and upon which a population-based surveillance system could be based: (1) death certificate files collected and maintained by the state health department; (2) hospital discharge data collected and maintained by the state hospital association, a designee, or a state agency charged with health planning; and (3) motor vehicle crash data collected and maintained by the registry of motor vehicles or highway patrol. Any of these sources can provide data at a community level. If there is a centralized statewide trauma registry or a statewide system for emergency medical services reports or emergency department visits, you will also want to examine the data contained there.

In all likelihood, most existing data sources may not have been analyzed at the level of detail you need for injury prevention program planning purposes. For example, state publications of residents' deaths may have data tables that aggregate injury into five standard categories: total injury deaths, total motor vehicle–related deaths, homicides, suicides, and all other unintentional injury deaths. You will need to determine whether you can acquire more detail from these data, for example, disaggregating bicycle and pedestrian from all motor vehicle, disaggregating falls, fire and burns, drownings, and suffocations from all unintentional, or aggregating all firearms-related deaths regardless of intent. You will also want to determine whether age groupings can be obtained that are more specific than global aggregations of all children ages 19 and under.

Discuss your data needs with data generators and owners. You will be amazed at what accommodations to your needs people will consider making once they are convinced that you will really use the data for the benefit of the community (for example, by developing a smoke detector giveaway program in ZIP code areas identified from the data as being at unusually high risk). Unfortunately, many local and state health departments are still not making use of readily available data sources. One of the only injury-related surveys of state health agencies showed that while 90% have examined vital statistics data, less than 60% have examined data from trauma registries, poison control centers, or emergency medical services.[32]

## STEP 5: CONDUCT PRELIMINARY DATA ANALYSIS

The finer nuances of data source completeness and adequacy rarely are evident until you actually try to carry out data analysis. Thus preliminary data analysis is an important step.

Obtain the big picture by examining the broader categories first. As the going gets tougher, you may want to ask for help from an epidemiologist. Is an epidemiologist included in your coalition? Is there an epidemiologist you can call on at the state health agency? Can you contract with someone from a university? Can you identify a graduate student looking for experience and able to receive guidance from a faculty member?

Whenever possible, request or use standard groupings that promote accuracy and comparability of injury data analyses and reporting across time or between jurisdictions. Use case definitions that have been recommended by others (e.g., traumatic brain injuries [head] and spinal cord injuries have been studied and defined by the CDC).[33] A particularly useful guide for such data grouping is provided by the recommended framework for presenting injury mortality data that appears in Appendix 3–A. These matrix tables for assignment of E codes provide a standardized approach to facilitate data comparisons among states.

## STEP 6: RE-EVALUATE OBJECTIVES FOR THE SURVEILLANCE SYSTEM BASED ON STEPS 3–5

Having made the attempt to gather and analyze data from existing sources, determine the feasibility of achieving your data collection objectives using these available sources. Can existing data sets and data collection processes be improved and integrated together to meet injury surveillance objectives? Can you work with existing data sources to maximize their utility? Can the existing data sources be enhanced? For example, several states have made attempts to increase the use of E codes in hospital discharge data and improve the quality of reporting by educating administrators about their importance to injury prevention, educating medical information specialists in E coding processes, and educating physicians and nurses about which details are essential to document. What are the costs of such improvements? How will they be brought into being? How many data providers will be included in the system? Can you reach consensus on case definitions for the surveillance system and on the data elements to be included as a minimum data set? Should you continue the systems as they are or should you attempt to upgrade them? Or should you modify the original objectives for your injury surveillance system? Now is the time to consider how to improve the integration of data among sources and whether expansion of an existing injury data system is required. In short, can your surveillance system be an outgrowth of existing systems or is it reasonable to create an entirely new and separate injury data collection system?

Addressing these questions will help you prepare a surveillance plan that will include the collection, analysis, and dissemination of the data you need. When you have an idea of the overall causes of injury in the community, you may want to go back and collect more detailed information on one or two of the leading causes.

## STEP 7: CONSIDER LINKING INFORMATION FROM EXISTING DATA SOURCES

No single data source will contain all the information you would like to have for your injury prevention program. Having identified and accessed potential data sources and analyzed their strengths and weaknesses, think about linkage issues—this means linking data from more than one existing data source or with some original data.

Linkage is a potentially effective strategy for generating more information without the expense and delays of gathering new data. For example, medically based data systems are essential for injury surveillance, but not sufficient in themselves. Police reports, on the other hand, contain information on the vehicle, crash, use of safety equipment, and involvement of alcohol, but contain little information on the injuries and their consequences and underestimate the number of injuries that occur. Police crash data alone are unable to convey the magnitude of the medical and financial consequences. There is a definite need to have medically based surveillance systems linked to those operated by police and fire departments so that injury events can be traced from the scene through the health care system. This is accomplished by linking the prehospital emergency medical provider form with the police report and the hospital emergency department or admitting form. Linking police and medical reporting systems can provide outcomes on the frequency of occurrence, severity, disability, and medical costs associated with vehicle design characteristics, airbags, or alcohol-impaired driving as well as the effects of changes in legislation. It can help you target interventions by determining who is at risk for increased severity and high health care costs and which locations are likely to cause the most expensive injuries. Linking also provides some understanding of the significance of missing information in police and medical reports and can be used to improve the quality of data used for linkage and analysis.[34] The advantages of linking also include improved data quality (e.g., improving data validity through cross-checking of data elements found in more than one source), increased data comprehensiveness, and expansion of the usefulness of data sources.[35]

In an ideal world, key elements from existing data sources could be merged into one data bank, but in reality it is a challenge to retrospectively identify and link individuals and events from different sources of data. Often data are released without case identifiers (e.g., date of incident, date of birth) or are only provided in aggregate form. And the potential misuse of identifiers such as social security numbers cannot be ignored. Because of confidentiality requirements, information access will be constrained, especially for some of our most vulnerable populations. For example, records kept by police and by child protective services that may be subject to the criminal justice system are often aggregated. Despite initial fears that confidentiality problems make effective data linkage impossible, many areas have made great progress in linking data without compromising confidentiality. North Carolina was one of the pioneer states in this regard.

Other obstacles to linkage can include different storage media (making it difficult to download data), noncomputerized data, poor data quality (which may lead to invalid matches), and interagency politics. Successful data linkage requires collaboration between the owners and users of data. Those who have performed the most successful data links have used sophisticated computer systems, software, and staff, sufficient funding and time, and familiarity with relevant national, state, and institutional confidentiality requirements. One recent example of successful data linkage, with funding from NHTSA's Crash Outcome Data Evaluation System (CODES) project, involved model projects in Hawaii, Maine, Missouri, New York, Pennsylvania, Utah, and Wisconsin. Each project received large grants to link statewide data sets (police motor vehicle crash reports, emergency medical services run reports, hospital discharge data, and state mortality files) and obtain the crash and injury outcome information needed to prepare a report for Congress on the benefits of safety belt and motorcycle helmet usage. The NHTSA projects employed probabilistic linkage techniques, wherein individual cases are identified across different data sources without exact matches on the identifiers being required. This enables linkage in a short amount of time and at a relatively low cost, as determined by the availability and quality of the state level data. As a result of the CODES project, NHTSA assistance is now available to all states on how to obtain the requisite state data, resolve barriers related to confidentiality, prepare data files for linkage, and institutionalize such linkage.

Linkage is always possible and need not be difficult unless data sources are incomplete or unedited. Date of birth, last name, and social security number are the usual identifiers for linkage. But linkage is not an end in itself. Think about why you want to do linkage and make sure it will be truly useful to your situation.

## STEP 8: PERFORM VALIDATION STUDIES TO EVALUATE THE INJURY SURVEILLANCE SYSTEM

How accurate is the reporting and recording of the data? Is the system meeting its objectives and serving the needs of both the producers and users of the data? Is the system operating efficiently? Could data collection objectives be achieved with less information? What other improvements could be made? To effectively answer these questions, there should be a mechanism to continually monitor the quality of the system.

Validation of an injury surveillance system requires attention to data specificity and sensitivity. As Graitcer notes:

> The development of injury surveillance systems for local and state programs is crucial in providing detailed data on injury trends, clusters, and program intervention effectiveness. . . . An injury surveillance system should collect data that are *representative* of a defined population. . . . The *sensitivity* of an injury surveillance system is a measure of the system's ability to correctly identify all of the true cases of injury in the surveyed population. *Specificity* is a measure of how noncases are misclassified as cases. . . . As sensitivity and specificity approach 100%, the surveillance system is more likely to be representative of the populations of interest. Efforts to increase sensitivity and specificity tend to make a surveillance system more complex, potentially decreasing its acceptability, timeliness, and flexibility.[3(pp192,197)]

The reader interested in learning more on this aspect of surveillance may wish to consult the CDC's Guidelines for Evaluating Surveillance Systems,[31] as well as Teutsch and Churchill's *Principles and Practice of Public Health Surveillance*.[36]

## STEP 9: DEVELOP A DISSEMINATION PLAN FOR SHARING DATA

It is critically important for people to know why you have asked them to collect and share data, how the data will be used, and why they will be important in preventing injuries. The most effective way to do this is to disseminate local injury data back to the providers of the data, as well as to target audiences in the community, so that they can all see that the data are being appropriately analyzed and used. This will motivate them to continue supporting data collection.

Put the data you have uncovered to good use. Inattention to the dissemination of injury surveillance reports has limited the potential value of many injury surveillance efforts. An annual report with yearly tabulations is an important and realistic goal. (More frequent reporting will be overly ambitious unless you have immense resources or a very small geographic area.) Disseminate the data in different formats and for different target groups. It is a good idea to disseminate data through other organizations—

such as in their newsletters—and through presentations, workshops, and staff training.

Data and information are not synonymous. It makes absolutely no sense to give a detailed report with a lot of tables to a policy maker who will never read it. You will immediately be labeled as an impractical number cruncher. Injury epidemiology data must be converted into useful information relevant to local people and nonscientists. Determine what different audiences need to know and keep it simple. While having more detailed reports available, you may also want to develop a two- to five-page report that summarizes your findings and includes a few simple graphs emphasizing the points you are trying to convey. Ask data providers and users to generate a wish list of products that will help them. As nice as it may be to see in print, a peer-reviewed journal is not the type of publication that will get to a policy maker or a community-level person who develops injury prevention programs.

Data do not have to be perfect to be used. If you have documented 38 spinal cord injuries annually to children in your state, but know this is most likely an undercount, you may wish to disseminate the information nevertheless. Given the implications of spinal cord injuries, you have a fairly costly and serious problem regardless of missing cases, but make sure you disclose the imperfections as part of the dissemination. Any data reports should include a list of limitations or biases that need to be taken into consideration in interpreting the data. These should be sufficiently detailed in an appendix for epidemiologists and researchers, while expressed in a summary fashion as a cautionary note in the introduction for lay audiences.

## STEP 10: TIE SURVEILLANCE TO ACTION AND FUNDING

Translating the data into action is not a small feat. Data are never the end product—they are only the means to an end. Now that you have diagnosed a problem, it is critical to take the next step and determine changes that need to be made to counteract the defined problem.

## CONCLUSION

Injury surveillance is the critical precondition to effective injury prevention. Surveillance makes it possible to understand and assess an injury problem, develop prevention approaches, and guide and monitor action.

Injury prevention efforts have too often been hampered by the lack of appropriate databases, but this is not an inescapable problem. In fact, using the 10 steps to injury surveillance outlined in this chapter, you should be well on your way to laying the groundwork for successful surveillance and prevention.

---

## NOTES

1. Guyer B, Gallagher SS. An approach to the epidemiology of childhood injuries. *Pediatr Clin North Am*. 1985;32:5–15.

2. Malenga B. Consent and dissent: Reaction from the farming community to recommendations for childhood agricultural injury prevention. Presented at the American Public Health Association Annual Meeting; New York City; November 1996.

3. Graitcer PL. The development of state and local injury surveillance systems. *J Safety Res*. 1987;18:191–198.

4. Committee for the Study of the Future of Public Health, Institute of Medicine. *The Future of Public Health*. Washington, DC: National Academy Press; 1988:114.

5. Gallagher SS, Finison K, Guyer B, Goodenough S The incidence of injuries among 87,000 Massachusetts children and adolescents: Results of the 1980–81 statewide childhood injury prevention program surveillance system. *Am J Public Health*. 1984;74:1340–1347.

6. Barancik JI, Chatterjee BF, Greene YC, et al. Northeastern Ohio Trauma Study: I. Magnitude of the problem. *Am J Public Health*. 1983;73:746–751.

7. Fife D, Barancik JI, Chatterjee BF. Northeastern Ohio Trauma Study: II. Injury rates by age, sex, and cause. *Am J Public Health* 1984;74:473–478.

8. Baker SP, O'Neill B, Haddon W Jr, Long WB. The injury severity score: A method for describing patients with multiple injuries and evaluating emergency care. *J Trauma*. 1974;14:187–196.

9. Committee on Injury Scaling. *The Abbreviated Injury Scale*. Park Ridge, IL: American Association of Automotive Medicine; 1980.

10. Baker SP. Current status of trauma severity indices. *J Trauma*. 1983;23:193–196.

11. Champion HR, Sacco WJ, Copes WS, Gann DS, Gennarelli TA, Flanagan ME. A revision of the trauma score. *J Trauma*. 1989;29:623–629.

12. Cales RH. Injury severity determinations: Requirements, approaches, and applications. *Ann Emerg Med*. 1986;15:1487–1496.

13. Boyd CR, Tolson MA, Copes WS. Evaluating trauma care: The TRISS method. *J Trauma*. 1987;27:370–378.

14. Copes WS, Champion HR, Sacco WJ, et al. Progress in characterizing anatomic injury. *J Trauma*. 1990;30:1200–1207.

15. Kaufmann CR, Maier RV, Kaufmann EJ, Rivara FP, Carrico CJ. Validity of applying adult TRISS analysis to injured children. *J Trauma.* 1991;31:691–697.

16. Tepas JJ III. Update on pediatric trauma-severity scores. In: Haller JA Jr. *Emergency Medical Services for Children.* Columbus, OH: Ross Laboratories; 1989.

17. Annual editions published by the National Safety Council, Itasca, IL.

18. Fingerhut LA, Warner M. Injury chartbook. In: National Center for Health Statistics. *Health, United States, 1996–97 and Injury Chartbook.* Hyattsville, MD: U.S. Public Health Service; 1997.

19. *Healthy People 2000: National Health Promotion and Disease Prevention Objectives.* Washington, DC: U.S. Department of Health and Human Services; 1990 (Public Health Service publication 91-50212).

20. http://www.cdc.gov/epo/mmwr/mmwr.html

21. Combs DL, Parrish RG, Ing R. *Death Investigation in the United States and Canada.* Atlanta, GA: Centers for Disease Control; 1992.

22. Dave Barry column, *Boston Sunday Globe*, May 28, 1995.

23. Guyer B, Lescohier I, Gallagher SS, et al. Intentional injuries among children and adolescents in Massachusetts. *N Engl J Med.* 1989;321:1584–1589.

24. Davidson LL, Durkin MS, O'Connor P, et al. The epidemiology of severe injuries to children in Northern Manhattan: Methods and incidence rates. *Paediatr Perinat Epidemiol.* 1992;6:153–165.

25. Grisso JA, Wishner AR, Schwarz DF, et al. A population-based study of injuries in inner-city women. *Am J Epidemiol.* 1991;134:59–68.

26. Wishner AR, Schwarz DF, Grisso JA, et al. Interpersonal violence related injuries in an African-American community in Philadelphia. *Am J Public Health.* 1991;81:1474–1476.

27. Schwarz DF, Grisso JA, Miles CG, et al. A longitudinal study of injury morbidity in an African-American population. *JAMA.* 1994;271:755–760.

28. Scheidt PC, Harel Y, Trumble AC, Jones DH, Overpeck MD, Bijur PE. The epidemiology of nonfatal injuries among U.S. children and youth. *Am J Public Health.* 1995;85:932–938.

29. Agran PF, Winn DG, Anderson CL. Surveillance of pediatric injury hospitalizations in Southern California. *Inj Prev.* 1995:1:284–287.

30. Barancik JI, Fife D. Northeast Ohio Trauma Study IV: Discrepancies in vehicular crash injury registry. *Accident Analysis Prev.* 1985;17:147–154.

31. Centers for Disease Control. Guidelines for evaluating surveillance systems. *MMWR.* 1988;37(Supplement No. S-5):1–18.

32. Harrington C, Gallagher SS, Burgess LL, Guyer B. *Injury Prevention Programs in State Health Departments: A National Survey.* Boston: Harvard School of Public Health, Childhood Injury Prevention Resource Center; 1988.

33. Thurman DJ, Sniezek JE, Johnson D, et al. *Guidelines for Surveillance of Central Nervous System Injury.* Atlanta, GA: Centers for Disease Control and Prevention; 1995.

34. *Why Data Linkage? The Importance of CODES.* Washington, DC: National Highway Traffic Safety Administration; October 1996, DOT HS 808 461.

35. Johnson S. Where do we go from here? Presented at the Uniform Pre-Hospital EMS Data Conference, Washington, DC; August 1993.

36. Teutsch SM, Churchill RE. *Principles and Practice of Public Health Surveillance.* New York: Oxford University Press; 1994.

# An Injury Surveillance Example

One state's example illustrates how several of the issues discussed in this chapter were actually addressed. In 1993, the Massachusetts Department of Public Health (MDPH) implemented the first statewide surveillance system in the country based on emergency department reporting. Entitled the Weapon-Related Injury Surveillance System (WRISS), it is a second-generation surveillance effort. The first, a pilot project known as the Sentinel Injury Surveillance System, began collecting data in 1990 from hospitals in two geographic areas. In November 1993, all remaining hospitals in the state began participating in the system. Both surveillance systems have focused solely on collecting data on gunshot wounds (intentional and unintentional) and sharp instrument wounds (intentional only). The systems have collected data to describe the injury problem, target risk groups, and measure the impact of interventions. Such information is analyzed for use by injury professionals internal and external to MDPH. Reports profiling injuries also are made available to the general public.

Both surveillance systems have relied on an automated emergency department log, which the MDPH designed (according to the standards defined by the Joint Commission for the Accreditation of Healthcare Organizations). The computerized *Logbook* "covers all standard [ED] log variables; for injuries, variables captured include injury cause [coded into collapsed E code categories], diagnosis, intent, job-relatedness, and basic demographics . . . the program is designed largely to serve ED management needs and patient care needs." The *Logbook,* in addition to creating a surveillance tool for all types of injuries treated in the emergency department, has computerized the WRISS.

Courtesy of Morrison Institute for Public Policy, Tempe, Arizona.

The WRISS is undergirded by a Massachusetts law requiring all physicians to report (by phone or in writing) gunshot and stabbing wounds to the Department of Public Safety (DPS). WRISS data are collected manually and entered in a computerized emergency department log. The DPS form requires the victim's name, street address, city of occurrence, age, type of wound, date of incident, name of attending physician and hospital, and name of investigating agency. The WRISS form collects additional elements, such as the type of incident (e.g., self-inflicted, violence related), precipitating circumstance, victim/offender relationship, race, medical record number, location of incident, mode of arrival to ED, suspected alcohol or drug use, and discharge disposition (such as patient expired, patient was transferred to home, skilled nursing facility, or other). The patient's name, street address number, month and date of birth, and attending physician are not transferable to the WRISS portion of the form. The top two pages of the three-page form are sent to DPS; the third page is sent to MDPH on a monthly basis for entry into a computer database.

The emergency department secretary is responsible for entering all cases treated in the emergency department into the *Logbook*. Data are transmitted by disk to the MDPH, where the data are assessed for quality, aggregated, analyzed, interpreted, and prepared for dissemination. Assessing the quality of data—compliance, accuracy, completeness, and so forth—is a key feature of both the manual and computer reporting systems. "For the paper reporting system, compliance is measured by comparing reports filed with MDPH against actual cases identified during periodic record reviews by WRISS staff at each participating hospital. System compliance averages about 70 percent." For the computerized system, "[t]he potential problems are incorrect coding of injuries. WRISS staff periodically compare a sample of the ED's injury medical records to the codes assigned in the *Logbook* data. Coding accuracy exceeds 95 percent for each injury variable," and less than 10% of intentional injury cases are estimated as being missed by the system.

The WRISS has met its objective as an ongoing, low-cost system that provides data at the community level for the development of effective violence prevention strategies. WRISS data are available to public health, violence prevention practitioners, injury control professionals, and local groups through timely newsletters, presentations, staff training, and workshops. MDPH is credited with having "transformed a passive criminal justice reporting requirement into an active public health intentional injury surveillance system."

Lessons learned from the Massachusetts study include the following:

- Mandated physician reporting of intentionally inflicted firearm and knife injuries and a manual reporting form can be used successfully to create the foundation for this cause-specific surveillance system.
- The minimum data set being collected can be limited to ensure the entire form can be completed within one to two minutes.
- WRISS focuses on compelling and emotional injuries; "less compelling issues may have met with less success." Consequently, the data collected have specific utility. For example, while WRISS is limited to only two types of violent injuries (intentional firearm and knife injuries), results from the *Logbook* program show the majority of violent injuries treated in EDs do not involve weapons. This is a case where the public's interest in an emotional issue overrides other data that may be more compelling in numbers but which have less appeal to the general public.
- MDPH credits a measure of their success in obtaining and retaining hospital participation to their efforts to "give something back" to EDs, such as staff training or data.
- WRISS data are collected manually, and even though commitment to the program appears high, it is dependent on the memory and motivation of ED providers. Reporting would be enhanced by connecting injury reporting to the ED log (which all hospitals are required to maintain) or by expanding the computerized ED log to include software that codes injury information (e.g., E codes).
- Surveillance information has assisted in the design and monitoring of community programs, which have been shown to be effective in reducing violence-related injuries due to firearms and knives.
- As noted earlier, results from the *Logbook* program show that the most violent injuries do not involve weapons. According to one hospital's data, the number of patients who were assaulted with a sharp instrument was equal to the number who were assaulted with other weapons such as a bat or club. By far the most frequent victims of assault seen in the ED are those who are punched, kicked, or shoved. Such assaults outnumber victims of knife and other weapon assaults by a ratio of 3.2 to 1. Data further reveal that for every firearm homicide, a minimum of 123 assaults are treated and released in EDs.

# CHAPTER 13

# Real World Evaluation Techniques

"The only way to determine if something works is to try it, in a way that lends itself to reliable evaluation."

Panel on the Understanding and Control of Violent Behavior, *Understanding and Preventing Violence*, 1993

## WHAT THIS CHAPTER IS ABOUT

The effectiveness of injury prevention programs should be evaluated routinely, but for many injury prevention practitioners the term "evaluation" conjures up reactions of fear, loathing, and onerous chores. Evaluation is often equated with research and thought of as being narrowly focused on morbidity and mortality outcome measures. But measuring effectiveness is only one type of evaluation activity. In fact, evaluation is an essential tool for program management. Funders increasingly require that funded programs conduct evaluations, not just to measure success levels but, perhaps more important, to more effectively guide program implementation, particularly decisions as to how to prioritize resource allocations.

Evaluation should be an integral part of any injury prevention effort. Practitioners need to understand the process and realities of evaluation and make the most of existing evaluation methods and tools, fitting them into a real world, community setting.

There are multiple perspectives on evaluation depending on whether you are an epidemiologist, a researcher, or a program developer. This chapter is about real world program evaluation—evaluation in circumstances in which one does not have the luxury of engaging in carefully designed and controlled studies, where resources for conducting evaluation may be very limited, where nonresearch staff carry out the evaluation

309

and may not be accustomed to adhering to protocols, and where it may not be possible to carry out all of the desired evaluation steps.

For many professionals, "evaluation" can be an intimidating concept. In this chapter, we will try to make it less intimidating by reviewing the purposes of evaluation, some of the difficulties in conducting evaluations, the importance of clearly defining what you are evaluating, the different kinds of evaluation, the steps in the evaluation process, and common constraints on evaluation.

## INTRODUCTION

Why perform an evaluation? We want to know which injury prevention interventions work best, yet we often do not do the necessary evaluation ourselves. We want to see changes in outcome measures (e.g., reduction in injuries, behavioral changes) yet we don't allow enough time to demonstrate measurable changes. It is not so easy to show effectiveness directly attributable to an intervention program, especially in a short period of time. But the pressure is there to do so, nevertheless. Funding agencies want to see evaluation conducted, but are often reluctant to supply sufficient resources to carry it out. Injury prevention programs tend to be evaluated based on processes (e.g., tracking the number of individuals served or the number of materials disseminated), rather than on satisfaction on the part of target audiences. Rigorous and multilevel evaluation of injury prevention interventions that encompass both process and outcome measures are rare in the literature.[1-6] And the generalizability of evaluation results are severely limited by variability in implementation or differences in populations.

Why is there so little evaluation of injury prevention programs? What are some of the rationales for not doing it? Comments on evaluation include: "It's boring," "It is unnecessary and wastes precious resources," "We know our program is worthwhile and is well received by the community," "The community is ready to roll with the program . . . we can't hold them back and take the time to make baselines measures," "We don't have any money to do an evaluation," or "What if we come out looking bad?" These are valid concerns regarding evaluation as it is often practiced.

If you work in a government agency or in a politically charged atmosphere, you often need to respond to crises, demonstrating through action that you are doing something about problems. Public image is what counts, not proven effectiveness.

Even if a program or strategy can be shown to be effective, decision makers may pick other strategies because they seem easier to implement or more popular and acceptable to the community. Evaluation challenges policy decisions and calls into question the validity of a program's or an organization's existence.

It is not enough to say you have a program and are doing something. The real questions should be: Are the injury prevention strategies being employed demonstrably effective? Have organizational or behavioral changes been made? Have you been able to gauge your progress? What can be done to increase program effectiveness? Evaluation deals with methods for developing programs and for assessing program implementation and effectiveness. It does not mean doing academic research, although you may use such methods and tools. Traditional research methods do not usually fit into an action or real world community setting where one cannot control all the variables.

Evaluation is an essential tool for program management and is conducted to measure the impact of a program. Evaluation can also inform current decision making by identifying implementation problems (which will undoubtedly occur, no matter how well planned the program). Evaluation can help decision makers craft corrections to their implementation programs. And evaluation can be very useful in marketing programs. Do not wait until the end of a program to have some convincing successes. Evaluation is one way to justify program costs and fulfill demands for accountability, especially to funding sources. And finally, evaluation can provide the documentation to facilitate efficient replication at a later date, helping to advance knowledge for the field and guide future program development.

A study of state health agencies found that 41% conduct some level of process evaluation for their injury prevention programs and 23% conduct evaluation using outcome measures. In the same study, only 50% of the states listed evaluation of existing injury programs as a future priority.[7] There may not be enough resources to evaluate every program with equal vigor, but as public health practitioners, we can and should do better.

## EVALUATION STEPS

Evaluating programs may seem difficult, but with proper groundwork to establish clear program and evaluation goals, collect evaluation data, and examine the data on a regular basis, useful evaluation is achievable. A good design that is built into the program from its inception is at the core of a good evaluation.

In developing a good evaluation plan there are several clear-cut steps that can help ensure success. The following pages lay out 15 basic steps that experience has shown characterize effective real world evaluation of injury prevention programs. The steps are

1. Develop specific, measurable, and written goals and objectives for your injury prevention program.
2. Specify and define a set of activities that can be implemented to accomplish program goals and objectives.
3. List questions to be answered for formative, process, and outcome evaluation.
4. Identify resources needed to carry out your evaluation and compare these with the resources available.
5. Set realistic priorities for the evaluation given the resources and time available.
6. Identify a specific individual responsible for overseeing the evaluation.
7. Select methods appropriate to the evaluation questions.
8. Identify potential data sources and develop specific data collection forms.
9. Develop an evaluation schedule.
10. Conduct formative evaluation of materials.
11. Collect baseline data.
12. Analyze and interpret the data.
13. Use the findings to provide feedback to improve the program.
14. Communicate the findings, both positive and negative, in a timely manner.
15. Continue the evaluation process.

Some of these steps are overarching in application while others are closer to being process tips. Some are discussed at length, others only briefly. But all can help facilitate an effective real world evaluation process. They should be used as a guide, not followed rigidly. The discussion of these steps is followed by a discussion of constraints encountered when implementing real world evaluations. Remember that a good evaluation design that is built into a program from its inception is at the core of a good evaluation. And to state the obvious, any evaluation expertise that is available to you should be consulted from the very beginning of evaluation planning.

### Step 1: Develop Specific, Measurable, and Written Goals and Objectives for Your Injury Prevention Program

Poorly defined goals and objectives often hamper evaluations. Before implementing an injury prevention program, you must have a clear idea of what you are trying to accomplish. Be realistic. Define what you want to change—and define your objectives in a measurable way. Most programs are overly ambitious and overestimate what can be achieved, which then also makes for unrealistic evaluation. It is important to lay out, *in writing*, what your program is intended to achieve. If you can't put it in writing, how can you evaluate it? Writing forces you to clarify your ideas and tends to make your goals manageable.

Goals are usually broad statements with an expectation of the improvement expected for the long term. Goal examples might include: To decrease motor vehicle–related occupant injuries to the young. To decrease deaths and injuries related to fires. To implement a smoke detector give-away program in a high-risk area. Goals can be measured over the long term, but it is more important to measure objectives.

Objectives specify a program's approach, are more specific and time limited, and describe how the program will achieve its goal. Objectives should be measurable. Components might include: Who will do what to carry out the program implementation? What measurable results are expected? How large an effect is necessary to demonstrate success? How much time is required for change? Examples might include: To increase the correct use of child car restraints among children 0 to 4 years of age in low-income families and rural communities by at least 20% by January 2000. To pass a state law eliminating four loopholes in the current child passenger safety law by June 1999. To increase the installation of smoke detectors in households in four ZIP codes by October 2001. By December 1999, to bring together key groups in the community for a series of at least three monthly meetings to collaborate on the development of a comprehensive youth violence prevention plan for the community.

A good program manager will continually reassess goals and objectives, as well as monitoring progress in meeting them. Flexibility is a prerequisite to improvement and evolution of a program.

## Step 2: Specify and Define a Set of Activities That Can Be Implemented To Accomplish Program Goals and Objectives

Exactly what will you try to do to bring about a reduction in injury rates or a change in policy? You must clearly define key activities if you are eventually to assess their contribution to meeting program objectives. Activities may range from one-on-one counseling on injury prevention during clinic visits, to a media campaign, to training of sanitarians in safety inspections of playgrounds, to developing a coalition to push for passage of bike helmet legislation, to changing organizational practices to have questions about domestic violence be part of routine prenatal visits, to making it a policy that children who ride their bikes to school must wear bike helmets.

Define activities that can be connected to intermediate evaluation measures. An example might be increased police enforcement of violations of the child passenger safety law, as measured by the number of citations issued. How are you going to do it? A seemingly simple task, like storage of car seats for a child passenger safety loan program, could be the program's downfall if not factored into the implementation plan and tracked along the way. If one of your goals is to develop a coalition of organizations in favor of changes in the current child passenger safety laws, what linkages need to be made and how? If one of your goals is to distribute smoke detectors to households in low-income areas, how are you going to do it? Exhibit 13–1 details the steps that might be involved in achieving one such objective.

## Step 3: List Questions To Be Answered for Formative, Process, and Outcome Evaluation

This is the major evaluation step and will be discussed at much greater length than any of the other steps. There are several types of evaluation to consider for each intervention program: formative, process, and outcome. These can complement one another, as illustrated in Figure 13–1.

### Formative Evaluation

Formative evaluation can be used to refine a program's implementation before full-scale implementation. It is a way of examining program appropriateness and potential reception on a small, preliminary scale. This usu-

**Exhibit 13–1** Activities for Meeting an Injury Prevention Objective: An Example

**Objective:** To increase the correct use of child car restraints among children 0–4 years of age in low-income families and rural communities by at least 20% by January 2000.

Activities (in no particular order):

- Identify geographic areas with low-income rural families to be targeted.
- Determine where such families access services.
- Determine incidence of correct car seat usage in the target population (parking lots of service providers, fast food restaurants, grocery stores, discount stores).
- Identify volunteers to perform observation studies.
- Train volunteers.
- Publicize the results and set target rate 20% higher.
- Develop educational and promotional materials for the target population.
- Identify participants for a focus group.
- Determine site for a focus group.
- Obtain donated items as incentives for participation in a focus group.
- Conduct focus group to determine parental attitudes regarding need for child safety seats, barriers, and incentives.
- Develop protocol to follow in conducting observations.
- Train providers to teach parents proper installation and use of car seats.
- Determine incentives to get providers to attend a training (e.g., on-site).
- Develop protocol for providers.
- Provide list of car seat loaner programs in the area.
- Provide educational materials.
- Encourage hospitals with services for newborns to develop policies regarding discharge of newborns in approved child car restraints and reinforcement of message whenever a service is delivered.
- Survey current hospital practices.
- Meet with key informants in the community to obtain support for a change in hospital practice.
- Develop protocol for hospital staff regarding discharge procedure.
- Make available convertible car restraints for families with infants and young children.
- Locate convenient storage area for child car seats.
- Develop application form for child car seat loans.

*continues*

**Exhibit 13-1** continued

- Provide information on child car seats at point of purchase sites (e.g., used car dealers, retailers).
- Provide information at day care settings and with day care licensers.
- Provide information at childbirth education and postpartum settings.
- Repeat observations at targeted sites.
- Use the findings to alter the program.

ally includes pretesting, pilot studies, and focus groups to determine the likely response of target audiences and program deliverers. With formative evaluation, information is collected and fed back to program developers early in the course of implementation in order to enhance the program and maximize its chances of success. For example, questions might include: Are the service deliverers satisfied with the materials? Were materials perceived as being useful by the target population? (These questions may be repeated again during the process evaluation stage.)

Focus groups can be an especially useful part of formative evaluation.[8] Small groups of people are convened for in-depth interviews to obtain their opinions about messages to be delivered, methods of delivery, acceptability of materials, and other reactions to an injury prevention program. Focus groups allow a fuller understanding of potential target audiences and the pretesting of materials to ensure that they are appropriate for—and appeal to—that target audience. This is especially important when the backgrounds and experiences of a target audience are distinctly different from that of the program staff; target audience and staff may respond to messages in significantly different ways. This could be the case with programs aimed at teenagers, low-income populations, or recent immigrants. When such groups are the targets of an injury prevention program, they should definitely be represented in your focus group sample. You can use focus groups to test recall, aesthetic appeal, message credibility, comprehension, relevance, acceptability, language style, and readability. Focus groups are also used to help generate ideas and develop hypotheses for research of a quantitative or qualitative nature.

In conducting focus groups, you should have a trained moderator who can skillfully handle a group process to lead the discussion. The moderator does not need to be an expert in the subject matter under discussion. You should also have a note taker or start-to-finish tape recording of the discussion for later review. Materials should be at a suitable readability level and

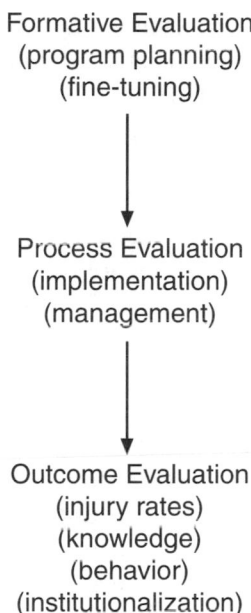

Formative Evaluation
(program planning)
(fine-tuning)

Process Evaluation
(implementation)
(management)

Outcome Evaluation
(injury rates)
(knowledge)
(behavior)
(institutionalization)

**Figure 13–1**  The Interrelationship of Evaluation Approaches

should be culturally appropriate to the target population. Focus groups are relatively inexpensive and can generate large amounts of information in a short period of time. Costs include a moderator's time, facility rental for a comfortable meeting room, refreshments, and a stipend to participants. Drawbacks of this method include difficulty in the recruitment of participants, peer pressure for acceptance and conformity (especially in responses generated by adolescents), single-participant dominance if a seasoned moderator is not present, and participants who are not representative of your total population. A detailed case study of a process evaluation of a community-based injury prevention program is presented in Appendix 13–A at the end of this chapter.

### Process Evaluation

Process evaluation can document the degree to which an injury prevention program is being implemented as designed. The assessment is not of program results but of whether program activities and their delivery are being carried out as planned; thus process evaluation is necessary, but not sufficient, in evaluating a program's results.

Process evaluation should be ongoing and examine each element of the total program being evaluated. What was actually done, where and when was it done, how often was it done, by whom, with whom, and for whom? Process evaluation can focus on the amount and range of content delivered, number and places where delivered, consistency of implementation across locations and agencies, and quality of program delivery. For example, an evaluation might be conducted of the appropriateness and quality of training, numbers referred for follow-up counseling, and numbers who follow through with the referral. Process evaluation can be used to assess exposure to components of an intervention, materials and equipment, implementation, and costs.

Under some circumstances, process evaluation data can be used to better understand program effects. When process data can be linked to outcome data, analysis may provide a more sensitive way to detect program effects. Those participants who had the longest exposure to the truest implementation of the program should receive the greatest benefit and demonstrate the largest impact—a kind of dose-response relationship.

The following types of questions can be asked and answered using process evaluation.

*Exposure.* Is the community aware of the program? Is the target population being reached? Has the target population been trained? How many teachers have been trained? How many schools and hospitals have participated? Who attended community meetings? What percentage of the target population actually received materials or safety equipment? These questions provide an estimate of the penetration rate of the program in the population.

*Materials and Equipment.* What quantity has been distributed? Are these available in accessible locations to the target population? Did people receive them? Did people use them?

*Implementation.* What has been the extent of implementation? Is the protocol actually followed in the field? Do providers comply and provide referrals? Do police enforce the law and write citations? What joint activities are being carried out with community organizations? How many coalition meetings have been convened? What linkages have been established among organizations?

*Costs.* What has been the program implementation cost? What in-kind services have been provided? What additional funds have been forthcoming from the community? How many staff and volunteers are needed to carry out each component of the program? What has been the cost per smoke detector distributed?

Process evaluation is a management tool that is used to ensure that a program is proceeding as expected and at the right pace. Program staff should use the information derived to adjust program implementation. Much of process evaluation depends on accurate record keeping, which can consist of simple record keeping (e.g., making an addition to an existing record in the clinic to determine if counseling on injury prevention is given) or complex record keeping (e.g., introducing a new form that will have to be filled out for each interaction). The completion of different log forms by community members on a monthly basis is an excellent tool for monitoring events, ongoing services provided, media coverage, and resources generated. It is essential for categorizing the work of coalitions in a community. Evaluation data collection may include direct counts of participation made as the program is being implemented or surveys conducted after the program is completed to determine exposure to the program. When exposure is limited or less than anticipated, it may not be possible to get an expected outcome.

Many epidemiologists and researchers neglect this area of evaluation, focusing instead on outcomes only. They may correctly conclude that a program wasn't effective, but have no understanding of why the program didn't work. Maybe the program design was flawed or inappropriate, maybe the problem was intractable or misunderstood, or maybe the program wasn't implemented as planned and didn't reach enough of the target audience. Without process evaluation, a useful approach could be abandoned, when—if it was delivered properly—it would have had the desired effect. With process evaluation, implementation problems can be discovered early on and corrective modifications put into effect.

### *Outcome Evaluation*

Have the objectives of a particular injury prevention program been achieved? Outcome evaluation can document a program's effectiveness in producing expected outcomes related to program goals. An assessment might be made of whether there has been a change in the number and severity of injuries, of a particular risk factor, or of knowledge, attitudes, and policy. For example, has there been an increase in the number of children wearing bike helmets?

Outcomes can be measured using a variety of methods, ranging from short questionnaires to self-reports to independent observations to a complex epidemiological study with pretests and posttests. Choosing an appropriate outcome indicator to measure is critical to determining program effects. Indicators may include knowledge, attitudes, self-reported behavior, observations of behavior, hazard reduction in the home or on the playground, morbidity, mortality, changes in public policy and practice, and cost-effectiveness. Mortality and morbidity are obviously among the most significant indicators of program outcome, while changes in knowledge would be a poorer indicator because such changes may not lead to altered behavior and reduced injury rates. Changes in policy and organizational practices can also be important outcome measures, although they are not measures of individual change. Examples might include establishing a memorandum of understanding between two state agencies to share information or the provision of car seats to be kept in the cars of social workers who deal with children in foster care. Practitioners and researchers often neglect these policy and organization measures, even though in the long run they may have a greater impact in bringing about individual change.

How will you recognize success when you see it? Success should not be defined solely by reduced injury rates, even if you have the luxury of a long-term program to accomplish this goal. Proxy or surrogate indicators are often used to demonstrate program effectiveness. These are often needed because of the difficulty in showing reductions in injury morbidity or mortality over a short time period or in a small population. Proxy indicators measure intermediate outcomes, such as changes in behavior or in public policy that relate to changes in injuries. For example, the literature has already shown that child car seats are effective in reducing both deaths and injury to children; therefore, it is not necessary to measure injury rates for every injury prevention program. It is totally acceptable to measure use of child safety seats or a change in their correct usage as an intermediate measure, which would ultimately lead to a reduction in the injury rate.

There are at least eight questions to address in order to trace potential impacts of a program and identify intermediate variables that also need to be evaluated.

- What is the goal of the program?
- What are the objectives to accomplish the goal?
- What activities need to occur to reach the goals and objectives?

- Who do the activities need to reach (children, parents, providers, teachers, legislators, law enforcement, or other agencies)?
- How are these groups related to the goals of the program?
- What do we want these groups to do and how will they be affected?
- What actions should happen as a result of their activity?
- How long should it take for this to happen?

A flow chart may be useful in determining process and outcome linkages and the sequence of effects leading from one to the other. By working through the pathways in a flow chart, you obtain better clarity on who and what your target for intervention really is.[9]

Changes in risk behavior are an acceptable and legitimate intermediate outcome measure, especially if the change is documented through on-site observation rather than as a self-reported measure. Examples of other types of proxy indicators include seatbelt use, helmet use by bicyclists and motorcyclists, use of mouth guards and other protective sports equipment, proper storage of firearms, installation of an operating smoke detector, reductions in "dart out" behavior of child pedestrians, and increases in sales of bike helmets or firearm trigger locks. Changes in public policy and practice that have been shown to affect the injury risk environment are also acceptable proxy outcome indicators. An example would be an increase in law enforcement citations for nonuse of seatbelts. A decline in revenue from alcohol taxes could suggest that community groups are having an impact on alcohol consumption, a very important risk factor for injury.

Outcome evaluation is more rigorous and requires more technical data collection than process evaluation, but this does not mean it is synonymous with a major research effort, although it could have all the characteristics of a research study if you have the resources available. A full-fledged outcome evaluation would include randomized assignment to an intervention group or a no-intervention control group as a source of comparative information. Using comparison groups is a challenge because they require (1) a set of circumstances similar enough to the target group to provide valid comparisons, (2) measurements in a population with whom you are not working, (3) using additional resources, and (4) incentives for participation even though no program is offered. There is also an ethical issue involved in withholding a promising intervention from members of a comparison group. More typical than randomized assignment is outcome evaluation using time series measurement, such as measurement of seatbelt use before a law is implemented, shortly after a law is implemented, and one year later.

It is unwise to have reduced injury rates be the sole outcome indicator, even though this is the ultimate goal of injury prevention. Decreased injury rates can be accurately measured only with a very large sample and only over the course of many years. If you want to evaluate your program's effect in this way, you should consider obtaining assistance from skilled epidemiologists, statisticians, and educational researchers.

### Step 4: Identify Resources Needed To Carry Out Your Evaluation and Compare These with the Resources Available

The difficulties and costs of program evaluation should not be underestimated. Investments of talent, time, and financial support and planning are required. Routine monitoring of program implementation need not be very expensive, but outcome measures that require collection of new data can be quite costly. Printing forms, travel time to collect evaluation data, consultants for planning the evaluation or analyzing resulting data, a focus group facilitator—all these costs need to be factored into your choice of an evaluation approach. Always keep in mind the other side of the cost equation: Program implementation that is off-base and ineffective is a tremendous waste of resources. The earlier you can discover and correct such wasteful efforts, the better—and more cost-effective—your program will be.

### Step 5: Set Realistic Priorities for the Evaluation Given the Resources and Time Available

Include some process measures and some form of outcome measurement. Choose outcome measurements carefully, limiting these to the minimum necessary unless you have outside resources to help you carry out the evaluation.

### Step 6: Identify a Specific Individual Responsible for Overseeing the Evaluation

A staff person must be assigned specific responsibility for monitoring and evaluation. This person will ensure that the evaluation is kept on schedule. You do not need an epidemiologist, researcher, or social scientist to fill this role. What you do need is someone with a good understanding of the program, its goals, and its objectives. You could choose to use an outside evaluator, although this is likely to be more costly. In any case, the person responsible for evaluation should build a relationship with the community so as to implement the evaluation process in an understanding and accurate manner.

## Step 7: Select Methods Appropriate to the Evaluation Questions

Potential methods include the use of comparison groups, interviews, surveys, observations, ratings by staff or experts, knowledge tests, institutional and administrative record review, government statistics, and financial records. Evaluation protocols and timelines should be developed as part of the method selection process.

## Step 8: Identify Potential Data Sources and Develop Specific Data Collection Forms

Cast a wide net. Who are the frontline people that interface with your target audience or deliver the injury prevention program? Who could collect the kind of information you need? Will they need training? Are there agencies that keep the type of records you need or that could readily add an evaluation item onto an existing method of collection?

Evaluation data must be collected systematically. Anecdotes are not sufficient for convincing funders and policy makers of your success. Observational studies, self-reports of behavior, and household, provider, or hospital record surveys require standard data collection, as do program documentation and other routine monitoring (e.g., indicating program counseling on a medical record, obtaining baseline perceptions of coalition members, or recording of requests from and linkages to community organizations). You will need to design simple forms with ease of data entry, tabulation, and analysis. Keep it simple and eliminate unnecessary information that may cost more to process than it is worth or which will discourage data collectors. During the design process, be sure to involve as many people who will be filling out the form or providing written documentation as possible. Data collection must conform to the demands of the setting. If it is too tedious and lengthy, completion will be sporadic. Be creative. Determine incentives for buy-in. For example, in one anticipatory guidance project that required added paperwork, medical providers were able to receive continuing education credit for their participation.

## Step 9: Develop an Evaluation Schedule

Timing is everything. Make sure you are clear on exactly when a program or activity will be initiated in different settings or different communities. Determine the intervals at which different measurements need to be performed. Then stick to your schedule. Plan ahead. If you are going to need reviews and approvals, make sure that you leave enough time to do so. Most things take longer than you think.

## Step 10: Conduct Formative Evaluation of Materials

Make sure that materials are suitable for and acceptable to the target audience and those involved in program delivery. This does not have to be a big process; you only need a small number of participants. Use a formative evaluation approach—such as focus groups—to carry out this step.

## Step 11: Collect Baseline Data

Baseline data collection should be built into the program's design. It must be done *before* you initiate your program. This requires careful planning and a rigid schedule. Without appropriate baseline data, the evaluation will suffer.

## Step 12: Analyze and Interpret the Data

Recognize the limitations in the information you will collect. If necessary, seek assistance from a consultant to guide you to determine appropriate analytic techniques. It is helpful to display the information you collect graphically. In presenting your analysis, clearly explain how the data were analyzed and interpreted, why you selected the approaches you used, and what key assumptions and possible weaknesses you think exist in the analysis.

**Step 13: Use the Findings To Provide Feedback To Improve the Program**

The focus is program guidance and more rational decision making. It is never too late to enhance your program. Use the identified strengths and weaknesses to improve program delivery.

Make modifications to the program. A program should not be static. It should be evolving with adjustments made based on evaluation findings. The modification process may also be a way to increase community involvement. The following description from *Injury Prevention: Meeting the Challenge* describes one example of using evaluation findings to modify a program.

> One program in Massachusetts illustrates well how efforts can evolve as new data emerge. In response to a growing concern among pediatricians and parents, the Child Passenger Safety Resource Center (CPSRC) was established in 1979 at the Massachusetts Department of Public Health. CPSRC's original goal was to "decrease the incidence of premature death and disability in children under 14 through the increased safe and consistent use of child automobile restraint devices."

> During its first year, the program focused on increasing safety seat use among Massachusetts children under the age of 5, in particular newborn infants leaving the hospital obstetrics ward. This decision was based on national data and the assumption that children so protected will progress to regular use of safety belts later in life. Activities centered on establishing safety seat loaner programs (especially in hospitals with obstetrics wards) and training loaner program staff to inform new parents about child safety seat use.

> In 1980 new data from a statewide observational survey became available, and CPSRC began to expand its focus. The data indicated a 50% safety seat use rate among children under the age of 1, an 18% rate for ages 1–4, and a 5% safety belt use rate among 5- to 9-year-olds. Former CPSRC assistant director Cindy Rodgers commented, "We learned that infant seat use was fairly commonplace. Adults seemed to be a lot more hesitant, however,

to use toddler seats for older preschoolers and to convince their school-age children to wear safety belts. . . ." CPSRC refined its activity to focus on children between the ages of 1 and 10 and their parents.

The program's efforts were given a boost in January 1982 by the state's new child passenger safety law, which covered children from birth to the age of 5. Concerned that the law was not being fully enforced, Rodgers surveyed local police departments and learned that enforcement of the law was minimal. So CPSRC developed and disseminated materials to familiarize law enforcement officers with the law and provide suggestions for enforcement.

In 1984 CPSRC evolved into the Massachusetts Passenger Safety Program (MPSP), a comprehensive program focusing on all age groups. New developments since then have been based on data from outcome and/or process evaluations. For example, 1984 statewide observational data on high rates of child safety seat misuse led to the provision of special training sessions and educational materials for parents and service providers. In 1985 observational data on safety belt use and a new mandatory safety belt use law caused the program to focus on teenagers, the elderly, and blue collar workers.

Although the safety belt law was repealed in late 1986, 6 months later the state's child passenger safety law was expanded to cover children up to the age of 12. This has provided a new focus for MPSP's public education efforts, as well as outreach to police departments about enforcement. Thus we see how the ongoing use of outcome and process data enabled this program to modify its goals, objectives, and interventions in order to address the issue of motor vehicle safety more effectively.[10(p95)]

### Step 14: Communicate the Findings, Both Positive and Negative, in a Timely Manner

Communication should be directed toward a wide range of key audiences, such as funders, local and state legislators, the media, health professionals, academics, and the public. Remember that evaluation is intended to identify strengths as well as weaknesses. Showcase your efforts and celebrate early successes. Translate the findings into nontechnical terms.

### Step 15: Continue the Evaluation Process

Evaluation should not be a one-shot process. It should be part of the program cycle and involve the continual generation of information and data to make decisions, modify program activities, and reassess effectiveness. Improvement requires measurement. You need to keep asking questions to improve and maintain the quality and success of a program.

## CONSTRAINTS ON "PERFECT" EVALUATION

Despite the best intentions and commitment, you will encounter a number of constraints on evaluation.[1] We have already referred repeatedly to the problem of limited resources. Another major constraint on evaluation can be unrealistic expectations. As one commentator has posed it, "Can you really expect a usually brief, relatively inexpensive public health intervention to produce medium or large effects?"[11(pp1075–1076)] In the for-profit field, manufacturers spend billions of dollars on advertising to increase product sales and a 1% to 4% sales increase is deemed a huge success. Yet an injury prevention program that increases a behavior by such a percentage might be considered a failure.

There are several other factors that add to the complexity of evaluation. These include sample size, program exposure, contamination, the outcome measures used, attenuation of effect, and duration of the program and of the evaluation.

### Size of the Sample

The size of the sample used for evaluation affects not only the number of incidents you are likely to encounter, it also affects your ability to draw statistical conclusions—what is often referred to as the power of the design or test. A meaningful, albeit small, change in injury rates or other outcomes may go undetected because of insufficient sample size. Especially for practitioners working in a small community or setting, there will be few injuries in the target population and consequently it may be impossible to show a reduction in injury rates. Rarely are we given the resources to develop a program that will reach a large enough population to make small—or even medium—effects detectable. The use of intermediate measures, as discussed earlier, may help to overcome some of this limitation.

## Amount of Exposure

The amount and intensity of exposure to an intervention program will vary considerably according to program site, community, fidelity of implementation, and program duration. In an injury prevention program carried out in Massachusetts in the early 1980s, the overall population in nine communities receiving a set of childhood injury intervention programs was approximately 140,000, of which 42,500 were children. Of these, 12,000 were within the targeted age group of 5 years and under. Over a 20-month period, only 25% to 30% of households with children were exposed to an intervention. Of these households, a smaller percentage (5%) received a home visit considered to be a high-intensity exposure, a larger percentage (21%) received counseling by a pediatrician during a routine office visit, and a moderate percentage (10%) received the same messages through meetings for parents held at libraries, schools, and day care centers. The program elements considered to be most powerful reached the fewest people. Telephone surveys and other process measures aimed at evaluating participation were critical in helping the program director understand the reasons for lack of dramatic reductions in injury outcome.[1]

## Contamination in Comparison Settings

No matter how carefully you may pick a comparison or control group for a population in a community or a school classroom, the comparison site may still be exposed to injury prevention activities you cannot control. In the Massachusetts study just described, the initiation of specific injury prevention activities at the program sites occurred at the same time as spontaneous injury activities in the comparison sites. The media promoted childhood safety, as did literature aimed at the pediatric community; schools introduced safety curricula into their health education programs; the Massachusetts legislature debated a highly publicized child auto safety seat bill; and a boy scout troop chose community child safety as the focus of badge activities. These simultaneous injury prevention efforts were de-tected through process evaluations and a telephone survey. It is all but impossible to eliminate such unplanned exposures that introduce an element of contamination into any comparison measures undertaken for purposes of evaluation.

## Selection of an Outcome Measure

Matching the injury prevention program to be implemented with an appropriate outcome indicator is not easy. Stringent outcome measures lower the chance of showing success. Although we may want to ultimately reduce morbidity and mortality, the most appropriate outcome measure for a program will usually be a measure of behavior, not a measure of injury. But as one commentator asks, is it fair to view an individual who reduces a high-risk behavior from 100 to 10 as no more of a success than someone who reduces such acts from one to none?[11] Outcome measures must be sensitive to the purpose of the program. What is it you want to measure? Be specific. For example, what do you want a health care professional to do following attendance at training about youth suicide? Talk to parents of young children and adolescents about increased risk where there is access to firearms? Discuss proper storage of firearms? Discuss barriers to removing firearms from the home? How will you measure these? Before you think about measurement, you may need to take a step back and use focus groups to identify the barriers to getting participants such as health care professionals to do what you would like them to do. Select some key measures that reflect the relative emphasis on corresponding program objectives. You may even want to obtain outside consultation to define possible outcome measures.

## Attenuation of Effect

An education program may succeed in increasing knowledge, but its effect on behavior—and on injury rates—will usually attenuate over time. It is therefore important to consider and measure each of the several factors that connect educating people regarding injury and the actual reduction in injuries. Evaluation at each step of the knowledge-to-behavior process will be crucial for understanding why injury prevention behaviors do or do not get adopted. For example, in a burn prevention intervention, it was one thing to expose people to the message "hot tap water can cause a severe scald burn," but quite another for people to remember the message and behave differently, modifying their daily routine (testing the tap water with a thermometer before bathing a young child), and reacting instantly in an emergency to prevent a burn injury or reduce its severity (immediately putting cold water on a burn).[12] Also, it is necessary to view the target population as distinct groups—innovators, early adopters, the middle majority, the laggards, and the refusers or hard to reach. Each will vary in their adoption of new behaviors. And each may require different methods and messages in an education program.[13]

Once you realize that this attenuation of effect process is to be expected, you can set up your evaluation program to track its progress, measuring results at each level. Most important, you will not have unrealistic expectations dashed as you see the results narrow downward along the reverse pyramid of attenuation of results effect.

### Duration of the Program

The length of time a program is in place has a great deal to do with its success—and with the success of the evaluation process. There must be enough time for the benefits of changed knowledge and behaviors to manifest themselves to show an effect. It is not clear how long is long enough. A review of seven community-based injury prevention programs with durations of 3 to 24 months concluded that "given the scope and complexity of what many programs may be expected to achieve in terms of changes in knowledge, behavior, environment, and ultimately injury rates, such time frames are clearly inadequate."[2] Evaluation may require a longer follow-up than the traditional amount of one to three years provided by most program and research funders.[14]

## CONCLUSION

Evaluation is a critical part of successful intervention efforts. Evaluation helps guide, correct, and document interventions, steering these efforts closer to the ideal. It is a mistake to view evaluation as simply an academic exercise or as something only academics can do; rather, it is a basic tool of effective management and, as such, should become familiar to all injury prevention practitioners. The following short "tips" may help incorporate evaluation into your injury prevention activities:

- Establish some level of evaluation.
- Allocate somewhere between 10% and 20% of your budget for evaluation.
- Build some form of evaluation into your program planning—at the initiation stage, not after the fact.
- Be realistic in setting goals and objectives. Do not promise unrealistic outcomes you cannot deliver in the specified time period.
- Choose outcome measures that best suit your needs and resources.
- Make sure that objectives are quantifiable, so that you can measure your success.
- Perform multilevel evaluation (i.e., some combination of formative, process, and outcome evaluation).
- Collect the best possible information under real world circumstances.
- Keep asking questions and refining your program. Evaluation should not be a one-time occurrence.
- Identify multiple change points that occur in what seems to be a simple intervention. Ask for help from others in brainstorming possible change points.
- Remember that an epidemiologist is not the same as an evaluation specialist. There is much more to evaluation than outcome measures such as morbidity and mortality.
- Consider that the evaluation of a community intervention program of two or three years' duration requires more than an injury surveillance system, it requires an individual who can oversee, push, monitor, and interpret the evaluation, someone who realizes it is their job to ascertain whether or not the intervention is working.
- Make sure your evaluator interfaces with community needs and is understood by the target audience.
- Consider hiring an outside evaluation consultant, but realize that you can accomplish much in the way of helpful evaluation on your own. Stretch your resources by collaborating with a local community college or university to conduct community surveys or observation studies as part of a class project.

---

**NOTES**

1. Guyer B, Gallagher SS, Chang BH, Azzara CV, Cupples LA, Colton T. Prevention of childhood injuries: Evaluation of the Statewide Childhood Injury Prevention Program (SCIPP). *Am J Public Health.* 1989;79:1521–1527.

2. Gielen AC, Collins B. Community-based interventions for injury prevention. *Fam Community Health.* 1993;15:1–11.

3. DiGuiseppi CG, Rivara FP, Koepsell, TD, Polissar L. Bicycle helmet use by children: Evaluation of a community-wide helmet campaign. *JAMA.* 1989;262:2256–2261.

4. Rodgers LW, Bergman AB, Rivara FP. Promoting bicycle helmets to children: A campaign that worked. *J Musculoskeletal Med.* 1991;8:64–77.

5. Rivara FP, Thompson DC, Thompson RS, et al. The Seattle children's bicycle helmet campaign: Changes in helmet use and head injury admissions. *Pediatrics.* 1994; 93:567–569.

6. Powell KE, Dahlberg LL, Friday J, et al. Prevention of youth violence: Rationale and characteristics of 15 evaluation projects. *Am J Prev Med.* 1996;12:3–12.

7. Harrington C, Gallagher SS, Burgess LL, Guyer B. *Injury Prevention Programs in State Health Departments—A National Survey.* Boston: Childhood Injury Prevention Resource Center, Harvard School of Public Health; 1988.

8. Kreuger RA. *Focus Groups: A Practical Guide for Applied Research.* Beverly Hills, CA: Sage Publications Inc; 1988.

9. Brink S, Gallagher SS. Working paper on evaluating injury prevention programs. Children's Safety Network, 1992. Derived from Green LW, Lewis FM. *Measurement and Evaluation in Health Education and Health Promotion.* Palo Alto, CA: Mayfield Publishing Co; 1986.

10. National Committee for Injury Prevention and Control. *Injury Prevention: Meeting the Challenge.* New York: Oxford University Press (Published as a supplement to the *Am J Prev Med.* 1989;5:95).

11. Fishbein M. Editorial: Great expectations, or do we ask too much from community-level interventions? *Am J Public Health.* 1996;86:1075–1076.

12. McLoughlin E, Vince CJ, Lee AM, Crawford JD. Project Burn Prevention: Outcome and implications. *Am J Public Health.* 1982;72:241–247.

13. Rogers E. *Diffusion of Innovations.* 3rd ed. New York: Free Press; 1983.

14. Lescohier I, Gallagher SS, Guyer B. Not by accident. *Issues Sci Tech.* 1990;6:35–42.

# An Evaluation Case Study

The Protecting Young Workers Project (PYWP) is a community-based injury prevention program in Brockton, Massachusetts. It is an ongoing, multiyear project. The program had a modest amount of start-up funding. The target city was chosen because of its rate of injuries to teen workers and because of an existing network of agencies collaborating to implement a school-to-career program. There were three primary target groups: teens, parents, and employers.

Evaluation of the program combined several methods, including qualitative information obtained through administrative forms and site visits and some quantitative before-and-after measurements. Random assignments and use of controls were not deemed feasible. The evaluation component required approximately 25% of the overall program budget and included an extensive pre- and postintervention survey of high school students, a small subcontract with a university to analyze the results, focus groups with teens, parents, and employers to assist in the design of the program and materials development, surveys of parents and health care providers, process measures, and outcome measures. The evaluation specialist was involved in the design of the program at its inception, was a primary writer of the proposal that funded the project, oversaw the community needs assessment, was an active participant in community advisory board meetings, and spent a considerable amount of time in the community. A new project activities database was designed to capture much of the information for the process evaluation.

The ultimate project goals were (1) reduction of workplace injuries to teens aged 14 to 17 and (2) preparation of young workers to become lifelong advocates for safe and healthful workplaces. It was recognized early on that given the available resources and time frame, it would be unrealistic to use reduction in injuries as the outcome measure. Also, it was believed that the introduction of the program would actually improve the hospital reporting of such injuries and increase the rate. Raising awareness is an essential first step toward reaching the ultimate goals. To reflect this, the goals were redefined: Enhance the safety of teen workers by developing a model community-based program that will (1) increase the knowledge of teens, parents, and employers about safety risks in the workplace, and (2) stimulate community organizations to modify existing practices and programs to include teen worker safety issues.

Activities developed for the program included exercises that integrate health and safety information within a variety of high school classes; training for employers participating as school-to-work mentors; inclusion of teen worker safety as an aspect of a teen helpline; training of teachers, peer leaders, helpline staff, and restaurant supervisors; development of a trigger video and accompanying curriculum guide; development of teen, parent, and employer informational materials; training of school-to-work mentor staff; regular meetings of a community advisory board comprised of 35 agencies; inclusion of sections on health and safety within community resource guides; development of criteria for a "best practices" award for employers; and development of learning activities for teens including hazard mapping, role-playing to resolve workplace problems, and a fast-paced prevention strategies game for teams of students.

To achieve these goals, objectives were developed at a variety or levels using a six-tiered model that integrates individual and environmental change. Process and outcome measures and data collection tools were developed for *each* of the program objectives. The primary outcome proxy measures were to be collected via pre- and postproject student surveys and work permit applications. Pre- and postproject community telephone surveys were not deemed feasible because of the expense and because the program staff did not believe that exposure to the intervention activities on a communitywide basis during the one full year of implementation of the program would be sufficient to create large-scale change.

What follows are the six levels of program objectives for the PYWP and their associated evaluation factors.

## LEVEL 1: STRENGTHEN INDIVIDUAL KNOWLEDGE (ONE-ON-ONE INSTRUCTION)

*Objectives*: To increase the knowledge of teens ages14 to 17 about child labor laws, hazards at work, and actions that can be taken to protect oneself by September 1997 and to increase the number of actions taken by teens to protect themselves while working between Spring 1996 and Spring 1997.

*Process measures of exposure:*
- the number of high school classes incorporating health and safety information (teacher reports)
- the number of students receiving targeted information in class (teacher reports)
- the number of teens participating in peer-led workshops (peer leader reports)
- the number of students receiving teen work packets

*Outcome measures:*
- changes in knowledge and attitudes about risks at work, changes in knowledge, attitudes, and compliance with child labor laws, changes in response to hazards encountered on the job (comparison of responses to student survey administered at school at beginning and end of the project)
- changes in the number of calls by teenagers to the teen helpline (teen helpline phone contact forms)
- changes in the number of students obtaining a work permit between Spring 1996 and Spring 1997 (school records)

*Objective*: To increase parental awareness of child labor laws, potential hazards to teen workers, and their role in protecting their child's health and safety at work by September 1997.

*Process measure:*
- the number of teen worker packets distributed to parents of high school students (activities database)

*Outcome measures:*
- changes in the number of parent calls received by the teen helpline (teen helpline phone contact forms)
- self-report by parents of receipt of parent brochure, what they learned, whether they talked with their teen about hazards at work, and what issues were discussed (written responses to parent survey)

*Objective*: To increase employer's knowledge of child labor laws, risks to teen workers, and prevention strategies.

*Process measure:*
- the number of employers who attend School-to-Work Mentor Trainings and Public/Private Partners Trainings (trainer reports of number of trainings offered and number of employers participating)

*Outcome measures:*
- changes in knowledge of participants in School-to-Work Mentor and Public/Private Partners Trainings (comparison of pre- and postproject responses to employer survey administered in class)
- changes in knowledge, hazards, and strategies identified on-site (comparison of pre- and postproject walkthroughs in participating restaurants by project staff; to be done with additional funding by the state Department of Industrial Accidents)

## LEVEL 2: PROMOTING COMMUNITY EDUCATION (POSTERS, NEWSPAPERS, COMMUNITY MEDIA OUTLETS)

*Objective*: To increase the awareness of health and safety at work, child labor laws, and where to go for help among the target audience and the broader community members by September 1997.

*Process measures:*
- number of posters put up (staff counts for activities database)
- number of teen helpline resource guides disseminated (teen helpline records)
- number of "Are You a Working Teen" brochures disseminated in Brockton (staff counts for activities database)
- number of newspaper articles on the project or the topic of teen worker safety (activities database)

- number of public service announcements on local media—radio and cable television (activities database)
- numbers of articles on the project or the topic of teen worker safety appearing in the newsletters of community groups (activities database)

*Outcome measure:*
- number of callers to the teen helpline who became aware of the issue, called the helpline, and reported seeing the poster, resource guide, brochure, media (teen helpline telephone contact forms)

## LEVEL 3: EDUCATING PROVIDERS (TRAINING TEACHERS, HEALTH CARE PROVIDERS, PEER LEADERS, COMMUNITY ADVISORY BOARD PARTICIPANTS)

*Objectives*: To increase the knowledge of occupational hazards to teens and prevention strategies on the part of professionals and others who teach and counsel teens by September 1997, and to increase the number of professionals who provide health and safety information to teens.

*Process measures:*
- number of peer leaders trained and the number of hours of training (activities database)
- number of teachers in high school trained and the number of hours of training (activities database)
- number of staff of the MY Turn program for high-risk youth trained and the number of hours of training
- number of teen helpline information and referral staff trained
- number of Brockton health care providers who receive packet on occupational health and safety of teen workers (Massachusetts Department of Public Health [MDPH] intern's records)

*Outcome measures:*
- number of trainings delivered by the teen helpline peer leaders (activities database)
- number of classes delivered by teachers and by the MY Turn staff (activities database)
- number of times community providers give unsolicited suggestions for outreach to project staff (activities database)

- changes in health care provider practices such as counseling teen patients and their parents, distributing brochures, showing videos (comparison of pre- and postproject provider survey being conducted by MDPH intern in both the target community and a comparison community)

## LEVEL 4: FOSTERING COALITIONS AND NETWORKS (SCHOOL-TO-WORK PARTNERSHIP, COMMUNITY ADVISORY BOARD)

*Objective*: To develop informal linkages among community agencies and other groups around the issue of health and safety for working teens by January 1996.

*Process measures:*
- number and types of agencies joining the community advisory board (activities database)
- number of coalition meetings and number of participants at each (activities database)
- number of meetings between project staff and coalition members (activities database)

*Outcome measures:*
- number of subcommittees formed, especially related to employer outreach (activities database)
- number of connections made and working relationships developed among community agencies (survey of advisory board members)
- provision of workplace health and safety materials to other towns in the partnership (report from executive director)

## LEVEL 5: CHANGING ORGANIZATIONAL PRACTICES (AGENCIES, ORGANIZATIONS, AND BUSINESSES)

*Objective*: To integrate the promotion of health and safety for working teens into the ongoing practices of community agencies, the School-to-Work Local Partnership, and the Community Health Network Area (CHNA) by December 1996.

*Process measures:*
- number of meetings with agencies to discuss possible changes in practice (activities database)
- number and type of contacts with agencies to provide materials, training, and other consultation (activities database)
- number of contacts with two community hospitals to encourage reporting of teen occupational injury data (activities database)

*Outcome measures:*
- inclusion of workplace health and safety information in school-to-work curricula developed by the partnership (activities database)
- inclusion of occupational health and safety information in school-to-work mentor training developed by the partnership (report from executive director)
- examination of teen occupational health and safety data on an annual basis by the CHNA (MDPH records)
- comparison of activities reported by organizations in year 1 and year 2 of the project (Community Group Interview Form)
- changes in practices reported by members of advisory board (survey)
- decisions by community organizations to take the lead in training a target group, such as youth or employers (activities database)
- changes in reporting of teen occupational injury data by hospitals (MDPH records)

*Objective*: To integrate the promotion of health and safety for working teens into ongoing practices of employers of youth by September 1997.

*Process measure:*
- number of meetings held with employers to describe model "Best Practices" Employer Program

*Outcome measures:*
- number of employers agreeing to participate in model program
- number of best practices added by employers
- number of requests for health and safety walkthroughs and Occupational Safety and Health Administration (OSHA) consultations (activities database, OSHA records)
- number of "best practices" awards given out

*Objective*: To integrate health and safety for teen workers into programs at the Brockton high school.

*Process measures:*
- number and content of meetings with department chairs to discuss current courses and integration of health and safety for teen workers into the existing curricula (activities database)
- number and content of contacts with job placement staff to discuss ways they can promote health and safety for teen workers (activities database)
- number and content of contacts with work permit office staff to discuss the work permit process and ways to integrate health and safety information when the permit is given out (activities database)
- number of contacts with other school personnel regarding integrating occupational health and safety in other generic activities at the school (activities database)

*Outcome measures:*
- changes in school curriculum in years 2 and 3 (school reports)
- changes in practices of job placement office, inclusion of display of posters and dissemination of informational packets (activities database)
- changes in practices of work permit office, inclusion of display of posters and dissemination of informational packets (activities database)
- inclusion of occupational health and safety information in other school programs (activities database)

## LEVEL 6: DEVELOPING AND ENFORCING POLICY AND LEGISLATION (THE WORK PERMIT SYSTEM)

*Objective*: To influence local and state initiatives to reform the work permit system for teens and the child labor laws.

*Process measures:*
- number and content of meetings between advisory board and attorney general's State Task Force on Reform of Child Labor Laws (activities database)

- number of advisory board members writing letters and providing other input to the State Task Force (activities database)
- number of advisory board members providing input to the school system on changes needed in record keeping for work permits (activities database)

*Outcome measures:*
- changes made to work permit record keeping system (survey)
- changes in child labor laws and work permit system that relate to input from the advisory board (report from state-level task force chaired by project principal investigator)

# CHAPTER 14

# Barriers to Injury Prevention

"The risk of [injury] is one of the clearest instances of health inequality in our society."

Allison Quick, *Unequal Risks*, 1991

## WHAT THIS CHAPTER IS ABOUT

The previous chapters have emphasized three primary points: (1) injury is a major public health problem, (2) injury is highly preventable, and (3) governmental injury prevention programs are an essential part of successfully reducing injury in America. But if we know so much about how to reduce the deadly toll of injury, why are current injury prevention programs so limited relative to the magnitude of the problem? Here is where practical realities rear their ugly heads.

Why don't policy makers jump at the opportunity to save lives—and money—by implementing proven programs? Why do injury prevention advocates often feel like their messages are falling on deaf ears? What can be done to overcome organizational and political barriers to injury prevention? Why are injury prevention initiatives so politically sensitive? And, most important, how can one most effectively navigate through organizational, political, and other practical realities to implement meaningful injury prevention programs?

This chapter will seek to illuminate the broader, real world context within which injury prevention efforts exist. We will discuss the hard and constraining barriers of the actual world, the world of limited funding, organizational difficulties, turf battles, limited scientific and policy information, and economic and political constraints. We wish to emphasize how important the public policy arena is for injury prevention and will attempt to make it understandable.

## INTRODUCTION

From technical as well as theoretical perspectives, injury is highly preventable. And yet injury prevention efforts have limited support. Why is this so? Even proven and cost-effective successes are constantly under assault, as evidenced by periodic attempts—led by the National Rifle Association—to abolish the Centers for Disease Control and Prevention's (CDC) National Center for Injury Prevention and Control. No matter how optimal the approach, all efforts to reduce injury are limited by the fact that they take place within the real world, not the safe confines of a textbook. In an ideal world the identification of an injury problem would logically be followed by the implementation of the most effective intervention program. But we do not live in an ideal world.

Successful injury prevention intervention requires more than simply alerting policy makers to key problems and promising solutions. There are a variety of barriers to the rational implementation of prevention programs. Even the most able program administrator cannot repeal the laws of physics, change the economic system, or transform the political world into something it is not. Effective policy input on injury problems requires an understanding and consideration of the financial, organizational and political context within which solutions must be undertaken, as well as a willingness to make compromises. Failure to do so means wasting time in trying to change the unchangeable or in missing the opportunity to realistically tailor strategies that may be viable and successful.

The following pages, then, will explore

- funding limitations
- organizational difficulties
- turf battles
- scientific and policy analysis and data
- economic and political aspects of injury prevention
- advocacy for injury prevention

## FUNDING LIMITATIONS

As was discussed in Chapter 11, funding is a central problem. Health departments have limited resources available to them and most of those resources are already committed to well-established public health programs with existing staff, a support network, a public image, and the inertia of the status quo—all favoring their continuation against the "threat" of a redirection of funds to a new program initiative, such as injury prevention.

All reviews of the state of injury prevention in America have identified inadequate funding as a critical barrier. A review of the Statewide Childhood Injury Prevention Program in Massachusetts listed among the barriers to injury prevention efforts a "lack of both private and public resources in terms of informational sources and start-up funds."[1] And a conference on Barriers to Injury Control sponsored by the CDC and held at the Johns Hopkins University concluded that: "Resources must be redirected to injury control."[2(p9)] By this the conference participants explained that they meant that

- The cost of injury control is assumed to be great. This assumption is often not valid, but it still serves as a barrier in the competition for public resources.
- Public and private resources must be reallocated toward injury prevention.
- Better ways to compare the injury problem to other public health problems are needed.
- Public health agencies have not had the time, data, interest, training, and legislative support to deal effectively with injury control.[2]

So how do injury prevention advocates achieve a redirection of resources to injury prevention programs? This is obviously a case-by-case task, but some general advice can be offered.

- Emphasize the cost efficiency of such interventions. Prevention is often cheaper than the medical and rehabilitative care, lost productivity, and other costs resulting from injury.[3] (Injury prevention is cost-efficient at all levels. For the individual, the relatively small amounts spent on prevention are a minuscule fraction of the costs in medical care, rehabilitation, and lost wages that would accompany a serious injury. For health care providers, such as health maintenance organizations and hospitals, injuries are expensive because risk takers—such as unrestrained motor vehicle occupants—are more likely to be uninsured.[4] And for society as a whole, as reflected in social service support for the injured and loss of productivity, injury is especially costly.)

- Compare the cost-benefit ratio to that of other health problems and other areas of public expenditure, demonstrating that relative to the problem very little is currently spent on injury prevention.
- Focus particularly on the needs of children.
- Remember the oft-noted fact that society can have any level of good health and injury avoidance it is willing to publicly pay for.

## ORGANIZATIONAL DIFFICULTIES

As with any new endeavor within a bureaucratic framework, injury prevention faces a variety of organizational hurdles beyond the basic lack of funding. To begin with, injury prevention has not generally been recognized as a distinct field of endeavor and therefore has not had an established model that could serve as a standard organizational guide for new programs. Nor has injury prevention developed as a profession to the point that assigning organizational responsibility for injury programs to someone with no background in the area would seem odd or inappropriate. This means new programs have little to draw on in terms of either an organizational template or credentialed staff. Nor do they have much in the way of an existing infrastructure tailored to the needs of injury prevention programs.

These organizational constraints are further complicated by the historical pattern of injury prevention, which has been one of dealing with different aspects of the same overall pattern under different governmental agencies. Thus, for example, occupational injuries are within the purview of departments of labor, and motor vehicle injuries are within the purview of departments of transportation, even though the leading cause of occupational deaths is motor vehicle injury. To those untrained in the field, the multiple dimensions of the challenge posed by injury make the overall set of injury problems seem much more diverse than is really the case.

Perhaps the best way to illuminate some organizational deficiencies that can plague agency injury prevention programs is to look at those factors that characterize successful health department programs of any type, characteristics that, unfortunately, tend to be weak or missing in injury prevention programs. In a successful program

- Key members of the leadership within the agency are involved in program planning.

- There is a comprehensive program plan.
- The program is integrated with other health department programs and there is effective communication with other programs within the health department.
- There is an established practitioner training effort.
- Cooperative arrangements have been developed with community groups and organizations.
- There is an ongoing program evaluation system in place.

If any of these organizational components are lacking, it will be extremely difficult to initiate injury prevention programs, no matter how clear the need. Appendix 14 A presents a fuller listing of some of the organizational factors that can act as barriers to injury prevention programs.

## TURF BATTLES

Turf battles refer to situations in which the programmatic prevention goal may be clear and agreed on but the question of who is responsible for implementation is at issue. Injury prevention has not been generally recognized as a technical field or area of expertise, which makes it much more likely that a variety of agencies and skill areas will claim expertise and ownership of injury issues. It also makes it less likely that public health officials can claim the mantle of primary responsibility and expertise in the way they might regarding vaccination advice or outbreaks of foodborne diseases.

There are no inevitable or insurmountable turf problems. If handled well, the involvement of many agencies in dealing with an injury problem can be positive and synergistic. But if handled poorly, turf battles can become political squabbles in which everyone loses—especially the public. A wide spectrum of public and private agencies may be involved with injury prevention efforts, ranging from those that clearly have injury prevention as a mandate and view themselves as being involved in injury prevention (such as a public health agency), to those that deal with the aftermath of injury (acute care, rehabilitation, and law enforcement), to those for whom injury prevention is a tangential, perhaps unconscious, concern (such as courts and judges or municipal departments of public works and sanitation).

## SCIENTIFIC AND POLICY ANALYSIS AND DATA: MYTHS VERSUS REALITY

There is a body of knowledge to apply to injury prevention. Some of it is purely scientific, such as the epidemiology of injury and biomechanics, and some is policy oriented, such as studies of how policy makers perceive injury risk. In an ideal world this body of knowledge would lead us toward identifying and implementing those injury prevention interventions most likely to reduce the number or severity of injuries. But often there are important weaknesses in how data are acquired and used. The result can be distortions in knowledge that influence what is done or not done to deal with injury issues. Why do such distortions exist? In the area of injury prevention science, the four main factors are

1. lack of affordable, ongoing surveillance
2. gaps in epidemiological data
3. gaps in information regarding the efficacy of interventions
4. lack of access to current research

In the area of injury prevention policy analysis, the four main factors are

1. lack of agreement on appropriate policy analysis tools
2. lack of policy analysis studies
3. lack of evaluation, during implementation, and of outcomes
4. lack of understanding of the scientific process and the ambiguities of science

These deficiencies are not only unfortunate in themselves, but they also have the effect of making it much more difficult to respond to many of the negative myths that impede injury prevention programs. These include

- Myth #1: Injury interventions don't work; they aren't feasible.
- Myth #2: Injury interventions cost too much; they are economically inefficient.
- Myth #3: Individual behavior and uncontrollable, random events lie at the heart of most injuries.

Not only the general public, but key decision makers as well, can harbor these myths, which affects their support (or lack of it) for injury prevention programs. To overcome this problem, we need to increase our informational arsenal to be able to effectively respond to misperceptions. This in itself takes money, money to undertake the epidemiological studies and policy analyses to evaluate the effectiveness of various intervention programs.

Injury prevention interventions require policy choices, which in turn requires policy studies to support and guide the policy choices and to defend against challenges to proposed and existing intervention programs. Such studies may draw on cost-benefit and cost-effectiveness analysis, decision analysis, risk analysis, after-the-fact program evaluation, and the like. It is important the injury prevention practitioners are familiar with these various analytical approaches. And as discussed later in this chapter, it is also important that injury prevention practitioners know how to effectively frame and communicate the results of their studies to the public, the media, and policy makers in ways that will ensure maximum impact.

## ECONOMIC AND POLITICAL ASPECTS OF INJURY PREVENTION

Injury and injury prevention are extremely political, even more so than is the case with disease and disease prevention. This point should not be overstated, since tobacco-caused illness, chemical carcinogens, AIDS, and other important disease areas can also be quite political. But the fact is that injury prevention can only be properly understood within a political, economic, and sociohistorical framework. A full explication of this framework is beyond the scope of this book. Such a discussion would require exploring the various components of one's political-economic world view: Where does social control (i.e., power) lie in our society? Do we have a pluralistic, elitist, or class system? These questions lie behind the discussion in this chapter, but they will not themselves be explored. Each requires its own volumes, not merely a lone chapter in one book.

To understand any social issue, it is necessary to understand who pays for and who benefits from any change in the status quo, and who has the power to control the situation. Injury is very costly for our society. As discussed in Chapter 1, the estimated annual cost of injury and its consequences for the United States currently ranges from $224 to $325 billion. Because of these negative cost consequences, injury prevention has the potential to benefit society and be cost-effective for government. Certainly the individuals who escape injury or who suffer less severe consequences from injury events benefit from injury prevention programs. So does society as a whole, both in terms of an enhanced community in which individuals are less likely to experience the negative consequences of injury and in terms of economic savings. From government's perspective, the same logic would seem to apply. As the National SAFE KIDS Campaign has pointed out:

> Injury prevention is health care—the best kind—that is proven to save money and prevent suffering. Just as childhood immunizations prevent costly and deadly diseases, investments in childhood injury prevention can save the health care system billions of dollars.

> Injury prevention saves money because it employs inexpensive, low-tech interventions to avoid the most costly types of care—emergency room treatment and hospitalization.[5]

For example, Ted Miller and colleagues have calculated that for children ages 0 to 4, every dollar spent on child safety seats saves $33, including $2 in medical costs, $6 in future earnings, and $25 in avoided pain, suffering, and lost quality of life.[6] For children ages 4 to 15, every dollar spent on bicycle helmets saves $25 to $31, including $2 in medical costs, $6 to $7.50 in future earnings, and $17 to $21.50 in avoided pain, suffering, and lost quality of life.[7]

As to who pays for injury prevention, however, the question is more complicated than simply who bears the direct costs of specific intervention programs. As has been suggested in previous chapters, the most effective injury prevention efforts are those that affect the very environment in which injury occurs. Most injury is the result of human-created environments, and what women and men design and create they can presumably redesign and re-create for greater safety. But environmental modifications, such as the Motor Vehicle Safety Standards, affect major economic interests within the society and may not be cost-effective from industry's perspective alone. These federally mandated standards may contribute to increased prices for automobiles, which may reduce the demand for new cars, reduce travel and the economic gain generated by such travel, and serve as the incentive for communities to switch to other forms of transportation that may be safer modes—mass transit—or less safe modes—motorcycles.[8]

Thus injury prevention efforts that may seem almost self-evidently positive from a public health perspective may engender powerful opposition.

And if this opposition comes from powerful interests, promising injury prevention ideas will often be delayed or derailed. Note, for example, the 20 years of resistance to airbags by the automotive industry (see Exhibit 14–1), resistance motivated by fear of competitive disadvantage, resistance for which the nation is still paying a price because some automakers have complied with the airbag requirement by using inadequate technology that injures as well as protects. And this is just one example of money triumphing over safety. The firearms industry has successfully blocked almost all efforts to reduce gun violence by regulating guns. Alcohol taxes have risen insignificantly and have not kept up with inflation, despite the well-known price sensitivity of alcohol and the prominent role of alcohol in both unintentional and intentional injury.

To understand the political economy of injury prevention, it is necessary to understand that there are two basic approaches to dealing with societal problems such as injury. Rely on the market to reduce injuries or make use of government and regulation to reduce injuries.

## The Market Approach

According to neoclassical economics, the marketplace within which goods and services are exchanged is the best mechanism for maximizing social goals. As applied to injury, this view suggests that consumers will make calculations regarding how much safety they want and how much they are willing to pay for it. Manufacturers who do not correctly respond to consumer demand, either by marketing products that are too unsafe or by marketing products for which safety comes at too high a price, will lose out to those manufacturers who provide the combination of safety and cost that most consumers want. In addition, several markets can exist simultaneously, allowing consumers who are willing to pay more for safer products to satisfy their desires alongside those consumers who are willing to trade away enhanced safety for lower prices. This approach, it is argued, is better than a heavy-handed, "one-size-fits-all" governmental regulation approach.

An important part of the market approach is that consumers have adequate information to make cost versus safety tradeoffs and that manufacturers be held accountable for misleading consumers. The latter has generally meant that consumers can recover damages for injuries resulting from a manufacturer's failure to warn about product hazards it knew about but

**Exhibit 14–1** "The Regulatory Equivalent of War"

---

The first airbag was patented in 1952. In 1966 Congress enacted the National Traffic and Motor Vehicle Safety Act, authorizing the Department of Transportation to propound occupant protection regulations, such as requiring seatbelts and/or airbags. In 1969 the Department proposed a passive restraint requirement. In 1971 Chrysler and Ford filed lawsuits challenging the requirement, while Henry Ford II and Lee Iacocca met secretly with President Nixon to win a delay in implementing the requirement. After additional delays, new regulations, rescission of those regulations, and a U.S. Supreme Court decision declaring the rescission arbitrary and capricious and thus unconstitutional, airbags did not begin to become available in significant numbers until the 1990s. In ruling on the airbag issue, the Supreme Court observed that "For nearly a decade, the automobile industry waged the regulatory equivalent of war against the airbag and lost—the inflatable restraint was proven sufficiently effective."[a]

[a]*Motor Vehicle Manufacturers Association v. State Farm Mutual Automobile Insurance Company*, 463 U.S. 29, 1983.

---

hid from the consumer, such as a motor vehicle likely to overturn or have its gas tank rupture in low-speed collisions or highchairs that are unsafe because they lack safety straps.

## Government Regulation

Advocates of governmental approaches to injury prevention argue that the marketplace does not and cannot adequately protect the public from injury. In the first place, consumers do not have satisfactory information or the means to discover hidden risks and defects. In the second place, experience has shown that the "choices" are often not really there (for example, safe workplaces, automobile occupant restraint systems, self-stopping power lawnmowers, adequate mass transit, none of which have been provided through the market). Third, reliance on the market means only those with sufficient wealth can afford safety: Many people buy and drive smaller cars rather than safer, larger, and heavier vehicles because the latter are simply not affordable to them. Fourth, the deterrent effect of lawsuits against harmful products is diminishing as it becomes harder to bring such lawsuits due to legislative restrictions. These restrictions have been imposed despite the fact that only a fraction of injuries lead to claims—let alone awards—and that most of the lawsuits "clogging" the courts are contract and divorce disputes. Moreover, an increasing number of meritorious lawsuits and settlements are sealed so they cannot serve as a warning to the public regarding defective products. Finally and most important of all, the economic marketplace has functioned for hundreds of years without producing the injury reducing results its advocates tout. Revealingly, the unrestrained free markets fostered by the North American Free Trade Agreement and the General Agreement on Tariffs and Trade seem to have reduced safety by allowing, for example, trucks and truckers from Mexico who would not otherwise meet our safety standards to travel on U.S. highways.

It has been the regulatory efforts of recent decades —the actions of the National Highway Traffic Safety Administration, the Food and Drug Administration, the Consumer Product Safety Commission, the Occupational Safety and Health Administration, and similar federal and state agencies—that have produced reductions in injury rates. For example, using data from the Fatality Analysis Reporting System, Leon Robertson estimated that from 1975 through 1982 the Motor Vehicle Safety Standards saved between 85,000 and 125,000 lives.[9-12] On the other hand, it is in unregulated areas with free markets, such as the poorly regulated area of firearms sales, where injury problems remain the worst. Thus, it is argued, it is only the authority of government that can protect the public from avoidable hazards by enforcing community safety requirements on those with the power to control risks: manufacturers, employers, landlords, and the like. These requirements can take the form of standards, such as local building codes or federal Motor Vehicle Safety Standards, or can be laws affecting how products are used, such as seatbelt use laws or gun control laws.

Reliance on government regulation to protect the public from harm is an approach that goes back at least 4,000 years to the Code of Hammurabi. Even in these ancient times, government regulated the safe construction of houses and the safety of food and medicinal products. Thus the idea that community values should encompass governmental protections of health and well-being are hardly new, nor do they lack in public support.[13] In fact, it is hard to see how threats to the public's safety, such as drunk driving, can be dealt with without governmental involvement in terms of laws, law enforcement, and incentives.

The argument for governmental intervention rather than reliance on markets was made forcefully a century and a half ago in a classic newspaper editorial, which commented on the responsibility of government to protect the public from injury:

> How can the passengers in a steamboat foresee the bursting of a boiler? Or those on a railroad the neglect of a switch? Or those in a street the falling down of a new wall from bad mortar? But engineers and architects can foresee such things, inspectors can provide against them, and executions for murder and fines and imprisonment for manslaughter or mayhem or other injury, will make managers more vigilant. "Oh! But such precautions interfere with free trade; there would be a relapse into the dark ages, when the world is already governed too much. Leave everybody to regulate his own business, and let consumers take care of themselves. Demand and supply will regulate everything, and those who *offer* the best article cheapest will get all the custom." Yes! And after they are blown up, run over and crushed, knocked down dead, or poisoned to death, they will discover they have made a mistake. . . . The proverb says that a burned child will dread the fire. But of what use for safety is its dread, after it has burned to death?[14(p19)]

Governmental policies—or lack of them—are indeed a key determinant of our injury rates. At present, these policies are in retreat as the interests of the poor and disadvantaged take seats in the back of the governmental bus. Corporations are in ascendancy, with enhanced political effectiveness at both the federal and state governmental levels. Because injury prevention issues can present significant threats to these powerful interests, anything more than Band-Aid approaches to the injury problem have an uphill fight. Injury prevention interventions threaten to have serious economic implications, taking resources from the well-to-do and directing them to the advantage of the less well-to-do. For example, a switch to greater governmental support for public transportation could mean fewer people relying on private cars. This would reduce the number of motor vehicle injuries (public transportation being a much safer mode of transport) but it would reduce the sales of motor vehicles.

Opposition to injury prevention is more complex than a matter of the rich and powerful simply not wanting to pay for anything that does not directly contribute to profit. Rather, truly effective injury prevention interventions challenge the structural underpinnings of the status quo. Effective injury prevention means things like worker participation in production decisions, community involvement in land use policy making, equitable distribution of risk, and meaningful compensation for injury harms. These are dangerous ideas; they challenge unbridled free-market competition. Yet they are necessary for long-term, meaningful advances in injury prevention.

An approach wherein consumers simply bear the trauma and costs of injury seems to be increasingly the direction in which corporate-dominated politics is taking the United States. And since injury does not occur randomly within our society, this means that its impact falls most heavily on the poorest, the most disadvantaged, and the politically weakest segments of society. As Allison Quick points out in her book *Unequal Risks* "[p]overty, unemployment, dangerous working conditions, bad housing, overcrowding, and a poor environment all make [injury] more likely. The risk of [injury] is one of the clearest instances of health inequality in our society."[15]

Unequal risk is more than a matter of greed and selfishness. Rather, social policy choices regarding injury prevention are grounded in the structural needs of an economic system that—especially in these days of out-of-control competition—cannot afford the luxury of safety for its entire population. It is necessary to understand this reality in order to deal with it. As Quick points out, the basic goal of injury prevention—maximizing the quality of life for all citizens—cannot be achieved by leaving the task to technical experts who tinker at the margins. The public health practitioner can point to a problem and its possible solution (a role played quite effectively by individuals such as former U.S. Surgeon General Dr. C. Everett Koop and Tennessee child restraint advocate Dr. Robert Sanders). But unless there is an open discussion of underlying economic and political issues—including who benefits and who pays for action or inaction—the policy debate will be artificially and narrowly constrained.

## ADVOCACY

Protecting the public from injury is a just and good cause, but it is not without opposition. This may not be much of a problem when the intervention of choice is education or voluntary standards, but it is a major problem for more intrusive interventions. Such interventions, such as motor vehicle or consumer product safety standards, are governmental mandates. They are most readily established with the support of the public that is being protected. Ideally, getting that support would not be difficult: Safety advocates would make the case that such interventions are justified by the savings in death and injury and the public would be persuaded. But this assumes a free, open, and fair discourse, which is not the playing field that exists in the real world. Public relations manipulation has reached incredible heights, mixing computer and communications technology with psychological insights and considerable amounts of money to create effective political barriers to any interventions that challenge moneyed interests. Safety advocates must therefore be prepared to find themselves faced with well-financed opposition campaigns. Indeed, there are firms that specialize in creating pseudo "grassroots" organizations to block governmental efforts that impinge on their clients.

Does the fact that powerful interests have the means, motive, and opportunity to block injury prevention measures mean that significant progress in injury prevention is impossible? The answer is no, provided that injury prevention advocates appreciate the self-interest and power relationships involved. These realities have important implications for the direction injury prevention advocacy should take. Ignoring economic and political realities means consigning injury prevention to a side arena, where only truncated "safe" options are viable. Thus it is critical for injury prevention that these economic and political issues be widely discussed. A classic model for effectively bringing realities out into the open is Ralph Nader's *Unsafe at Any Speed*, which presented safety data and policy arguments in a popular format, focusing on a particularly egregious injury risk to create political pressures for a larger governmental role in automotive safety.

Advocating for injury prevention is as important as surveillance, epidemiology, and program design. Each is critical to effective prevention; however, this is often a difficult concept for practitioners who are new to what Abraham Bergman—a master of the art—refers to as "political medicine."[16(pvii)] Injury prevention practitioners more often than not lack experience in the public policy and media arenas,[17] but this does not need to be the case. As the examples presented at the end of this chapter illustrate, injury prevention efforts can be effectively pushed through the policy process. To do so, there are several important things to keep in mind.

First, it is necessary to continually highlight for all who will listen both the extent of the injury problem and the costs of that problem, while pointing out who bears those costs (i.e., not only the injured individuals themselves but also the larger society in general, including small businesses and others who might normally support the corporate viewpoint over that of the faceless "consumer").

Second, deal directly with concerns people may have regarding the legal and philosophical appropriateness of using legislation and public programs to reduce injury, rather than leaving things to the individual.

Some additional advocacy tips include

- Start with a focus on children, the group that needs the most protection and for which programmatic support is easiest to achieve.
- Emphasize the fact that success is achievable, that examples of winning injury prevention interventions abound.
- Use data, anecdotes, and statements from respected individuals to highlight the importance of injury prevention efforts.
- Do not lose the opportunity to highlight ways in which preventive measures could have avoided highly publicized tragedies.

How can these messages be conveyed and directed? We are talking here about citizen advocacy and coalition building. Public health agencies cannot be directly involved in efforts to influence legislation, but they can work cooperatively with advocacy groups that can, groups such as Mothers Against Drunk Driving, Parents Against Tired Truckers, National SAFE KIDS Campaign, or Citizens for Reliable and Safe Highways. On any particular injury prevention issue, it is important to develop political alliances, bringing together all those with a stake in injury prevention changes, not only those whose major concern is injury prevention. It also includes citizen groups that focus on other issues. An outstanding example here is the environmental movement, since—to use our recurring example—increased reliance on public transportation would not only lower injury rates but would also contribute significantly to reducing pollution. Also, it is important to maintain alliances so that different citizen coalitions are not turned against one another or find their messages confused by statements from industry-sponsored "astroturf" efforts (i.e., phony grassroots organizations).[18] Some well-known advocacy groups that work on injury prevention issues are listed in Exhibit 14–2.

How can injury prevention specialists, citizen groups, and others concerned with the injury problem have an impact, both on the general public and on key policy makers? A critical factor is the careful use of the media. Unfortunately, as the city editor of the *Boston Globe* told participants at a

**Exhibit 14–2** Selected Injury Prevention Advocacy Groups

- Alcohol Control Network
- Marin Institute for the Prevention of Alcohol and Other Drug Problems
- Center for Science in the Public Interest (alcohol)
- Center for Auto Safety
- Trauma Foundation (burns/fire-safe cigarettes/helmets)
- Coalition to Stop Gun Violence
- Mothers Against Drunk Driving
- Parents Against Tired Truckers
- Citizens for Reliable and Safe Highways
- Advocacy Institute
- National SAFE KIDS Campaign
- American Academy of Pediatrics
- Consumer Federation of America

conference on publicity and advocacy for injury prevention, "It's a shame we don't know each other better." As the conference report noted, "Unlike politicians, injury prevention professionals do not have an ongoing relationship with the media."[17(p2)] Developing alliances with the media is a critical aspect of all advocacy efforts. A valuable guide to how to do this is *Media Advocacy and Public Health: Power for Prevention* by Lawrence Wallack et al.[19] These authors note that:

> Media advocacy reflects a public health approach that explicitly recognizes the importance of the social and political environment and defines health problems as matters of public policy, not just individual behavior.[19]

They lay out an approach that involves the following components, which they explain in some detail.

- *Legitimization* of the problem in terms of root causes rather than personal behaviors.
- *The Importance of Drama* to get the attention of the media.
- *Opportunism* to take advantage of events as they happen.
- *Anticipating the Reaction of Adversaries* and responding pre-emptorily.
- *Creating a Protest Controlled Communication System* to develop strategies in a timely fashion and respond quickly to breaking issues.[19]

Part of proficient advocacy and media efforts is the effective use of injury data. It is important that you relate data to the day-to-day lives of individuals and the needs of the community. Often the use of tables and charts to capture and encapsulate the data will make it more understandable and have more of an impact.

It is also important to cultivate relationships and advocacy on the part of physicians, trauma surgeons, and nurses. These professionals can be very influential in the community. Legislators listen when they present testimony on the "human side" of injury based on their working daily with injured patients. These professionals can form partnerships with injury survivors and their families and become a strong influence on the public debate. Major successes that have made effective use of this approach include brain injury programs, drunk driving laws, and gun control laws.

Finally, the media is most likely to get your information and message across if you can frame things in a way that grabs attention. The AIDS quilt has been extremely effective in dramatizing the magnitude of the human tragedy wrought by this disease. The quilt personalized the AIDS epidemic in a way that mere statistics—even with the best of tables and charts— simply would not. Despite the even greater overall impact of injury, as advocates we have not been nearly as successful in conveying the human tragedy involved.

It would be wrong, however, to characterize advocacy success as merely being a matter of a good sell. More important is how the debate is framed and limited. What is on the table and what is not. It is not just a matter of how much money is to be spent on government programs or what injury prevention laws will be enacted—although, along with health care costs, this is clearly one of the most critical governmental concerns for public health practitioners. No, the question is one of options offered: How extensive an array of interventions will be used to reduce the injury toll? For example, as Quick explains, in Great Britain—as in the United States:

> Road safety efforts have . . . not focused on the basic cause of accidents—traffic—and have instead concentrated on minimizing the number of accidents and injuries caused by such traffic. . . . Current policy gives priority to the mobility of car users, who are predominantly fit, reasonably well-off adults, particularly men. They have been the beneficiaries of considerable public expenditure in road building and maintenance, at the expense

of the mobility of less privileged members of the population. . . . [Yet] those excluded from the benefits of car-based transport suffer disproportionately from the accidents it causes. . . . [Moreover, fewer] people on the streets leads to a reduced feeling of "street safety", more opportunities for street crime and burglary, and less casual contact with neighbors and sense of local community.[15(pp16,20,21)]

Quick argues that "a potentially effective approach to accident reduction is to encourage a switch from cars to public transport, to get freight off the roads where possible, and to discourage unnecessary journeys. Fortunately, these aims correspond well with wider concerns."[15] Thus, for example, a good public bus system is not only safer than automobile travel, it is also more accessible for children, the elderly, and the poor, and is more protective of the environment.

Is it proper for employees of public health agencies to involve themselves in advocacy efforts? As to professional appropriateness, the history of public health and safety protection has been one of policy choices since the days of Snow and Virchow. Still, there are some, such as epidemiologists Kenneth J. Rothman and Charles Poole, who argue that public health researchers should not involve themselves in policy making or policy advising: "The time for a scientist to be a political and social mover is after hours."[20(p341)] Sylvia Tesh, on the other hand, argues that "There is no science uninfluenced by politics."[21(p177)] According to Tesh, injury is socially caused; the very concepts of causation are ideological constructs.[21(p167)] Both sides in this debate would seem to agree that effective prevention requires policy analysis and advocacy. The only questions are whether individual researchers weaken their credibility by publicly revealing the policy conclusions they have derived from their scientific work and whether it is even possible to remain aloof from policy issues.

What about legal limitations on such involvement? Public employees cannot be involved in partisan political activity or fund raising, but can provide expert input into the legislative process. This input can include information, including testimony, made available to legislators, legislative committees, legislative reference bureaus, and other participants in the legislative process. If called on by legislative or administrative authorities to provide expert input, public health practitioners can present information on injury problems and on what is known about possible interventions to deal with the problems. In addition, unless specific limitations exists—for example, limits on the Consumer Product Safety Commission regarding release of manufacturer-specific information—agency employees are free to make information available to the public and to meet with the public.

## EXAMPLES

### Hot Water Heaters

In the late 1970s, pediatricians became aware of the injury threat posed when new hot water heaters were routinely shipped from the factory preset at 150° F. Although these devices could easily be reset to a lower temperature, few people did so. The result was tap water scald burns to those unable to move quickly enough out of the stream of overly hot water (particularly young children and the elderly). At 140 to 150° F, full-thickness burns will occur in adults in 2 to 5 seconds of exposure, even faster in children. At 120° F, it takes 10 minutes of exposure to produce such a burn. In two states, Washington and Florida, laws were enacted requiring that hot water heaters sold in the state be set at lower temperatures. This requirement in no way prevented the purchaser from immediately resetting the heater to a higher temperature.

In Madison, Wisconsin, pediatrician Murray Katcher, working with the medical profession, senior citizen groups, pharmacists, the local health department, and utility companies, began an education program for practitioners and the public. Educational pamphlets about tap water scalds were included with utility bills and distributed to primary care practitioners and senior citizen groups. Pre- and postprogram evaluation of this effort found it had increased awareness of the danger of tap water scalds, but without any associated increase in the lowering of hot water heater temperature settings. Katcher therefore concluded that a law similar to those in Washington and Florida would well serve the people of Wisconsin. The proposed law would have heaters sold in Wisconsin preset at 125° F, labels warning of the dangers of tap water scalds would be placed on the heaters, and landlords would have to reset heaters at 125° F before reletting a rental unit.

Enactment of such a law seemed easy: The American Academy of Pediatrics had developed a model bill, there were virtually no enforcement or administrative costs to the state, and the legislation was supported by the state medical society, state chapter of the American Academy of Pediatrics, the Wisconsin Public Health Association, and the Wisconsin Maternal and Child Health Coalition (an advocacy organization consisting of representatives of more than 40 organizations). Despite this support and the logic of the proposed legislation, the law barely survived the legislative process and the threat of a veto. This was largely because of opposition from an industry group, the Gas Appliance Manufacturers Association, apparently induced by their aversion to any restrictions that might serve as incentive and precedent for future regulatory interventions.

When the governor signed the bill into law in late 1987, he stated that letters from many citizens and organizations overcame his "natural inclination not to sign the bill." That it was eventually signed was the direct result of organized and unrelenting efforts by a dedicated coalition of health professional and children's advocacy groups. Their role was to uncover and respond to the concerns of legislators and the governor, providing information and arguments supporting the bill.[22]

After the Wisconsin bill passed, the water heater manufacturers wanted no further state legislation. Katcher then participated in a national coalition, including the American Academy of Pediatrics, the National Safety Council, and the Consumer Federation of America, to develop a consensus agreement. Water heaters are now set by the manufacturers at a safe temperature of 120° F, at which temperature it takes almost 10 minutes of exposure to result in a full-thickness burn. Reduction in the number of tap water scald burns has been demonstrated in Seattle, following the passage of a law requiring water heaters to be set at 120° F.

### Motorcycle Helmets

California is the only state that did not pass a helmet law between 1966 and 1975, the period during which the promise of federal highway funds induced other states to do so. In 1985 a mandatory helmet law that applied only to riders under 15½ years old took effect in the state. Two years later a helmet bill that would have covered all ages was lobbied through to passage in the State Assembly by Mary Price, whose 18-year-old helmetless son had died in a motorcycle crash, but the bill failed in the State Senate. The following year the same bill was approved by both houses of the legislature but vetoed by the governor as being "unfair" to "responsible, mature operators." Several additional frustrating years followed until helmet use law advocates finally succeeded with a law that took effect in 1992.

In a description of this prolonged legislative effort, Elizabeth McLoughlin drew several key advocacy lessons from the prolonged battle.

- Select the bill's author carefully.
- Identify obstacles to the bill's passage.
- Build organizational and grassroots support, with particular attention to constituents of key legislators.
- Use the emotional and symbolic elements inherent in the helmet issue to advantage. This is inextricably linked with media coverage.
- Learn the principles and practices of media advocacy and pursue them vigorously during the campaign.
- Know your facts thoroughly and accurately. This includes general facts about the issue and state and local data on crashes, deaths, injuries, and current use rates.
- Use the authentic voice of survivors and family members who have been affected by motorcycle crashes in support of a helmet law.
- Estimate the potential cost savings if your state had a full-use helmet law.
- Acknowledge that politics has a life of its own, essentially unrelated to the merits of any particular bill.
- Be prepared, on a regular basis, for the roller coaster of emotions that follows your bill's victories and defeats.[23]

## Pickup Trucks

Pickup trucks are increasingly being used for personal transportation. The share of pickup trucks serving as household vehicles has approached one in five, and pickup trucks have also come to account for about one in five vehicles involved in fatal crashes. A significant portion of these fatalities involves people riding in the cargo areas of pickup trucks. The cargo area of pickup trucks is a nonpassenger location of the vehicle and, as such, is not required nor designed to meet occupant safety standards applicable to passenger locations. Yet many people do ride in this area. The result each year is some 200-plus deaths nationwide to occupants riding in the back of pickup trucks.

Tragedies associated with passengers—often young passengers—riding in the cargo areas of pickup trucks has led the American Medical Association and the American Academy of Pediatrics to focus on this safety issue by developing policy statements regarding the transport of passengers in cargo areas. This concern has also led to legislative initiatives in most, if not all, of the 50 states. In California, a bill to restrict the transport of passengers in the cargo areas of pickup trucks was introduced into the State Assembly early in 1991. The bill was backed by a variety of child advocacy groups and had the support of law enforcement officials. The motor vehicle manufacturers, who potentially face lawsuits from victims, also provided support. On the other hand, agricultural interests provided the main opposition to the bill. Because of the public appeal of this safety issue, the opposition was behind the scenes, never public.

Despite the organized support, and the logic and emotional appeal of the issue, the effort to enact legislation had a rocky road to success. The bill failed in the Assembly, but after a well-publicized pickup crash that killed one child and injured four others, the bill was reconsidered and passed. The bill passed the State Senate shortly after another pickup crash killed eight young people, ages 15 to 21. But the behind-the-scenes opposition was more effective, and the legislation was vetoed by the governor.

A similar pattern occurred in 1993, after reintroduction of a similar bill. This time, however, legislative passage was followed by the governor's signing the bill into law. There are several useful lessons to be drawn from this legislative effort. Developing broad support is obviously critical to success. This includes, in particular, persons whose loved ones have been victims of the type of tragedy to be prevented, along with health professionals and law enforcement officials. Educating the press on the issue, so that they may rally the public, is also critical. And being able to compromise is a part of achieving victory; the successful bill had been "watered down" with the inclusion of an exception for those riding in camper shells, although there are no data to justify such an exception. Supporters of the bill concluded that a less-than-perfect law was better than no law at all.

Legislative successes in the injury prevention arena often hinge on tragedies occurring at critical times in the legislative process. It is unfortunate that this has to be the case, but it is also why the legislation is being sought in the first place. It would be even more unfortunate if these misfortunes were not effectively used to help in the injury prevention effort. It is important, therefore, that spokespeople for injury prevention initiatives adeptly use the media when such human tragedies occur, pointing out what needs to be done to prevent similar tragedies in the future and tying this lesson directly to pending injury prevention efforts such as state legislation or funding requests.

## Survivors

In many campaigns to enact injury prevention legislation, the advocacy effort can be helped significantly through the involvement of survivors of the type of injury involved or from friends and family of victims. Well-known and effective examples include

- Mothers Against Drunk Driving, which has played a prominent role in promoting more effective drunk driving legislation and enforcement
- former Presidential press spokesman James Brady, who, with his wife Sarah, spearheaded the effort that resulted in the federal "Brady Bill" requirement of a waiting period and background check prior to firearm purchases
- various state brain injury associations, which have been influential in advocating on both the state and national levels in behalf of the needs of brain injury victims

## CONCLUSION

Social choices must be made after thorough and open discussion. Too often this does not happen. Instead, as in the infamous history of U.S. automobile companies buying up public transport systems in the early part of the century to destroy competition to automobiles, we have behind-the-scenes policy making. Injury protection practitioners can best work to alter this situation by providing the public and policy makers with a steady stream of effectively presented information and policy options on injury risks and injury prevention.

---

### NOTES

1. Gallagher SS, Messenger KP, Guyer B. State and local responses to children's injuries: The Massachusetts Statewide Childhood Injury Prevention Program. *J Soc Issues.* 1987;43:149–162.
2. Johns Hopkins School of Hygiene and Public Health. *Report of the National Conference on Injury Control.* Atlanta, GA: U.S. Centers for Disease Control; 1981.

3. Haddix AC, Teutsch SM, Shaffer PA. *Prevention Effectiveness: A Guide to Decision Analysis and Economic Evaluation.* New York: Oxford University Press; 1996.

4. Clyde AT, Hemenway D, Nagurney D. Seat belt use, insurance status and hospital bad debt. *J Trauma.* 1996;41:100–104.

5. *Reform That Works: Preventing Childhood Injuries Produces Real, Documented Health Care Savings.* Washington, DC: National SAFE KIDS Campaign; undated (circa 1995).

6. Miller T, Demes J, Bovbjerg R. Child seats: How large are the benefits and who should pay? In: *Child Occupant Protection.* SP-986. Warrendale, PA: Society of Automotive Engineers; November 1993:81–90.

7. Miller T, Douglass J, Galbraith M, Lestina D, Pindus N. Costs of head and neck injury and a benefit-cost analysis of bicycle helmets. In: *Head Neck Inj.* P-276. Warrendale, PA: Society of Automotive Engineers; September 1994.

8. Hemenway D. *Prices and Choices: Microeconomic Vignettes.* 3rd ed. Lanham, MD: University Press of America; 1993:218.

9. Robertson LS. Automobile safety regulation in the United States. *Am J Public Health.* 1981;71:818–822.

10. Orr LD. The effectiveness of automobile safety regulations: Evidence from the FARS data. *Am J Public Health.* 1984;74:1384–1389.

11. Robertson LS. Automobile safety regulation: Rebuttal and new data. *Am J Public Health.* 1984;74:1390–1394.

12. Robertson LS. *Injury Epidemiology: Research and Control Strategies.* 2nd ed. New York: Oxford University Press; 1998:172–183.

13. Bellah RN, Madsen R, Sullivan WM, Swidler A, Tipton SM. *Habits of the Heart: Individualism and Commitment in American Life.* New York: Harper & Row; 1985.

14. *Philadelphia Public Ledger*, August 28, 1852. Who benefits? Reprinted in the *New York Times*, March 24, 1981; 19.

15. Quick A. *Unequal Risks: Accidents and Social Policy.* London: Socialist Health Association; 1991. (Quick unfortunately uses the term "accident" throughout her otherwise excellent book. We have changed all of her uses of this word to the more appropriate—for U.S. readers: "injury.")

16. Bergman AB, ed. *Political Approaches to Injury Control at the State Level.* Seattle: University of Washington Press; 1992.

17. *Publicity and Advocacy for Injury Prevention.* Newton, MA: Education Development Center; 1988.

18. For descriptions of industry campaigns to resist regulation, see Stauber J, Rampton S. *Toxic Sludge Is Good for You: Lies, Damn Lies and the Public Relations Industry.* Monroe, ME: Common Courage Press; 1995.

19. Wallack L, Dorfman L, Jernigan D, Themba M. *Media Advocacy and Public Health: Power for Prevention.* Newbury Park, CA: Sage Publications; 1993:201–208.

20. Rothman KJ, Poole C. Science and policymaking. *Am J Public Health.* 1985;75:340–341.

21. Tesh SN. *Hidden Arguments: Political Ideology and Disease Prevention Policy.* New

Brunswick, NJ: Rutgers University Press; 1988.

22. Katcher ML. Efforts to prevent burns from hot tap water. In: Bergman AB. *Political Approaches to Injury Control at the State Level.* Seattle: University of Washington Press; 1992:69–78.

23. McLoughlin E. The almost successful California experience: What we and others can learn from it. In: Bergman AB. *Political Approaches to Injury Control at the State Level.* Seattle: University of Washington Press; 1992:57–67.

# Developing a Comprehensive Injury Prevention Program: Selected Factors Contributing to Health Systems Problems

| System Component/Problem | Contributing Factors |
|---|---|

*Analysis/Assessment*

| System Component/Problem | Contributing Factors |
|---|---|
| Lack of data on injury rates, inadequate surveillance | • Staff unaware of all the data sources that are available<br>• E codes not mandated—policy makers unaware of their importance; hospitals not supportive; cost a barrier<br>• Various data sources not coordinated and collected in one place<br>• Hospital, emergency medical service, police records uncomputerized<br>• Poor documentation in hospital records<br>• Lack of trained epidemiologists; others in department lack expertise in data analysis |
| Failure to adequately examine social/political/economic environment | • Unaware of the importance of this analysis; unaware of the extent of ethnic, political changes in local communities<br>• Staff in office become insulated |

- Lack of staff to do time-consuming assessment
- Travel restrictions inhibit staff from visiting and becoming familiar with other parts of the state

### *Design and Development*

Lack of a comprehensive plan

- Lack of awareness among policy makers of importance of comprehensive planning in injury control
- Staff lacks the time to step back and plan, pressured to initiate interventions
- Planning not valued

Most at-risk populations and injuries not targeted

- Data not accessed—unaware of how, where to get it
- Tendency to target groups and injuries with which staff is familiar regardless of data on risk
- Lack of knowledge about effective interventions for certain injuries leads to reluctance to address them
- Intentional injuries are more complex, thus they often are not addressed

Key individuals at state and local levels not involved in program planning

- Staff insulated—unaware of potential collaborators
- Turf issues interfere with cooperation
- Lack of outreach to local communities
- Lack of time, overwhelmed with other responsibilities
- Personality conflicts
- Bureaucratic restrictions on collaboration among offices in health department

- Geographic isolation of potentially helpful individuals

Most effective and appropriate interventions not selected

- Lack of most recent information on effective interventions
- Inability to translate research into practice
- Failure to recognize that priorities of target populations may not be the same as those of program planners
- Political climate is antiregulatory
- Financial constraints on planners or target populations limit the purchase of effective safety devices

### *Implementation*

Staff and management insufficiently trained in injury content and program management

- Few professional and academic training opportunities
- Broad field; research constantly evolving
- Lack of access to current research
- Unclear career path in injury prevention programs
- Few injury professionals available for hire

Incomplete integration into other health department programs

- Not mandated or encouraged by decision makers
- Poor communication among various sections
- Lack of awareness of creative ways to fit injury into other programs
- Turf issues/isolation

Lack of collaboration with community groups

- Insulation of state agency, lack of familiarity with and linkages to community

|  | • Lack of community leadership |
|  | • Community has priorities other than injury |
| Inappropriate, insufficient implementation tools | • Effective, targeted materials are unavailable |
|  | • Intervention takes singular approach only, as opposed to incorporating education, technology, and legislation/regulation |
|  | • Staff is inexperienced in legislative advocacy |
|  | • Staff is inexperienced in using the media |
|  | • Inflexible plan, unable to adjust to changing situation |
|  | • Appropriate technology is unavailable |

### *Evaluation*

| Evaluation not built into plan from the beginning | • Unaware of need to develop evaluation plan/methods |
|  | • Unclear objectives |
|  | • Focus on program development rather than on evaluation |
|  | • Evaluation literature is weak |
|  | • Lack of staff time |
| Process evaluation not ongoing during implementation | • Practitioners uncomfortable with being evaluated |
|  | • No person assigned responsibility for tracking |
|  | • Lack of communication between lead agency and practitioners regarding the need for and use of data collection |
|  | • Lack of a computer for data collection and analysis |

| Lack of or incomplete outcome evaluation | • Data not collected consistently<br>• Lack of expertise in evaluation design<br>• Funding and staff inadequate<br>• Target population too small to demonstrate statistically significant results |

# Conclusion

This book has consisted of a few simple messages. Injury is a critical public health problem. Injury is preventable. Public health practitioners working to prevent injuries can maximize their effectiveness by learning from those who have gone before.

Not that it is easy. Funding limitations, political barriers, irrational attitudes—these and other factors conspire to make the prevention task a difficult one. But it is an exhilarating task, the more so now that public health as a profession is heading down the injury prevention path. It is no longer a matter of a few pioneering giants—the William Haddons—needing to proselytize in a conceptual wilderness. Injury prevention is now a crusade with numerous foot soldiers, a growing professional network, proven approaches, and significant resources. It is an exciting time to be involved.

In this book we have presented a brief introduction to the injury problem—its nature, magnitude, and epidemiology—and we have described the basics of injury prevention, including environmental, educational, and regulatory interventions. And we have explored programmatic efforts to reduce injury, focusing on how to be most effective in dealing with the injury problem and stressing practical knowledge, skills, and strategies. We have tried to emphasize the importance of surveillance, of a systems approach to developing programs, and of evaluation.

Our hope has been that the ideas and examples that we have provided will help the reader move injury prevention efforts forward an additional step. At a minimum, we need to work to

- Implement interventions that we know can work, adapting them for local application as appropriate.

- Tackle underaddressed areas of injury prevention, such as suicide and sports injuries.
- Improve our approaches with hard-to-reach high-risk populations.
- Integrate injury prevention more fully into the rest of public health.
- Bridge the gap between injury prevention research and practice.
- Constantly seek increases in injury prevention funding and support.

As long as injury prevention continues to move forward, ever expanding and improving its impact, we may be optimistic that injury, this leading public health problem, will be brought increasingly under control. After all, it is because the infectious diseases of the past have been effectively brought under control with the tools of public health that injury has moved into the lead as the number one cause of productive years of life lost in the United States. The public health approach—so effective with infectious diseases—can be used to reduce injury, protecting the public from a preventable source of mortality, morbidity, and misery. This is what public health is all about—a challenge and a cause that carries with it the potential to help create a safer, better, and more satisfying world.

# Injury-Related World Wide Web Sites

American Academy of Pediatrics
http://www.aap.org

American Association of Poison Control Centers
http://www.aapcc.org

American Association of Suicidology
http://www.cyberpsych.org/aas/index.htm

American Automobile Association
http://www.aaa.com

American Foundation for Suicide Prevention
http://www.asfnet.org

Association for the Advancement of Automotive Medicine
http://www.carcrash.org

Bike Helmet Safety Institute
http://www.bhsi.org

Brain Injury Association
http://www.biausa.org

Building Bridges between Health and Traffic Safety
http://www.edc.org/HHD/csn/buildbridges

Building Safe Communities
http://www.edc.org/HHD/csn/bsc

Bureau of Labor Statistics/Safety and Health Statistics
http://www.bls.gov/oshhome.htm

Bureau of Transportation Statistics
http://www.bts.gov/contents.html

Burn and Shock Trauma Institute—Injury Prevention Program
http://www.meddean.luc.edu/umen/DeptWebs/brnshock/preventi.htm

Canada Safety Council
http://www.safety-council.org

Canadian Automobile Association—Traffic Safety
http://www.caa.ca/CAAInternet/trafficsafety/frames13.htm

Canadian Centre for Occupational Health and Safety
http://www.ccohs.ca

Canadian Hospitals Injury Reporting and Prevention Program—Child
Injury Division
http://www.hc-sc.gc.ca/main/lcdc/web/brch/injury.html

CDC Wonder (CDC searches, queries, guidelines, and reports)
http://wonder.cdc.gov

Center for the Advanced Study of Public Safety and Injury Prevention
http://www.albany.edu/sph/injury_3.html

Center for the Study and Prevention of Violence
http://www.colorado.edu/cspv

Center for Violence Prevention and Control—University of Minnesota
http://www.umn.edu/cvpc

Child and Adolescent Emergency Department Visit Databook
http://cvic.edu/childed

Child and Family Canada—Safety
http://www.cfc-efc.ca/menu/eng012.htm

Child Maltreatment 1995: Reports from the States to the National Child
Abuse and Neglect Data System
http://www.acf.dhhs.gov/programs/cb/stats/ncands

Child Passenger Safety Web
http://www.childsafety.org/index.html

Children's Safety Network National Injury & Violence Prevention Resource Center
http://www.edc.org/HHD/CSN

Colorado Injury Control Research Center
http://www.ColoState.edu/Orgs/CICRC

Consumer Product Safety Commission
http://www.cpsc.gov

Crash Analysis and Reporting Environment (CARE)
http://care.cs.ua.edu

Crash Outcome Data Evaluation System (CODES)
http://cvic.edu/codes/

Creative Partnerships for Prevention—A Drug and Violence Prevention Resource
http://www.CPPrev.org

Department of Education
http://www.ed.gov

Department of Health and Human Services
http://hhs.gov

Department of Justice
http://www.usdoj.gov

Department of Labor (Safety and Health)
http://www.dol.gov/dol/asp/public/fibre/osha.htm

Department of Transportation
http://www.dot.gov

Disaster Epidemiology Applied Research Program
http://www.cdc.gov/nceh/programs/emergenc/disa_epi/disa_epi.htm

Early Prevention of Violence Database (Great Lakes Area Regional Resource Center)
http://www.csnp.ohio-state.edu/glarrc/vpdb.htm

E codes (workbook/spreadsheet-based listing of ICD-9-CM E codes and their associated mechanisms and intent groups)
http://www.pgh.auhs.edu/cvic/Ecode%20CDC%20matrix%20lookup.zip

Emory Center for Injury Control
http://www.sph.emory.edu/CIC/cichome.html

Family Health and Safety
http://www.twbc.com

Family Violence Prevention Fund
http://www.igc.apc.org/fund

Fatality Analysis Reporting System (FARS)
http://www.fars.idinc.com/fars95_96/fars.cfm

FBI's Supplementary Homicide Reports, 1980–1995
http://www.ncjrs.org/ojjdp/html/ezaccess.html#SHR

Gunfree Home (Coalition to Stop Gun Violence)
http://www.gunfree.org

Gun Info (Harborview Injury Prevention and Research Center)
http://guninfo.org

Handgun Epidemic Lowering Project (HELP Network)
http://www.childmmc.edu/help/helphome.htm

Harborview Medical Center—Injury Prevention and Research Center
http://weber.u.washington.edu/~hiprc/hiprc

Harvard Injury Control Research Center
http://www.hsph.harvard.edu/Organizations/hcra/hicc.html

Health Canada
http://www.hc-sc.gc.ca/english

Health, United States, 1996–1997
http://www.cdc.gov/nchswww/data/hus96_97.pdf

Indian Health Service
http://www.tucson.ihs.gov

Injury Control and Emergency Health Services Section of the American
Public Health Association
http://www.injurycontrol.com/ICEHS/

Injury Control Resources Information Network
http://www.injurycontrol.com/icrin/index.html#index

Injury Prevention (journal)
http://www.bmjpg.com/data/jip.htm

Injury Prevention Centre, Canada (and the Safe Community Support Centre)
http://www.med.ualberta.ca/acicr/

Institute for Preventative Sports Medicine
http://users.aol.com/wwwipsm

Institute of Transportation Engineers
http://www.ite.org

Insurance Institute for Highway Safety
http://www.highwaysafety.org

Interdisciplinary Pediatric Injury Control Research Center (University of Pennsylvania)
http://www.med.upenn.edu/trauma

International Society for Child and Adolescent Injury Prevention
http://weber.u.washington.edu:80/~hiprc/iscaip.html

Inventory of Federal Data Systems in the United States for Injury Surveillance, Research and Prevention Activities
http://www.cdc.gov/ncipc/pub-res/federal.pdf

Iowa Injury Prevention Research Center
http://info.pmeh.uiowa.edu/iprc/iprc.htm

Johns Hopkins Center for Injury Research and Policy
http://www.jhsph.edu/Research/Centers/CIRP

JOIN TOGETHER (community substance abuse and gun violence programs)
http://www.jointogether.org

Journal of Trauma
http://www.wwilkins.com/TA

Kentucky Injury Prevention and Research Center
http://www.kiprc.uky.edu

Kids Health (Nemours Foundation)
http://kidshealth.org/parent/safety/index.html

Maternal and Child Health Bureau
http://www.os.dhhs.gov/hrsa/mchb

Maternal and Child Health Bureau Kid's Place
http://158.72.82.84/kidspages

Minnesota Center Against Violence and Abuse
http://www.umn.edu/mincava/

Morbidity and Mortality Weekly Report
http://cdc.gov/epo/mmwr/mmwr.html

Mothers Against Drunk Driving
http://madd.org

National Association of Governor's Highway Safety Representatives
http://naghsr.org

National Bicycle Safety Network
http://www.cdc.gov/ncipc/bike

National Center for Health Statistics
http://www.cdc.gov/nchswww/default.htm

National Center for Injury Prevention and Control (CDC)
http://www.cdc.gov/ncipc

National Center for Statistics and Analysis (NHTSA)
http://www.nhtsa.dot.gov/people/ncsa

National Children's Center for Rural and Agricultural Health and Safety
http://marshmed.org/nfmc/children

National Clearinghouse for Alcohol and Drug Information
http://www.health.org

National Clearinghouse for Justice Information and Statistics
http://www.ch.search.org

National Committee on Uniform Traffic Laws and Ordinances
http://ncutlo.org

National Crash Outcome Data Evaluation System
http://www.cvic.edu/codes

National Criminal Justice Reference Service
http://www.ncjrs.org

National Data Archive on Child Abuse and Neglect
http://www.ndacan.cornell.edu

National Fire Protection Association
http://www.nfpa.org

National Group Rides and Designated Drivers
http://www.ntlgradd.w1.com/index.shtml

National Health Information Center
http://nhic-nt.health.org

National Highway Traffic Safety Administration
http://www.nhtsa.dot.gov

National Highway Traffic Safety Administration, Safety City
http://www.nhtsa.dot.gov/kids

National Injury Surveillance Unit (Australia)
http://www.nisu.flinders.edu.au/welcome.html

National Institute for Occupational Safety and Health
http://www.cdc.gov/niosh/homepage.html

National Institute on Disability & Rehabilitation Research
http://www.ed.gov/offices/OSERS/NIDRR

National Institutes of Health
http://www.nih.gov

National Network of Violence Prevention Practitioners
http://www.edc.org/HHD/NNVPP

National Pediatric Trauma Registry
http://www.nemc.org/rehab/nptrhome.htm

National Program for Playground Safety
http://www.uni.edu/playground

National Rehabilitation Information Center Home Page
http://www.naric.com/naric/index.html

National Safety Council
http://www.nsc.org

Occupational Safety and Health Administration
http://www.osha.gov

Oklahoma State Department of Health Injury Control Division
http://www.health.state.ok.us/program/injury/index.html

OSHA Statistics
http://www.osha.gov/oshstats/index.html

Pacific Center for Violence Prevention
http://www.pcvp.org

Partnership Against Violence Network
http://pavnet.org

Rehabilitation Services Administration
http://www.ed.gov/offices/OSERS/RSA/rsa.html#org

Research and Training Center in Rehabilitation and Childhood Trauma (Boston)
http://www.nemc.org/rehab/homepg.htm

Road Safety (Transport Canada)
http://www.tc.gc.ca/roadsafety/rsindx_e.htm

Rural Injury Prevention Resource Center
http://www.marshmed.org/nfmc/projects/csnriprc/csnriprc.htm

Safe Communities (WHO)
http://www.ki.se/phs/wcc-csp/main.html

Safe Communities Foundation (Canada)
http://safecommunities.ca/

SafeKids Campaign
http://www.safekids.org

Safe Start, USA, Inc. (drowning prevention)
http://safestart.org

San Francisco Injury Center
http://itsa.ucsf.edu/~sfic/INDEX.html

Scientific Data, Surveillance and Injury Statistics
http://www.cdc.gov/ncipc/osp/data.htm

Smartrisk Foundation (Canada)
http://www.smartrisk.ca

Southern California Injury Prevention Research Center
http://www.ph.ucla.edu/sciprc/sciprc1.htm

State and Territorial Injury Prevention Directors Association
http://www.stipda.org

State Health Departments—On-Line
http://www.cdc.gov/epo/mmwr/medassn.html#states

Suicide Awareness: Voices of Education
http://www.save.org

Texas Department of Health, Injury Prevention and Control Program
http://www.tdh.state.tx.us/injury

THINK FIRST Foundation
http://www.thinkfirst.org

Trauma Foundation at San Francisco General Hospital
http://www.traumafdn.org

Trauma.Org—Care of the Injured
http://www.trauma.org/trauma.html

United States Census Bureau
http://www.census.gov

University of Alabama Injury Control Research Center
http://www.uab.edu/icrc/icrc.htm

University of Iowa Injury Prevention Research Center
http://info.pmeh.uiowa.edu/iprc/iprc.htm

University of Michigan Transportation Research Institute
http://www.umtri.umich.edu/

University of North Carolina Injury Prevention Research Center
http://www.sph.unc.edu/iprc/

University of Otago Injury Prevention and Research Unit (New Zealand)
http://www.otago.ac.nz/Web_menus/Dept_Homepages/IPRU/home.html

University of Pittsburgh Center for Injury Research and Control
http://www.edc.gsph.pitt.edu/circl/index.html

University of Texas Health Science Center at San Antonio's Trauma
Home Page
http://rmstewart.uthscsa.edu

Violence Against Women Office, U.S. Department of Justice
http://www.usdoj.gov/vawo

WHO Helmet Initiative
http://www.sph.emory.edu/Helmets

Who's Who in Traffic Safety
http://www.edc.org/HHD/csn/buildbridges/whoswho

World Health Organization
http://www.who.int

Youth Violence Prevention (HUD and CDC)
http://www.spartacc.com/prevent/violence.html

## E-MAIL LISTS

Injury-L
  • subscribe at listserv@wvnvm.wvnet.edu
    (or access http://www.hsc.wvu.edu/crem/ncrem2.htm)

Alcohol and injuries
  • subscribe at Majordomo@igc.org

News and announcements from the Consumer Product Safety
Commission
  • subscribe at listproc@cpsc.gov

Child Passenger Safety Advocacy
  • subscribe at listserver@wildhack.com

CDC Injury list
  • contact seb2@cdc.gov

# Index

## G

# About the Authors

**Tom Christoffel** is a lawyer by training, with particular interest in the use of law to protect the public from injury. He has been an educator for most of his career, including 20 years on the faculty of the University of Illinois at Chicago School of Public Health. He has developed and taught courses on public health law, injury prevention, government regulation, health care politics, policy analysis, and related subjects, and is codeveloper of the Centers for Disease Control and Prevention's course modules on *The Legal Basis of Public Health*. He currently holds adjunct faculty appointments at the UIC School of Public Health, the Johns Hopkins University School of Hygiene and Public Health, and the University of Colorado School of Medicine. Professor Christoffel's previous books include *Health and the Law: A Handbook for Health Professionals* and, with Stephen P. Teret, *Protecting the Public: Legal Issues in Injury Prevention*. He is also the author of numerous book chapters and journal articles on law, public health, injury prevention, evaluation methodology, medical peer review, and other topics. Professor Christoffel is a Trustee of the Civil Justice Foundation, a member of the Editorial Board of the *Journal of Public Health Policy*, a member of the Massachusetts Bar, and past chair of the Injury Control and Emergency Health Services Section of the American Public Health Association. He is currently a consultant and freelance writer in Boulder, Colorado.

**Susan Scavo Gallagher** is a nationally recognized leader in child and adolescent injury prevention and in the development of injury prevention programs in state and local governmental agencies. She has 20 years of experience directing the development, implementation, and evaluation of injury prevention programs, surveillance system methods, research projects, and training initiatives at the national, state, and local level. She has coauthored more than 25 journal publications related to the epidemiology and prevention of injuries. Ms. Gallagher has been the Director of the Statewide Childhood Injury Prevention Program at the Massachusetts Department of Public Health, the Director of the Childhood Injury Prevention Resource Center in the Maternal and Child Health Department at the Harvard University School of Public Health, and is the founding Director of the Children's Safety Network (CSN) National Injury and Violence Prevention Resource Center. She serves on the National Academy of Sciences, Institute of Medicine Committee on Injury Prevention and Control, the Steering Committee of the National Children's Center for Rural and Agricultural Health and Safety, the Technical Advisory Board of the National SAFE KIDS Campaign, the Advisory Board for the Occupational Health Surveillance Program at the Massachusetts Department of Public Health, and chairs the Advisory Committee of the Harvard Injury Control Research Center and the Task Force on Unintentional Injury and Violence Prevention of the American School Health Association. She is also a founding officer of the International Society of Child and Adolescent Injury Prevention and is an Associate Editor of the journal *Injury Prevention*. She is currently a Senior Scientist and the Associate Director of the Center for Injury and Violence Prevention at Education Development Center, Inc. in Newton, Massachusetts.